MINORITY AND CROSS-CULTURAL ASPECTS OF NEUROPSYCHOLOGICAL ASSESSMENT

EDITED BY

F. RICHARD FERRARO, PH.D.

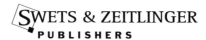

SWETS & ZEITLINGER PUBLISHERS

LISSE   ABINGDON   EXTON (PA)   TOKYO

Library of Congress Cataloging-in-Publication Data

Minority and cross-cultural aspects of neuropsychological assessment / edited by F. Richard Ferraro.
     p. ; cm. -- (Studies on neuropsychology, development, and cognition)
    Includes bibliographical references and indexes.
    ISBN 9026518307 (hardback)
    1. Neuropsychological tests--Cross-cultural studies. 2. Mental illness--Diagnosis--Cross-cultural studies. 3. Ethnopsychology. I. Ferraro, F. Richard, 1959- II. Series
    [DNLM: 1. Mental Disorders--diagnosis. 2. Neuropsychological Tests. 3. Ethnic Groups--psychology. 4. Ethnopsychology--methods. 5. Minority Groups--psychology. WM 145.5.N4 M666 2001]
    RC386.6.N48 M55 2001
    616.89'075'089--dc21

2001054188

Cover design: Magenta Grafische Producties, Bert Haagsman
Typesetting: Grafische Vormgeving Kanters, Sliedrecht, The Netherlands
Printed by: Krips, Meppel, The Netherlands

ISBN 90 265 1830 7

Contents

From the Series Editor

Dear Reader,

In keeping with our focus on contemporary issues which bridge the theoretical and practical aspects of Clinical Neuropsychology, we are proud to add: *Minority and Cross-Cultural Aspects of Neuropsychological Assessment* to our *Series on Neuropsychology, Development, and Cognition.* Edited by F. Richard Ferraro, this book is likely the first to cover aspects of neuropsychological issues dealing with a wide variety of cultural and ethnic issues. While some cultural and ethnic considerations (e.g., African/Black American issues, Hispanic/Latino issues) have been addressed in other venues, others, such as neuropsychological aspects of work with Asian/Pacific Islands, Native Americans, Rural Populations, and even work with Saudi Arabians have not been addressed in depth elsewhere. More general theoretical considerations are also included, including general guidelines for working with diverse populations and base rates to consider in looking for commonalities and differences between various ethnic groups.

As with the other texts in our series, we have attempted to assure that the information provided is theoretically current and practically useful. The guest authors all have recognized and relevant experience and have made contributions in their particular areas of expertise. References are also provided to guide the reader to relevant resources in conducting appropriately sensitive and fair clinical evaluations and/or research studies. In today's rapidly expanding world, with increasingly permeable geographic and cultural boundaries, we trust that this text will prove a ready reference to assist the Clinical Neuropsychologist in dealing with the realities of cultural challenge.

Linas Bieliauskas
Ann Arbor, May, 2001

Preface

In 1997, while going over thesis results from a recent student, I was stuck by the observation that relatively little, if any, good empirical research existed related to minority and cross-cultural aspects of neuropsychological assessment. In particular, this gap in the literature seemed especially large among Native American elderly individuals, which was the thesis topic. The thesis in question (which is actually detailed in the present book) had examined issues in neuropsychology in Native American elderly adults. What struck myself and the author of that thesis was that there was simply not very much in the professional literature regarding this topic. It was this situation that lead to the idea of the present edited book.

After examining and searching the relevant literatures, the idea of an edited book covering multiple cultures was generated. The notion of more than one culture being examined in the same book had not, to my knowledge, been performed. At that time, there were many books discussing specific individual cultures, but none that really combined cultures in a cross-cultural fashion. In my reading of the various literatures, I wanted to be consistent with some of the previous volumes that targeted a single culture or group, but also wanted to expand upon this notion, and include some groups that had not, in my searching, been documented. To this end, I submitted a proposal to Swets & Zeitlinger that was ultimately accepted.

I had other goals as I embarked on this project. In talking to many colleagues at various conferences, over email, and by phone it became apparent that a book such as this one you are holding was a true necessity. Many of these colleagues recounted to me that they would literally have to slap together articles, and book chapters to make a coherent collection covering multiple cultures. Hopefully, a major goal of this edited book will be to help colleagues overcome the potential problem of not having a concise, direct source at their disposal. I hope colleagues will use this book for their classes, their private practices and for their general education. The chapters that ultimately made it into the book are an attempt to achieve this specific goal. To some extent, this goal has already been met. Many of the authors as well as the ad-hoc reviewers have continually commented to me how relevant this book will be to them and that they only wished such a book were available to them only a few short years ago. Many of my private practice colleagues, especially, are seeing more and more culturally diverse populations in their clinics and practices and this book, they have said, will be an excellent addition. This is my goal and I hope this book makes some headway to achieve it.

The twenty chapters encompassed are current and up-to-date treatments of not only the typical groups studied, but some newer groups as well. Also, the combination of all these groups in one setting and in one edited volume is a unique contribution. I must also graciously thank the many ad-hoc reviewers who assisted in reading and commenting on these chapters:

Scott Hunter (University of Chicago)
Robert Widner (University of Colorado)
Robert Elsner (University of Georgia)
Lila Walker (Atlanta, Georgia)
Hajime Otani (Central Michigan University)
Douglas Faust (Children's Hospital, New Orleans)
Cathy Palmer (University of North Dakota)
Ruben Echemendia (Penn State)
P.W. Kodituwakka (University of New Mexico)
Lisa Brenner (Denver, Colorado)
Tim Makatura (University of Pittsburgh)
Andrea Zevenbergen (University of North Dakota)
Bonny Forrest (Columbia University)
Jason Olin (University of South Carolina)

I would also like to thank various people at Swets & Zeitlinger Publishers for their assistance (Martha Chorney, Beatrice Huisman, and especially Arnout Jacobs). In summary, it is hoped that this edited volume not only adds to the relatively scant literature in some of these cross-cultural groups, but also results in more questions being asked about neuropsychological assessment issues in these and other minority and cross-cultural groups. Thank you.

F. Richard Ferraro, Ph.D.
Department of Psychology
University of North Dakota

PART I

INTRODUCTION

Chapter 1

TRADITIONS AND TRENDS IN NEUROPSYCHOLOGICAL ASSESSMENT

Greg J. Lamberty, Ph.D. ABPP-CN
Noran Neurological Clinic, Minneapolis, Minnesota

Abstract

This chapter will cover a range of neuropsychological assessment approaches including traditional battery approaches, process-oriented approaches, and analytical/cognitive approaches. In addition, various individualized approaches that might be characterized as 'hypothesis testing' will be described. I will also present information on how neuropsychologist's batteries and approaches are evolving given changes in the current healthcare system.

Introduction

A chapter summarizing the movement and evolution of a field could scarcely begin without the assertion that there has been tremendous growth and progress during a time frame of interest. While this is a time worn sentiment, it is no less true for the field of clinical neuropsychology. The practice of neuropsychology has, in fact, evolved rapidly since its inception as a specialty area. Trends in clinical practice have generally followed advances in the research literature broadly, though this relationship has not always been as direct as it currently appears to be. Recent edited volumes provide accounts of the large number of ideologies and philosophies within the field of clinical neuropsychology (Goldstein & Incagnoli, 1997; Grant & Adams, 1996; Vanderploeg, 1994). Theories of neuropsychological function are obviously important, but in the context of a volume on minority and cross-cultural aspects of neuropsychological assessment it seems more relevant to focus on issues related to the assessment enterprise itself. Thus, rather than reconstitute the numerous accounts of clinical neuropsychology's growth and development in detail, this chapter will focus on the nature of practice and how it has evolved to its present day state. This will provide a context for understanding issues in the neuropsychological assessment of different groups as a function of their unique demographics, culture, and language.

Perusing a list of chapters on approaches to neuropsychological assessment in recent texts (Boll & Bryant, 1988; Goldstein & Incagnoli, 1997; Grant & Adams, 1996; Vanderploeg, 1994), one is left with the impression that perhaps there are formal blocks of neuropsychologists espousing a rigid adherence to a specific way of "doing" neuropsychology. This is in contrast to recent practice surveys that indicate "mixed battery" approaches as the predominant mode of practice in clinical neuropsychology today (Sweet & Moberg, 1990; Sweet, Moberg, & Westergaard, 1996; Sweet, Moberg, & Suchy, 2000). Of course, practicing neuropsychologists must make decisions about the most expedient way to practice and this often involves reconstructing batteries based on the exigencies of their practice, rather than on adherence to a formal neuropsychological ideology. This is where the real world and the theoretical world meet, or as some might contend, collide. For better or worse, the greatest influence on the *practice* of neuropsychology in the past ten to twenty years has probably been economic rather than theoretical.

Given the foregoing, it is very important to understand that theory-building and clinical practice in neuropsychology often proceed in a parallel fashion. That is, researchers (those who are employed primarily in the research, and not the clinical, enterprise) ask questions based on their knowledge and understanding of brain-behavior relationships. They may have external funding, or may be working in more traditional academic environs where profit considerations are relatively fewer than in the private sector. This is to say that they are more purely interested in the truth (with a capital 'T'). Most would agree that such a pursuit of knowledge and understanding is admirable, and in many cases, preferable to the manner in which a typical clinical examination of a patient is conducted. The clinical side of this equation has the clinician conducting an exam based on empirically validated measures that are preferably brief, powerful, and highly predictive of different forms of pathology or functional impairment. Clinicians are paid to proffer opinions or to know the answers, and to do so as efficiently as possible. Of course, this is an oversimplification for the purpose of understanding the difference between what we know and how we practice. Ideally, this gap should be small, but is often much larger than is comfortable for the practicing clinician. The following is a very brief summary of the evolution of ideas and practices in clinical neuropsychology. The chapter will conclude with what I regard as the most salient force in changing the way modern neuropsychologists practice. Namely, forging an understanding of how individual and group factors influence neuropsychological test performance and how this affects the judgments made by neuropsychologists. This is particularly important in a volume devoted to discussing minority and cross-cultural issues in neuropsychology.

Influences on Neuropsychological Theory and Practice

Historically, there have been two broad influences on neuropsychological theory and practice. One has its roots in behavioral neurology and psychiatry in the works of individuals such as Henry Head, J. Hughlings Jackson, and Sigmund Freud. These scientists and clinicians, through systematic and intensive observation of individual cases, came to posit various theories of mind and brain. The second path was through more traditional psychometrics and was pioneered by the likes of Francis Galton, Alfred Binet, and Charles Spearman. These individuals were not neuropsychologists in the sense that we would identify one today, but their thinking and theorizing provided foundations upon which current neuropsychological methods and theories are based.

Positing theoretical dichotomies is a veritable pastime in psychological science. As noted above, there is the traditional distinction between *qualitative* (observational) and *quantitative* (psychometric) approaches, but as neuropsychology has evolved other important distinctions have come to the fore. The qualitative and quantitative dichotomy is probably best represented in the differences between the *Boston Process Approach* (Kaplan, 1988) and the *Halstead Reitan Battery* (HRB; Reitan & Wolfson, 1996) – one emphasizing the careful description of intra-test behaviors and elements of performance, and the other emphasizing quantification via performances on a rigorously standardized battery of tests. Numerous other approaches to neuropsychological assessment rest at different points on the quantitative/qualitative continuum. For example, Benton's "hypothesis testing" model (Tranel, 1996) is known for applying a rigorous psychometric approach to assessing a range of higher cortical functions that were observed to be disrupted in neurologically impaired patients. Indeed, most extant approaches in neuropsychological assessment have incorporated both psychometric and observational methods to elucidate their models (COGNITIVE, etc. from Grant & Adams, 1996).

As the practice of neuropsychology became more entrenched in clinical settings, another major division occurred as a function of the kind of battery or method employed by practitioners. Russell (1997) described the fundamental distinction between current schools of thought as adhering to *hypothesis testing* or *pattern analysis* methods. Hypothesis testing assessments are driven by a series of individual hypotheses to be tested (appropriately enough) with regard to neuropsychological functioning in an individual patient. Unfortunately, the hypotheses generated are largely a function of the individual neuropsychologist's knowledge base and this can lead to a considerable lack of uniformity in the assessment end product. That is, if the individual administering the exam does not ask a question, it probably goes unanswered. The pattern analysis method is best represented by the Halstead Reitan Battery. Reitan refined Halstead's original battery of tests and added his own based on his observations that the relationship between tests differed in patients with different kinds of pathology. Therefore, in the pattern analysis method, the neuropsychologist is concerned with the interrelation of test performances as an index of neuropsychological functioning. One obvious limitation of such a method is exposed in unique cases for which there are no significant patterns of performance established.

Assessment Strategies in Present Day Neuropsychology

The actual composition of a neuropsychological test battery is yet another manner in which approaches to clinical neuropsychology can be distinguished. In actual practice, most every neuropsychologist uses a flexible battery. This is likely because, outside of the HRB and the Luria-Nebraska Neuropsychological Battery (LNNB; Golden, Purisch, & Hammeke, 1985), there are few widely validated "batteries" of tests. Furthermore, many users of the HRB and LNNB augment their assessments with other measures of specific cognitive functions (i.e., memory, attention, symptom validity, etc.). Thus, while some might argue that *ad hoc* or flexible batteries are difficult to validate, there seems to be agreement that the comprehensiveness of the cognitive domains assessed is probably more important than the ability to cite a validity statistic that may or may not bear relevance to a referral question. Longitudinal practice surveys conducted by Sweet and colleagues verify this trend in modern day practice. For example, Sweet, Moberg, and Westergaard (1996) noted that fully 85% of a sample of neuropsychologists reported using either a "flexible" or "flexible battery" approach in their practice. Only 14% of the same sample acknowledged using a uniform and invariant battery such as the HRB or LNNB. In a recent follow up of their 1996 paper Sweet, Moberg, and Suchy (2000) found that nearly 90% of board-certified (ABPP) neuropsychologists continued to use either flexible or flexible battery approaches, while 82% of APA division 40 member neuropsychologists espoused flexible or flexible battery approaches.

To be clear, the term "flexible battery" is used to convey the fact that a given practitioner uses a number of different measures in assessing a patient. It should be obvious that one neuropsychologist's flexible battery or flexible approach can be and often is quite different from that of another neuropsychologist. In this sense, the use of the flexible battery appellation is most unsatisfying in conveying what neuropsychologists actually do within their assessments. Nevertheless, the taxonomy of flexible batteries would be infinitely long and idiosyncratic to the user.

It is tempting to conclude that there are good reasons for the fact that mixed or flexible batteries are the most commonly used approaches in clinical practice today. Unfortunately, it is not clear that this is the case. A number of authors describing modern approaches to neuropsychological assessment suggest that individual practitioners may not have an adequate theoretical foundation upon which their flexible battery is built (Russell, 1997; Schmidt, in press). This is troubling because most practitioners would appear to give a *de facto* stamp of reliability and validity to the measures they use while not necessarily keeping a unifying theoretical rationale in mind when assessing patients. This is probably more troubling to neuropsychologists than it is to their patients or referral sources. Still, a conceptually coherent set of assumptions should underlie any assessment, no matter how brief or extensive it may be. It sometimes seems to be the case that interest in theories of brain function has taken a back seat to the standardization of specific instruments in today's neuropsychology. This is illustrated in the proliferation of instruments that purport to measure various cognitive skills by providing index scores on nicely organized record forms. This kind of descriptive approach is egalitarian in the sense that nearly anyone could administer the tests and describe the pattern of results. Whether or not the person administering the measure has a sense of the various kinds of dementia presentations they might be trying to distinguish, or the complexity of presentations following a traumatic brain injury is often not clear. Mentors and professors of today's aspiring neuropsychologists need to be mindful of the fact that neuropsychology is not simply an enterprise of test-giving and data collation.

Evolution of a Data-Based Science

As the science and practice of neuropsychology evolve, there is a need for empirical validation of the theories upon which the field has been built. This must be done through rigorous scientific inquiry and this is, indeed, the stage in which clinical neuropsychology finds itself today. Thirty to forty years ago neuropsychological tests were becoming recognized as tools that were impressive in their ability to detect the presence of "brain damage" and to localize pathology. The importance of these functions has decreased considerably over time as radiographic methods (e.g., CT, MRI) have evolved (though the detection of certain behavioral deficits continues to presage obvious structural damage in some dementias). The characterization of neurobehavioral strengths and limitations has become the primary focus of most assessments. Closely allied with this diagnostic purpose is the recommendation of different clinical courses of action (e.g., rehabilitation, psychotherapy, family interventions, etc.).

The success of neuropsychology in adapting to the changes in focus noted above is inextricably linked to the quality of the science supporting its methods. As such, issues of reliability and validity are vitally important. Most neuropsychologists would cite reliability and validity statistics as among the most important reasons for their use of a particular instrument. For example, the Rey Auditory Verbal Learning Test (RAVLT; Rey, 1964) is a serial word list learning and memory task that has been in wide clinical use for over three decades (Lezak, 1995; Spreen & Strauss, 1998; Mitrushina et al., 1999). Schmidt (1996) compiled a set of RAVLT norms based on many independent studies using the test and thus provided a very useful clinical tool for neuropsychologists. A similar wealth of normative data exists for a wide range of measures and provides a sound basis for clinical decision making. However, concern has been expressed regarding the validity of a collective set of measures used to assess a patient. By its nature, a flexible battery is not easily validated (as a battery) using traditional statistical methods. That is, because of the variable nature of the tests employed in a flexible battery, it may never be used more than once and validation would thus be very difficult. Garb (1998) reviews the relatively small literature on the validity of neuropsychological test batteries and concludes, "...neuropsychologists frequently make reliable and moderately valid judgments" (p. 170). He cautions, however, that validation studies of flexible batteries are essentially non-existent and the ability to draw firm conclusions about the reliability and validity of clinical judgment using such batteries is speculative.

Despite the lack of validity studies assessing batteries of neuropsychological tests, the neuropsychology literature abounds with reports of reliability and validity data for individual tests. Clinically oriented journals like *The Clinical Neuropsychologist* and the *Archives of Clinical Neuropsychology* are rife with studies that are essentially normative in nature. In addition, commercially available tests published by vendors like the Psychological Corporation and Psychological Assessment Resources are accompanied by extensive standardization and clinical data. There is widespread understanding that a test is often only as valuable as its supporting database. Thus, while some have argued that traditional batteries have greater empirical support because of a larger corpus of validity data, the approach of most clinicians involves identifying and using the most reliable and valid individual tests. There is an assumption that a battery of well standardized individual tests is more relevant and functional than a well validated battery in which some or many of the tests bear little relevance to the functions being assessed.

Neuropsychologists in clinical settings and research laboratories have clearly staked their future on empirical rigor. The wisdom of this approach is also being held up as a standard in the courtroom. The *Daubert versus Merrell Dow Pharmaceutical* (1993) ruling appears to have fueled the push for scientific validation of opinions about damages suffered in various personal injury contexts. In *Daubert* it was alleged by the plaintiffs, that exposure to an anti-nausea medication was responsible for birth defects in two children. The Court ruled that the evidence for teratogenicity in humans was essentially lacking and that expert opinions offered that were based on animal studies and re-analyzed human data were not appropriate as they did not constitute a sound basis for a scientific opinion. There will doubtless be vigorous debate as to how this ruling will or might affect neuropsychological testimony (Reed, 1999; Sweet, 1999). Nonetheless, to this date no *Daubert* challenges have been made to the admissibility of neuropsychological testimony in a federal lawsuit. The offshoot of the Daubert ruling appears to simply be serving as a wake up call to those who would offer expert testimony. It is becoming ever more crucial that opinions be based on scientific "facts," which typically means peer-reviewed articles and extensively validated tests.

It may seem unfair that the methods of clinical psychology and clinical neuropsychology come under the kind of scrutiny they do. Jensen (1998) points out that modern day intelligence tests generally have reliability coefficients that are in the .90 to .95 range and that this is more reliable than weight measurements taken in a doctor's office (p. 50). Other standard medical tests (e.g., blood pressure, serum cholesterol) that are presumably reliable and valid fare much worse in comparison. Yet it is seemingly without question that these data are accepted as scientifically sound. This is not to say that medical tests do not or should not bear the same scrutiny as neuropsychological tests, but they do appear to enjoy greater popular acceptance as valid and meaningful. While the scrutiny of the courts is often painful, it will serve as a catalyst for proving the scientific merit of our measures.

It seems that we are in the midst of a changing of the guard. Most clinicians would agree that careful observation of patients is an indispensable element of the neuropsychological evaluation. Much information can be collected in this manner and special insights can be gained. Nevertheless, regardless of the rich clinical and observational history that permeates our understanding of brain and behavior, we are by necessity, moving toward a more data based science. To some this is a disappointing indication that psychometric constructs are being reified, sometimes with too little clinical correlation. That is, data are beginning to take the place of clinical acumen and years of experience observing the nuances of patients with complex neurobehavioral presentations. While many hold fast in their beliefs about experience, clinical expertise, and credentialing as predictors of the quality of a neuropsychological assessment, the science of neuropsychology forges on, fueled by hard data. The corpus of Paul Meehl's work examining clinical diagnosis (e.g., Meehl, 1954; Meehl, 1973; Meehl, 1986) presaged neuropsychology's current dilemma. Briefly, Meehl has long contended that tests and measurement tools are easier to validate than are individual clinicians. This may take away from the mystique of a master clinician, but the ultimate goals of increasing diagnostic accuracy and providing better service and advice to our patients will be served in the end. Along these lines, it is interesting to see that the methods and wisdom of the Boston Process Approach are now being extensively standardized in measures like the WAIS-R NI (Kaplan et al., 1991) and the WISC-III PI (Kaplan, Fein, Morris, & Delis, 1999). Indeed the notion of standardizing Christensen's adaptation of Luria's methods via the LNNB was controversial (Adams, 1980). Nevertheless, these attempts speak to the larger issue of those factors that bolster any scientific endeavor – replicability of methods and findings, and the ability to make accurate interpretive statements. Rather than being a death knell for the observational tradition in neuropsychology, this should serve as a challenge to those whose keen observation provides special insights. Such observations should be standardized and made available to the field at large.

We needn't discard the notion of sage clinicians. Such individuals will always distinguish themselves with their breadth and depth of knowledge, their perceptive eye, and hopefully, their humanity. Perhaps these things cannot, after all, be taught. If this is the case, we are much better served by improving our craft with our knowledge of test construction and validation.

The Influence of Demographics on Understanding Neuropsychological Data

Part of the growth of clinical neuropsychology as a professional practice has involved increased recognition of special groups and their unique characteristics. Neuropsychology has combined the best of small and large group approaches to produce a scientifically based clinical practice that can accommodate the needs and characterize the uniqueness of a wide range of minority populations. It is probably safe to say that, as much as any one force, consideration of the influence of demographic factors on neuropsychological test performance has changed the face of practice in clinical neuropsychology. This is not to say that other approaches do not continue to exert influence on the collective thinking of the field, but the current trend and the shape of things to come are in the form of demographically matched comparison groups.

In the first edition of Grant and Adams' *Neuropsychological Assessment of Neuropsychiatric Disorders*, Heaton, Grant, and Matthews (1986; 1996) presented a chapter that looked at the relative influence of three demographic variables (age, education, gender) on the WAIS and HRB. In doing so, they galvanized a movement that would become one of the most rapidly and widely accepted approaches to understanding neuropsychological test performance. The influence of age and education on many different neuropsychological measures was well known (Seidenberg et al., 1984; Bornstein, 1986; Stuss et al., 1987), but the impetus for looking at such powerful demographic influences as a routine part of clinical practice was not well accepted, even 15 years ago. Cutting scores, impairment indices, and various "quotients" were the foundation on which our field was built and the brain damaged versus non-brain damaged distinction was viewed as a major goal of assessments.

It is perhaps not surprising that Reitan has vigorously opposed the use of demographically adjusted norms based on his argument that these variables exert little influence when examined in "brain damaged" populations (Reitan & Wolfson, 1996). The argument appears to be that the lack of stronger demographic effects within brain damaged groups begs the larger question of whether or not brain damage is apparent. The natural way to assess the presence of brain damage is, of course, to administer the HRB. While it is not my goal to critique the HRB model, it appears that a critique has already been thoroughly accomplished by virtue of prevailing professional standards. It simply is not necessary to administer a five to seven hour battery of tests to make this basic determination (i.e., the presence or absence of "brain damage"). Nonetheless, the field owes a debt of gratitude to the rigor of the HRB approach and its role in showing the importance of painstaking standardization. Moving back to the point, many of the questions that neuropsychologists are asked to address involve distinctions that are subtler than the old "functional versus organic" dichotomy that was the staple of referral questions 10 to 20 years ago. There is also ample evidence that demographic factors do, in fact, exert influence in brain damaged or dementing samples (Lamberty et al., 1993). Numerous recent studies have pointed to the influence of education as a "protective factor" by showing that those individuals with higher number of years of education typically show less impairment on traditional dementia screening tests and batteries. Whether education actually serves as a neuroprotective poultice, or perhaps simply as a cloaking device for neuropsychological test instruments, is still open for debate. The fact is, demographic factors assist in the detection of brain damage, for without appropriate knowledge of factors such as education and even general intellectual ability; false positive attributions are routinely made.

While actuarial or demographically corrected approaches have been very influential in the growth of clinical neuropsychology, reliance on such approaches without full understanding of the sampling procedures used and their implications could certainly be a "double edged sword." It is tempting to think that we can account for greater and greater proportions of test performance variability by improving the specificity of our sampling. However, appropriate norms for unique groups are probably only available on a "local norms" basis. Most clinicians have had to deal with patients whose background makes them unique, both from a humanistic and statistical standpoint. It may be that age, education and gender are solid blocking factors upon which to build a normative database, but the clinician must also be mindful of less universal variables that might also impact neuropsychological test performance. Again, this is where an understanding of the uniqueness of an individual's circumstances will assist in the accurate and appropriate diagnosis of neuropsychological dysfunction, and in turn, treatment recommendations.

As we have become more accurate and efficient in characterizing cognitive dysfunction, pressure to abbreviate our measures and overall exam times has been keenly felt. As noted earlier, this has been a largely economic issue with various payors at the center of the debate. It is common for individual practitioners to be played against one another by insurers to see who will provide the most cost effective services. In the insurance and managed care business, less is usually regarded as more or better. Thus, hungry providers are reduced to playing a game of "name that disorder" so that they might compete for the few dollars still allocated for the services we provide. Lest this be made to sound too desperate and unfair, the pressure to do more with less has really revolutionized the subfield of geriatric neuropsychology. A combination of actuarial methods and sane clinical practice has facilitated briefer dementia batteries that provide critical clinical input while preserving the dignity and peace of mind of dementia patients (Welsh, Butters, Mohs, Beekly, Edland, Fillenbaum, & Heyman, 1994; Randolph, 1998). There continue to be contexts in which briefer assessments are simply less. While screening evaluations have shown utility in a number of different acute settings, comprehensive neuropsychological assessments remain a standard in pediatric neurodevelopmental disorders, traumatic brain injury, presurgical epilepsy evaluations, and general adult referrals to name a few. Recent practice surveys continue to suggest that there is a lower limit on the amount of time needed to conduct and adequate assessment (Sweet et al., 2000; Camara, Nathan, & Puente, 2000). As with our general knowledge in neuropsychology, the parameters of adequate evaluations will eventually need to be determined via data collection and empirical assessment of what constitutes a good assessment. These are the issues on which the field will be reluctant to give ground. However, if we've learned anything from the past, it is that we are better suited to make these determinations than are insurance companies or healthcare administrators, so the time to take a dispassionate look at these issues is now.

Cross-Cultural Considerations

The remainder of this volume consists of a number of thoughtful discussions about factors involved in the neuropsychological assessment of minority populations. In the brief history just discussed, we have come to understand that neuropsychology is not a "one size fits all" enterprise. The scientific literature and clinical lore afford numerous examples of how well intended practitioners have erroneously assumed that tests that work for a typical North American cohort should be adequate for use with samples or individuals that differ in important ways. Artiola i Fortuny and Mullaney (1997) and others have been outspoken critics of those who would simply take existing measures and attempt to transform them into a foreign language measure without adequate understanding of the second language or the prevailing culture in which the test will be used. Translating measures is fraught with difficulties and is generally not recommended. While the work of developing and standardizing new, reliable and valid measures for different languages and cultures is demanding, it is essential if neuropsychology is to play an important role in other cultures and languages.

The foregoing account of the development of modern clinical neuropsychology will essentially have to be repeated in order to develop a reliable, valid, and functional practice of neuropsychological assessment in minority groups and different cultures. Fortunately, we can learn from our experiences in developing measures over the past 30 to 40 years. The application of demographic corrections provides a good model in accounting for factors that appear likely to exert influence on test outcomes. Neuropsychologists with a clear understanding of cultural issues and how they might affect performance on traditional measures must lead the charge. Indeed, such individuals have contributed widely to this volume and have started the process in earnest.

References

Artiola i Fortuny, L., & Mullaney, H. A. (1997). Neuropsychology with Spanish speakers: Language use and proficiency issues for test development. *Journal of Clinical and Experimental Neuropsychology, 19*, 615-622.

Boll, T., & Bryant, B. K. (Eds.) (1988). *Clinical neuropsychology and brain function: Research, measurement, and practice.* Washington, DC: American Psychological Association.

Bornstein, R. A. (1986). Classification rates obtained with "standard" cut-off scores on selected neuropsychological measures. *Journal of Clinical and Experimental Neuropsychology, 8*, 413-420.

Camara, W., Nathan, J., & Puente, A. (2000). Psychological test usage: Implications in professional psychology. *Professional Psychology: Research and Practice, 31*, 141-154.

Daubert v. Merrell Dow Pharmaceuticals, Inc., 113 S. Ct. 2786 (1993).

Garb, H. N. (1998). *Studying the clinician.* Washington, DC: American Psychological Association.

Golden, C. J., Purisch, A. D., & Hammeke, T. A. (1985). *The Luria-Nebraska Neuropsychological Battery Forms I and II manual.* Los Angeles: Western Psychological Services.

Goldstein, G., & Incagnoli, T. M. (1997). *Contemporary approaches to neuropsychological assessment.* New York: Plenum Press.

Grant, I., & Adams, K. M. (Eds.) (1996). *Neuropsychological assessment of neuropsychiatric disorders* (2nd ed.). New York: Oxford University Press.

Heaton, R. K., Grant, I., & Matthews, C. G. (1986). Differences in neuropsychological test performance associated with age, education, and sex. In I. Grant & K. M. Adams (Eds.), *Neuropsychological assessment of neuropsychiatric disorders.* New York: Oxford University Press.

Heaton, R. K., Ryan, L., Grant, I., & Matthews, C. G. (1996). Demographic influences on neuropsychological test performance. In I. Grant & K. M. Adams (Eds.). *Neuropsychological assessment of neuropsychiatric disorders* (2nd ed.). New York: Oxford University Press.

Jensen, A. R. (1998). *The g factor: the science of mental ability.* Westport, CT: Praeger Publishers.

Kaplan, E. (1988). A process approach to neuropsychological assessment. In T. Boll & B. K. Brynt (Eds.), Clinical neuropsychology and brain function: research, measurement and practice. Washington, DC: American Psychological Association.

Kaplan, E., Fein, D., Morris, R., & Delis, D. C. (1991). *The WAIS-R as a neuropsychological instrument: WAIS-R-NI manual*. New York: The Psychological Corporation.

Kaplan, E., Fein, D., Morris, R., & Delis, D. C. (1999). *The WISC-III as a process instrument: WISC-III-PI manual*. New York: The Psychological Corporation.

Lamberty, G. J., Bieliauskas, L. A., Chatel, D. M., & Holt, C. S. (1993). Effects of demographic factors and mental status on Wechsler Memory Scale performance in a geriatric clinic sample. *Developmental Neuropsychology, 9,* 271-281.

McKenna, P., & Warrington, E. K. (1996). The analytical approach to neuropsychological assessment. In I. Grant & K. M. Adams (Eds.) *Neuropsychological assessment of neuropsychiatric disorders* (2nd ed.). New York: Oxford University Press.

Lezak, M. (1995). *Neuropsychological Assessment* (3rd ed.). New York: Oxford University Press.

Meehl, P. E. (1954). *Clinical versus statistical prediction: A theoretical analysis and a review of the evidence*. Minneapolis: University of Minnesota Press.

Meehl, P. E. (1973). Why I do not attend case conferences. In P. E. Meehl (Ed.), *Psychodiagnostics: Selected papers* (pp. 225-302). Minneapolis: University of Minnesota Press.

Meehl, P. E. (1986). Causes and effects of my disturbing little book. *Journal of Personality Assessment, 50,* 370-375.

Mitrushina, M. N., Boone, K. B., & D'Elia, L. F. (1999). *Handbook of normative data for neuropsychological assessment*. New York: Oxford University Press.

Randolph, C. (1998). *Repeatable Battery for the Assessment of Neuropsychological Status (RBANS) manual*. San Antonio: The Psychological Corporation.

Reed, J.E. (1996). Fixed vs. flexible neuropsychological test batteries under the Daubert standard for the admissibility of scientific evidence. *Behavioral Sciences & the Law, 14,* 315-322.

Reitan, R. M., & Wolfson, D. (1996). Theoretical, methodological, and validational bases of the Halstead-Reitan Neuropsychological Test Battery. In I. Grant & K. M. Adams (Eds.), *Neuropsychological assessment of neuropsychiatric disorders* (2nd ed.). New York: Oxford University Press.

Rey, A. (1964). *L'Examen Clinique en Psychologie*. Paris: Press Universitaire de France.

Russell, E. W. (1997). Psychometric foundations of neuropsychological assessment. In G. Goldstein & T. M. Incagnoli (Eds.), *Contemporary approaches to neuropsychological assessment*. New York: Plenum Press.

Schmidt, M. (1996). *Rey auditory and verbal learning test: a handbook*. Los Angeles: Western Psychological Services.

Schmidt, M. (in press). *Test selection in clinical neuropsychology*. New York: Guilford Press.

Seidenberg, M., Gamache, M. P., Beck, N. C., Smith, M., Giordani, B., Berent, S., Sackellares, J. C., & Boll, T. J. (1984). Subject variables and performance on the Halstead Neuropsychological Test Battery: A multivariate analysis. *Journal of Consulting & Clinical Psychology, 52,* 658-662.

Spreen, O., & Strauss, E. (1998) *A compendium of neuropsychological tests: administration, norms, and commentary*. New York: Oxford University Press.

Stuss, D. T., Stethem, L. L., & Poirier, C. A. (1987). Comparison of three tests of attention and rapid information processing across six age groups. *The Clinical Neuropsychologist, 1,* 139-152.

Sweet, J. J. (Ed.) (1999). *Forensic neuropsychology: fundamentals and practice*. Lisse, Netherlands: Swets & Zeitlinger

Sweet, J. J., & Moberg, P. J. (1990). A survey of practices and beliefs among ABPP and non-ABPP clinical neuropsychologists. *The Clinical Neuropsychologist, 4,* 101-120.

Sweet, J. J., Moberg, P. J., & Suchy, Y. (2000). Ten-year follow-up survey of clinical neuropsychologists: Part I. Practices and beliefs. *The Clinical Neuropsychologist, 14,* 18-37.

Sweet, J. J., Moberg, P. J., & Westergaard, C. K. (1996). Five-year follow-up survey of practices and beliefs of clinical neuropsychologists. *The Clinical Neuropsychologist, 10,* 202-221.

Tranel, D. The Iowa-Benton school of neuropsychological assessment. In I. Grant & K. M. Adams (Eds.). *Neuropsychological assessment of neuropsychiatric disorders* (2nd ed.). New York: Oxford University Press.

Vanderploeg, R. D. (Ed.) (1994). *Clinician's guide to neuropsychological assessment.* Hillsdale, NJ: Lawrence Erlbaum.

Welsh, K. A., Butters, N., Mohs, R. C., Beekly, D., Edland, S., Fillenbaum, G., & Heyman, A. (1994). The Consortium to Establish a Registry for Alzheimer's Disease (CERAD). Part V. A normative study of the neuropsychological battery. *Neurology, 44,* 609-614.

Chapter 2

THE CROSS-CULTURAL NEUROPSYCHOLOGICAL TEST BATTERY (CCNB):

EFFECTS OF AGE, EDUCATION, ETHNICITY, AND COGNITIVE STATUS ON PERFORMANCE

Malcolm B. Dick, Ph.D.
Alzheimer's Disease Research Center, Institute for Brain Aging and Dementia, University of California, Irvine, California

Evelyn L. Teng, Ph.D.
Department of Neurology, Keck School of Medicine, University of Southern California, California

Daniel Kempler, Ph.D.
Department of Otolaryngology, Keck School of Medicine, University of Southern California, California

Deborah S. Davis, M.A.
Institute for Brain Aging and Dementia, University of California, Irvine, California

I. Maribel Taussig, Ph.D.
School of Gerontology, University of Southern California, California

Abstract

The Cross-Cultural Neuropsychological Test Battery (CCNB) was developed in response to the growing need for a culturally fair method of assessing cognitive functioning in minority populations. The CCNB includes 11 tests, takes approximately 90 minutes to administer, and has been given to 336 healthy older adults and 90 demented patients from five ethnic groups (African-American, Caucasian, Chinese, Hispanic, and Vietnamese). The participants' age ranged from 54 to 99 years ($M = 74.5$, $SD = 8.4$) and they had from 0 to 22 years ($M = 10.2$, $SD = 4.6$) of education. While education contributed significantly to performance on most of the tests, age affected scores on measures of recent memory and psychomotor speed. Ethnicity and language affected scores on measures of attention, category fluency, and visual-spatial functioning. As a whole, the demented patients scored significantly worse than their healthy peers on the entire CCNB. Tests of mental status and recent memory proved particularly useful in discriminating the two groups. Overall, the results demonstrated the effectiveness of the CCNB in identifying cognitive impairment in minority individuals and highlight the importance of considering education, age, and language when interpreting neuropsychological test findings.

Introduction

The field of neuropsychology is being challenged by the increasing ethnic diversity and aging of the United States population. Currently, 12% of all Americans are over age 65 and one in ten of these individuals is of minority background. By the year 2020, the 65-plus age group is expected to comprise 22% of the entire United States population, with a third of these seniors coming from diverse minority groups (U.S. Bureau of the Census & NIA, 1993). Despite the anticipated increase in the number of minority elders, relatively little work has been directed towards understanding the effects of age, culture, language, and education on neuropsychological test performance (Ardila, 1995; Gurland et al., 1992; Loewenstein et al., 1994; Taussig & Pontón, 1996). The lack of research on this issue is surprising as over a decade ago the National Institutes of Health, Consensus Development Conference, Statement on Diagnosing Dementias specifically noted the need for an "evaluation of results obtained with current neuropsychological instruments in populations that differ in age, education, ethnic composition, and social and cultural backgrounds" (NIH, 1987).

As the number of older adults continues to grow, the incidence of chronic conditions associated with aging, such as Alzheimer's disease (AD), can be expected to increase in minority as well as non-minority populations. The prevalence of AD has been estimated as ranging from 1-3% in the 65-74 age group, from 7-19% in those 75-84, and from 25-47.2% in those 85 and older

(Evans et al., 1989; U.S. Congress Office of Technology Assessment, 1987). Although the number of neuropsychological studies of AD has increased substantially over the past decade, most of these investigations have included primarily English-speaking Caucasian participants. There are relatively few published studies examining neuropsychological functioning in either cognitively intact or demented minority populations. Apart from a handful of studies (Ganguli et al., 1991; Glosser et al., 1993), most of the existing research contrasts the performance of English-speaking Caucasians on specific neuropsychological tests with either African-American (e.g., Fillenbaum, Huber, & Taussig, 1997; Ripich, Carpenter, & Zioli, 1997; Ross, Lichtenberg, & Christensen, 1995) or Spanish-speaking (e.g., Jacobs et al., 1997; Pontón et al., 1996; Taussig, Henderson, & Mack, 1992) individuals. To our knowledge, no published study has specifically compared the performance of elderly individuals from multiple ethnic groups on the same neuropsychological test battery.

Neuropsychological assessment has retained its key role in the diagnosis of dementia despite improvements in neuroimaging techniques, such as magnetic resonance imaging (MRI) and single photon emission computerized tomography (SPECT). According to the NINCDS-ADRDA criteria, a clinical diagnosis of possible or probable Alzheimer's disease (AD) can be based on a patient's neuropsychological test profile after all other possible medical, psychiatric, and neurological explanations for the individual's symptoms have been ruled out (McKhann et al., 1984). As noted by Loewenstein and Rubert (1992), NINCDS-ADRDA established stringent neuropsychological criteria, with the cutoff for impairment as the fifth percentile or lower in each of eight cognitive domains (orientation, memory, language, perceptual skills, praxis, attention, problem-solving, and functional status). Since cognitive impairment is the primary and most essential criterion for the diagnosis and staging of dementia, it is essential to have reliable and valid neuropsychological tools that are applicable across diverse cultures.

Identifying impairment, as defined by NINCDS-ADRDA, in individuals with different cultural, linguistic, and educational backgrounds is difficult without appropriate normative data. Clinicians may overestimate cognitive impairment in individuals with limited education, as these persons frequently score below the fifth percentile on neuropsychological tests (Ardilla, Rosselli, & Rosas, 1989; Ardila, Rosselli, & Puente, 1994; Taussig, Henderson, & Mack, 1992; Taussig & Pontón, 1996). For example, Pontón et al. (1996) found that nondemented Hispanic individuals with less than a sixth grade education scored up to two standard deviations below average when compared to persons with 16 years of schooling. These studies highlight the potential for misdiagnosis in the absence of appropriate tests or adequate normative data. In the absence of adequate norms, what is normal for one group (e.g., Caucasians) may be misinterpreted as pathological for another group. Consequently, the authors directed their efforts at compiling a set of relatively culturally fair neuropsychological measures with sufficient norms to allow accurate assessment of cognitive abilities in persons from a variety of ethnic backgrounds.

Method

Development of the Cross-Cultural Neuropsychological Test Battery (CCNB)

In 1991, the Southern California Alzheimer's Disease Research Centers (ADRC) formed a multi-disciplinary Language and Cultural Advisory Committee for the express purpose of addressing problems associated with diagnosing dementia in individuals from diverse educational, linguistic, and cultural backgrounds. Experts in dementia and cross-cultural research from several fields, including neuropsychology, linguistics, gerontology, and neurology, collaborated to develop a brief neuropsychological assessment battery with broad applicability across the various minority groups served by the ADRCs in the United States. The committee's goal was to compile a battery of tests that would accurately (1) characterize the primary manifestations of AD in minority individuals, (2) discriminate between cognitive changes associated with normal aging and those seen in dementia, and (3) measure the progression of cognitive impairment.

Several general guidelines governed development of the battery. First, the goal of minimizing administration time was achieved by limiting the CCNB to 11 instruments. Secondly, to facilitate comparisons between the wealth of existing data on English-speaking Caucasians and the performance of minority individuals, five well-established tests were included in the CCNB. Thirdly, the committee sought to reduce the effects of illiteracy or low education on performance, given evidence that even scores on a simple test involving continuous alternating finger movements show a high correlation with educational level (Rosselli et al., 1990). To achieve this goal, the committee employed several strategies, including using oral rather than printed instructions, requiring oral or nonverbal responses rather than written answers, and presenting pictorial rather than verbal stimulus information (Jensen, 1980) in the CCNB. Fourthly, as many minority families do not seek assistance until late in the course of a dementia (Elliott, Di Minno, Lam, & Tu, 1996), the committee included tests which can be performed by persons with moderate to severe cognitive impairment. Finally, to obtain valid data, the committee emphasized that the battery should be administered by a bilingual examiner in the patient's primary language rather than through a translator. Untrained translators may be unable to convey the nuances of cognition and affect (Sabin, 1975), normalize the patient's thought processes in an attempt to make sense of disorganized statements, and unintentionally distort test data through omissions, substitutions, and condensation (Marcos, 1979).

The committee identified tests for the CCNB through a multi-stage process, beginning with an extensive literature review. The limited number of instruments emerging from this review included Spanish (Escobar et al., 1986; Bird et al., 1987; Taussig et al., 1992), Chinese (Katzman et al., 1988; Yu et al., 1989), and Japanese (Hasegawa, 1983) versions of the Mini-Mental State Examination (MMSE; Folstein, Folstein, & McHugh, 1975);

the *Escala de Inteligencia Wechsler para Adultos* (EIWA; Green & Martinez, 1968) or Spanish version of the WAIS; the Hispanic Neuropsychological Battery (Valle, Hough, Cook-Gait, Lui, & Labovitz, 1991); and French, Spanish, Chinese, and Japanese (Demers et al., 1994; Feldman et al., 1997) translations of the test battery developed by the Consortium to Establish a Registry for Alzheimer's Disease (CERAD) (Morris et al., 1989).

Each of these existing instruments has certain limitations. First, global measures of cognitive functioning, such as the MMSE, yield only a single score and provide little information about the separate abilities impaired in dementia. Secondly, although the EIWA has extensive and carefully collected population-based norms, these norms have limited applicability to Spanish-speaking older adults in the continental United States (López & Romero, 1988). The EIWA normative sample, collected in the mid-1960s, is comprised of Puerto Ricans under age 65. Only 12% of Hispanic Americans, however, are of Puerto Rican heritage, while almost half are of Mexican background (U.S. Bureau of the Census, 1993). Thirdly, usefulness of the Hispanic Neuropsychological Battery is limited by the small normative sample of 42 non-demented and 30 demented individuals. Fourthly, although the CERAD neuropsychological test battery has been translated into multiple languages, normative data for non-Caucasian individuals is very limited. In addition, the CERAD battery includes tests, such as the Word List Memory task, that are of limited usefulness with illiterate individuals (Ganguli et al., 1991), as well as, instruments such as the Boston Naming test which is affected by both cultural/linguistic (Fillenbaum, Huber, & Taussig, 1997; Ross et al., 1995; Taussig et al., 1992; Valle et al., 1991) and educational (Rosselli et al., 1990) variables. While the instruments which existed at the time of the survey represented progress toward accurate neuropsychological assessment of minority individuals, the committee recognized that the approach of designing unique tests for every minority group would not only be too costly, but also hamper cross-cultural comparisons.

Given the handful of published instruments, the committee decided to survey 16 ADRC sites across the United States and California's nine Alzheimer's Disease Diagnostic and Treatment Centers (ADDTCs) as a means of identifying tests commonly used to assess dementia in English and non English-speaking populations. Of the centers contacted, only a few had tests for assessing minority individuals. Results of the survey, like the literature review, revealed the need for a battery of neuropsychological tests with true cross-cultural applicability. Consequently, the committee moved forward with the task of selecting and/or developing instruments for the CCNB based on the five governing principles described above.

Initially, the committee selected appropriate instruments from the pool of tests generated by the literature review and survey. The five commonly used tests which did not violate the guidelines were Trail Making Test Part A, WAIS-R Digit Span and Block Design, and the Animal Naming and Figure Drawing portions of the CERAD battery (Morris et al., 1989). Approximately 50% of the survey respondents used Trail Making Test Part A, 56% used Block Design and Figure Drawing, 62% used Digit Span, and 62% used animal naming as a measure of category fluency. Other frequently used tests were excluded in the selection process. For example, the Boston Naming Test, was not included in the CCNB although 94% of the survey respondents used this instrument to assess confrontational naming in English-speaking individuals.

While the five familiar tests made cross-cultural comparisons possible, these instruments did not cover the broader range of cognitive domains impaired in AD. To supplement these five tests, the committee developed five additional tests, including Body Part Naming, Auditory Comprehension, Read and Set Time, Modified Picture Completion, and the Common Objects Memory Test. Development of these tests involved (a) selecting and translating items, (b) adapting items as necessary for the five target groups (African-American, Caucasian, Chinese, Hispanic, and Vietnamese), (c) pilot testing and (d) final adjustments. First, items for each of the tests were selected and translated with the assistance of experts from each of the ethnic groups. Test items were translated and back-translated using the procedures outlined by Taussig et al. (1992). This standard process in cross-cultural research (Brislin et al., 1973) involves translation from English into the target language by one expert in that language, back translation by multiple individuals blind to the original English version, and comparisons of the back translations to ensure consensus and reconcile differences. During this process, the experts helped identify any biases or language-related issues in the test items. For example, as noted by Teng (1996), there are no words for certain body parts (*e.g.*, shin, instep) in the Chinese language. Consequently, only body parts for which names existed in all five languages were included in the Body Part Naming Test. Following the selection, translation, and adaptation process, the committee pilot tested the items on small samples of minority individuals. Based on this pilot testing, final adjustments were made to the instruments.

Using the standard translation process (Taussig et al., 1992), the committee also translated the five well-established tests into Vietnamese and Chinese. Existing Spanish language translations were used for the five tests. More specifically, instructions for Block Design and Digit Span were taken from the EIWA (Green & Martinez, 1968) and those for Trail Making Part A and the CERAD Category Fluency and Figure Drawing tests from Taussig et al. (1992). In addition to the ten measures of specific abilities, the committee included translated and adapted versions of the Cognitive Abilities Screening Instrument (CASI: Teng et al., 1994; Teng, 1996) as a global measure of cognitive functioning in the CCNB.

Measures of Neuropsychological Functioning
The CCNB taps six cognitive domains: recent memory, attention, language, reasoning ability, visual spatial skills, and psychomotor speed. The 11 tests

Table 1. Summary of tests comprising the cross-cultural neuropsychological test battery.

Cognitive Domain	Test
Mental Status	Cognitive Abilities Screening Instrument (CASI)
Recent Memory	Common Objects Memory Test (COMT) *
Language	Body Part Naming * CERAD Category Fluency for Animal Names Auditory Comprehension *
Visuospatial	Read & Set Time * CERAD Drawing WAIS-R Block Design
Attention	WAIS-R Digit Span
Reasoning	Modified Picture Completion *
Psychomotor Speed	Trails Making Test, Part A

* Denotes a new test developed by the authors.

comprising the CCNB are listed in Table 1, according to the cognitive domain being assessed. It should be noted that many of the tests measure several domains (*e.g.*, Digit Span can be considered a measure of working memory as well as of attention). The five well-established tests in the CCNB were administered using standardized procedures, as described in the references. The five new tests and procedures for their administration are described in detail here.

Mental Status. Overall cognitive functioning was evaluated with the CASI which taps ten cognitive domains commonly assessed in dementia: attention, concentration, orientation, short-term memory, long-term memory, language ability, constructional praxis, verbal fluency, abstraction, and everyday problem-solving skills. In most of these domains, scores range from 0 to 10 points, with the total CASI score ranging from 0 to 100. Designed for cross-cultural application, the CASI is easier to adapt for a variety of cultural/language groups than many of the screening instruments currently used with English-speaking individuals (*e.g.*, MMSE). Unlike these instruments, when direct translation of an item is inappropriate, the CASI provides a culturally fair alternative. For example, as the phrase "No ifs, ands, or buts" is meaningless to non-English speaking individuals, the CASI provides alternative versions of this item, using linguistically equivalent phrases from other languages.

Recent Memory. The authors developed *The Common Objects Memory Test* (COMT) as a culture fair measure of recent memory specifically for the CCNB. In this test, the examinee is shown a set of ten 3x5″ color photographs of common objects (*e.g.*, chair, scissors, leaf) across three learning trials at the rate of one picture every two seconds. The pictures are presented in a standard but different presentation order during each trial. The examinee is asked to name the objects aloud as they are shown and try to remember them for a later recall test. A test of free recall is given immediately after each trial. After the third trial, the examinee is engaged with a brief distracter task (*i.e.*, CERAD Figure Drawing) for three to five minutes and then asked once again to recall the items. This test of delayed recall is immediately followed by a recognition test in which the ten original objects are interspersed with ten distracters. The examinee is asked to indicate with a simple "Yes" or "No" whether an object was seen previously. The distracter items are similar to the original objects in terms of frequency of use and absence of distinctive details. Long-term retention of the original objects is assessed after a 30-minute delay using tests of recall and recognition, with a different set of ten distracters.

Language. Three tests are used to assess language abilities: *confrontational naming of body parts, auditory comprehension*, and *category fluency for animal names.* In body part naming, the examinee is asked to name ten body parts as they are pointed to or touched by the examiner. Body parts were selected as (a) all cultures and languages have specific names for parts of the human body (Anderson, 1978), (b) body parts provide a range of "difficulty" from common (*e.g.*, hand) to less common (*e.g.*, eyebrow, fingernail), (c) body part naming is relatively unaffected by education (Rosselli et al., 1990), and (d) this task does not require any additional materials (*e.g.*, pictures, objects) since the examiner's own body parts constitute the stimuli.

The Animal Naming test from the CERAD battery requires the examinee to name "all the animals you can think of in one minute." Examinees receive credit for naming general categories (*e.g.*, dog, cat) as well as specific exemplars (*e.g.*, poodle, leopard). Repeated responses are counted only once.

Finally, auditory comprehension is assessed by asking the examinee to execute ten verbal commands, which range from simple one-step actions (*e.g.*, open your mouth) to complex three-stage tasks (*e.g.*, put the watch on the other side of the pencil and turn over the card). The authors determined complexity of the commands by counting the number of "information units" contained in each statement. Grammatical complexity was specifically not manipulated since grammatical relationships vary markedly from language to language. The sentences in the comprehension section were translated into the target languages without altering the number of critical information units. The score on this test refers to the total number of informational units correctly responded to and can range from 0 to 25 points.

Visual Spatial Skills. The CCNB includes three tests which measure visual spatial functioning. The first, *WAIS-R Block Design*, is administered using standard procedures. The second test, *CERAD Figure Drawing*, requires the examinee to copy four figures of increasing complexity (*i.e.*, circle, four-sided diamond, pair of intersecting rectangles, and necker cube). There are specific criteria for scoring each figure, with a maximum total score of 11 points. The third test, *Read and Set Time*, involves having the examinee (a) read time on three clocks, set at 3:00, 7:10, and 4:45, and (b) draw the hands of a clock at three different times (*i.e.*, 9:00, 4:10, and 7:50). In the clock reading portion, the examinee receives one point each for the correct hour and the correct minute, for a maximum score of 6. In the clock setting portion, the examinee receives one point each for the correct positioning of the hour hand, the correct positioning of the minute hand, and the correct relative length of the two hands, for a maximum score of 9.

Reasoning. To assess reasoning ability, the authors complied a set of ten pictures which tap similar concepts to those measured by the Wechsler Picture Completion tests. The CCNB version includes line drawings of persons from various cultures involved in universal experiences, but with an important part missing (*e.g.*, a bearded man looking in a hand-held mirror, with the reflection missing the beard). The examinee is asked to identify the missing part in each picture either verbally or by pointing. Items are scored as either 1 (correct) or 0 (incorrect).

Attention. The *WAIS-R Digit Span* is included in the CCNB to measure attention and is administered using standard procedures.

Psychomotor speed. Part A of the Trail Making Test is used to assess psychomotor speed and administered using standard procedures.

Phase 1: Norming the CCNB

The normative sample included 336 healthy older adults from five ethnic groups: African-American, Caucasian, Chinese, Hispanic, and Vietnamese. To ensure representativeness of the sample, efforts were made to recruit an equal number of participants in the five ethnic groups from three age (*i.e.*, 60-67, 68-75, and ≥ 76 years) and education (*i.e.*, 0-8, 9-12, ≥ 13 years) ranges. Participants were recruited through senior centers, diagnostic centers, and the Los Angeles and Orange County chapters of the Alzheimer's Association as well as through public service announcements. Participants were reimbursed $20 for their involvement in this study.

Almost all of the participants in the Vietnamese, Chinese, and Hispanic groups spoke only their native language at home and the majority did not read English. Of the 61 Vietnamese participants , 97% spoke only Vietnamese and 56% did not read English. Of the 71 Chinese participants, 98% spoke only Chinese and 82% did not read English. Finally, of the 80 Hispanic participants, 81% spoke only Spanish and 63% did not read English. Median number of years in the United States was 3 for Vietnamese participants, 9 for Chinese, and 25 for Hispanic.

All of the participants were tested either at home or a local senior center by trained examiners. The examiners administered the entire test battery in one sitting and obtained demographic and medical information from each participant. More specifically, all participants were screened for the presence of major health problems, cognitive impairment, depression, and functional deficits. Participants who acknowledged a history of stroke, head injury, traumatic loss of consciousness, or psychiatric, speech, language, or memory problems on a health questionnaire were excluded. In addition, all participants had to be free of any physical disabilities (*e.g.*, movement disorders, uncorrected hearing or vision problems) that could interfere with neuropsychological testing.

To help rule out cognitive impairment, each participant was asked to have a family member complete (1) the Informant Questionnaire of Cognitive Decline in the Elderly (IQCODE) (Jorm & Jacomb, 1989; Jorm, Scott, Cullen, & Mackinnon, 1991) and (2) the Activities of Daily Living Scale (ADL) (Lopez & Taussig, 1991). The IQCODE is a 26-item rating scale that assesses cognitive decline in older adults independent of premorbid ability. A knowledgeable informant, usually the spouse, is asked to rate the degree of change in an older adult's memory and intellectual functioning over the previous ten-year period. Recent studies (Fuh et al., 1995; Jorm & Jacomb, 1989; Morales et al., 1995) have shown that the IQCODE accurately discriminates normal from cognitively impaired individuals in various ethnic groups and has little correlation with education. The 18-item ADL scale was used to exclude individuals with behavioral impairments in areas such as personal care, housekeeping, and management of finances from this study. In a comparison of English- and Spanish-speaking older adults, Lopez and Taussig found that their instrument accurately distinguished cognitively impaired from unimpaired elders regardless of language/cultural background.

Finally, the Center for Epidemiological Studies Depression Scale (CES-D) was administered to all potential participants. Individuals who scored over the cutoff of 16 for clinical depression were excluded from the study. Numerous studies have documented the validity and reliability of the CES-D in both community and clinical samples of Caucasians, Hispanics, and African-Americans (Roberts, 1980, 1981) as well as in Chinese (Ying, 1988) and other Asian-American groups (Kuo, 1984).

Data Collection and Analysis

A total of 14 examiners administered the battery to the 336 healthy participants. The three Chinese, three Vietnamese, and four Hispanic bilingual examiners administered the battery in each participant's primary language and dialect. One African-American and three Caucasian examiners administered the battery to the English-speaking participants. All of the examiners received 12-16 hours of training in administration and scoring of the CCNB.

All written responses and scores were reviewed by the authors for possible errors. Research assistants double entered individual item scores from all of the tests into a database under the supervision of the authors. Accuracy of data entry was maintained by having different research assistants review the data files and by checking outlying scores.

Hierarchical linear regression equations were used to examine the influence of age, education, and ethnic background on test performance. Preliminary regression analyses included each of the three variables of interest, as well as, all possible interaction terms. No interaction terms, however, were found to be significant. Thus, the analyses were repeated entering only the main variables. Education was entered into the regression equations first, as preliminary analyses indicated that Education had the greatest effect on performance. Age was entered second and Ethnicity variables was added last.

Results

Participants
Across groups, the healthy participants had a mean age of 73.2 (± 7.6) years and attended school for an average of 10.2 (± 5.0) years. More detailed demographic information on each of the five ethnic groups is shown in Table 2.

The groups differed significantly from one another on Age, $F(4,331) = 6.2$, $p \leq .001$, and Education, $F(4, 331) = 7.6$, $p \leq .001$. Tukey-HSD comparisons, evaluated at a Bonferroni adjusted .01 level of significance, revealed that the Caucasians were significantly older than participants in the other groups. In an effort to include enough data from low education Caucasians, the researchers ended up testing a greater number of older individuals, as they were more likely to have fewer years of schooling.

Test Scores
Mean and standard deviation scores for the 11 tests are shown in Table 3 for each of the five ethnic groups. Comprehensive norms for each of the CCNB tests according to age, education, and ethnicity are presented elsewhere (Dick, Teng, Kempler, Davis, & Taussig, in preparation; Kempler, Teng, Dick, & Davis, 1998).

The percentage of variance accounted for by Education, Age, and Ethnicity is reported separately for each test in Table 4. Analyses revealed that level

Table 2. Demographic background of the healthy participants.

Group	Age				Education			
	n	M	SD	Range	M	SD	Range	% male
African-American	54	72.7	9.1	59-99	11.6	4.7	0-22	23%
Caucasian	70	77.0	7.4	61-96	11.4	3.9	6-20	34%
Chinese	71	72.6	7.2	59-86	11.2	5.6	0-22	48%
Hispanic	80	71.9	7.4	54-89	8.3	5.3	0-20	20%
Vietnamese	61	71.5	5.8	62-87	8.6	4.1	0-16	57%
Total	336	73.2	7.6	54-99	10.1	5.0	0-22	36%

Table 3. Mean and standard deviation scores for healthy older adults on the CCNB according to ethnicity.

CCNB Test	African-American		Caucasians		Chinese		Hispanic		Vietnamese	
	M	SD	M	SD	M	SD	M	SD	M	SD
Mental Status										
CASI	84.5	10.3	91.4	5.2	88.3	10.7	84.4	10.7	85.7	11.0
Recent Memory										
COMT Trial 1	6.3	1.5	5.9	1.5	6.3	1.5	5.8	1.5	6.5	1.5
COMT Trial 2	7.5	1.3	7.3	1.0	7.7	1.6	7.5	1.6	7.6	1.7
COMT Trial 3	8.2	1.2	7.9	1.0	8.1	1.4	8.2	1.6	8.1	1.1
COMT 3-5 min. Recall	7.4	1.8	7.2	1.5	7.9	1.8	7.5	1.9	7.9	1.8
COMT 30 min. Recall	7.5	1.6	7.1	1.7	7.8	2.0	7.7	1.8	7.8	1.5
COMT 5 min. Recogn.	19.9	0.2	19.7	0.7	19.4	0.9	19.7	1.2	19.7	0.7
COMT 30 min. Recogn.	19.9	0.3	19.9	0.4	19.5	1.1	19.6	1.4	19.7	0.6
Language										
Body Part Naming	9.9	0.1	9.9	0.2	9.9	0.2	9.7	0.6	9.8	0.4
Animal Fluency	15.2	4.4	16.3	4.0	15.5	5.0	12.8	3.9	17.3	5.2
Aud. Comprehension	24.2	0.8	24.2	0.9	23.3	2.3	23.7	1.7	23.3	2.2
Visual-Spatial										
Read & Set Test	11.8	2.7	12.5	2.0	12.9	2.3	12.5	3.6	13.4	2.2
CERAD Drawing	8.3	2.1	9.3	1.7	9.4	1.9	9.2	1.9	9.9	1.8
WAIS-R Block Design*	13.7	7.1	20.8	7.5	22.3	9.5	17.2	9.9	18.9	9.3
Attention										
Digit Span Fwd.	8.4	2.1	7.8	2.1	8.7	2.4	4.7	1.9	9.1	2.8
Digit Span Bkw.	5.0	2.1	5.8	2.5	5.7	2.3	3.9	1.5	5.2	2.2
Reasoning										
Mod. Pict. Completion	7.3	2.1	8.8	1.1	7.2	2.3	7.5	2.2	6.6	2.7
Psychomotor Speed										
Trails Making, Part A	67.5	53.1	51.0	21.4	75.8	48.0	90.0	57.3	83.9	58.0

* Scores on the WAIS-R Digit Span and Block Design tests represent raw scores.

of education affected performance on almost all the tests and, on average, accounted for 15% of the variance in scores. Age was more important than education on the COMT and affected performance on recall but not recognition. Age also played a role in tests involving visual spatial functioning (*i.e.*, Drawing, Block Design) and psychomotor speed (*i.e.*, Trail Making Test, Form A). Overall, age accounted for 4% of the variance, while ethnicity accounted for 10%. Ethnicity affected performance primarily on tests of attention (*i.e.*, Digit Span), verbal fluency (*i.e.*, CERAD Animal Naming), and visual spatial functioning (*i.e.*, WAIS-R Block Design, CERAD Drawing, Read and Set Time). The Caucasians outperformed their African-American, Chinese, Hispanic, and Vietnamese peers on the Trail Making Test, CASI, and Modified Picture Completion test, but scored similarly to the other four groups on most of the remaining tests. The African-American participants had more difficulty than the other four groups on tests of drawing and visual-

Table 4. Percentage of variance accounted for according to education, age, and ethnicity for each of the CCNB tests.*

CCNB Test	Education	Age	Ethnicity
Mental Status			
CASI	27	3	5
Recent Memory			
COMT Learning Trials 1-3	--	9-16	--
COMT Delayed Recall	--	13	--
COMT Recognition	--	--	--
Language			
Body Part Naming	4	--	6
CERAD Animal Fluency	12	3	10
Auditory Comprehension	7	--	5
Visual-Spatial			
Read & Set Time	15	2	5
CERAD Drawing	10	3	9
WAIS-R Block Design	18	4	10
Attention			
Digit Span Forward	12	--	29
Digit Span Backwards	18	--	6
Reasoning			
Mod. Picture Completion	23	--	8
Psychomotor Speed			
Trails Making Test, Part A	15	7	6

* -- indicates less than 1% of the variance in test scores.

spatial constructional skills, while the Hispanics scored significantly lower than their African-American, Caucasians, Chinese, and Vietnamese peers on tests of category fluency and attention. Interestingly, there were no differences between the five ethnic groups on the COMT. All together, age, education, and ethnicity accounted for an average of 28% of the variance in test scores.

As the CCNB is comprised of multiple tests assessing a limited number of constructs, factor analysis was used to determine if the tests loaded onto the expected constructs. The results of a factor analysis using a Varimax rotation procedure revealed a four-factor solution. The tests comprising these four factors are shown in Table 5.

The five tests involving the processing of visual spatial information, namely Modified Picture Completion, Trail Making Part A, WAIS-R Block Design, CERAD Drawing, and Reading/Setting Time, all clustered closely together. Similarly, those tests assessing primarily language skills and/or requiring verbal responses (*i.e.,* body part naming, auditory comprehension, category fluency for animal names, and Digit Span) tended to group together. Interestingly, the two recognition tests formed a separate factor independent of the immediate and delayed recall portions of the COMT.

Table 5. CCNB factor analysis.

	Component			
CCNB Test	Visual-Spatial	Recall	Verbal	Recognition
Recent Memory				
COMT Learning Trials 1-3	.187	.843	.127	.068
COMT 3-5 min. Recall	.176	.857	.022	.036
COMT 30 min. Recall	.093	.865	.074	.015
COMT 5 min. Recognition	.007	.086	-.088	.876
COMT 30 min. Recognition	.046	.013	.140	.875
Language				
Body Part Naming	-.098	-.120	.770	.061
CERAD Animal Fluency	.321	.225	.573	.024
Auditory Comprehension	.097	.110	.568	.045
Visual-Spatial				
Read & Set Time	.702	.187	-.015	-.043
CERAD Drawing	.740	.128	.065	-.061
WAIS-R Block Design	.772	.169	.150	-.019
Attention				
WAIS-R Digit Span	.309	.051	.538	-.114
Reasoning				
Mod. Picture Completion	.722	-.036	.237	.165
Psychomotor Speed				
Trails Making Test, Part A	-.512	-.183	-.393	-.082

Extraction Method: Principal Component Analysis.
Rotation Method: Varimax with Kaiser Normalization.

Phase 2: Validation of the CCNB

In Phase 2, the researchers administered the CCNB to neurologically impaired patients in each of the five ethnic groups with the goal of determining how effective the battery would be at identifying cognitive impairment. A total of 117 cognitively impaired participants were recruited through the UCI and USC ADRCs. Twenty-seven individuals who scored at or near the floor on many of the CCNB tests were excluded from the validation sample. These individuals were all severely demented, with scores on the Clinical Dementia Rating (CDR) scale (Hughes et al., 1982) of 3 or higher. The final sample of 90 included four African-Americans, 20 English-speaking Caucasians, 18 Chinese, 39 Hispanic, and nine Vietnamese individuals. Barriers to service use created by language, cultural, economic, and educational differences interfered with the authors achieving the original goal of administering the CCNB to an equal number of AD patients in each ethnic group.

Eighty-four of the participants (93%) met the NINCDS-ADRDA diagnostic criteria for either probable or possible AD (McKhann et al., 1984). These participants evidenced mild-to-moderate dementia as indicated by CDR scores falling between 1.0 and 2.0. The remaining six individuals showed evidence of cognitive impairment on the clinical examination as well as the IQCODE and ADL measures, and scored 0.5 on the CDR (*i.e.*, questionable or borderline dementia). Limiting the sample to less impaired individuals made it possible to focus on determining the sensitivity of the battery to mild dementia. Finally, none of the participants had a history of major psychiatric illness, chronic alcoholism, other neurological disorders, or any physical impairment which would interfere with performance of the tests. The presence of multi-infarct dementia was ruled out through the patient's medical history, including neuroimaging data (*i.e.*, CAT and MRI scans) and a score of four or less on the Hachinski Ischemic Scale (Rosen et al., 1980).

The entire CCNB was administered to each cognitively impaired participant as part of the diagnostic evaluation. Although the 90 cognitively impaired participants were significantly older (M = 75.8, SD = 9.3 years) than their 336 non-impaired peers (M = 73.2, SD = 7.6), t (423) = 2.7, p < .01, the two groups were similar in level of education. More specifically, the cognitively impaired participants and healthy controls had completed an average of 10.4 (SD = 4.1) and 10.1 (SD = 5.0) years of formal schooling, respectively. As might be expected, the mean score on the IQCODE was significantly larger, t (341) = 18.2, p < .001, in the cognitively impaired participants (M = 4.3, SD = 0.6) than in the healthy controls (M = 3.1, SD = 0.4).

Results

Both ANOVA and logistic regression procedures were used to analyze the data. Given the small number of cognitively impaired participants in some of the ethnic groups, it was not possible to compare test sores for healthy and impaired individuals in each of the minority groups separately. Rather the data from the cognitively impaired participants were considered as a whole in the analyses. A series of ANOVAs compared the performance of the 336 healthy controls and 90 cognitively impaired participants on each of the 11 tests in the battery. Given the significant difference in age between the two groups, age was included as a covariate in all of the analyses. Age, however, did not turn out to be a significant factor in any of the analyses. As shown in Table 6, the healthy controls scored significantly higher than their cognitively impaired peers on all 11 tests in the CCNB. As might be expected, the difference between the 3-5-minute and 30-minute recall tests was significant in the cognitively impaired participants, t (88) = 3.6, p < .01, but not in the normal controls, t (332) = -0.4, p = .69. While the cognitively impaired participants scored significantly below their healthy peers on both of the COMT recognition tests, the difference in performance at 5 and 30 minutes was not significant for either group.

Although the performance of the cognitively impaired and healthy participants differed on all 11 instruments in the CCNB, the results suggest some of the tests may be more useful than others at discriminating between these two

Table 6. Mean and standard deviation scores for the 336 healthy controls and 90 AD patients on the CCNB tests.

CCNB Test	Healthy Controls		AD Patients		ANOVA	Adjusted R-Square
	M	SD	M	SD		
Mental Status						
CASI	87	10.1	59	21.1	F(1, 405) = 314.4*	.44
Recent Memory						
COMT Learning Trial 1	6.0	1.5	2.8	2.1	F(1, 419) = 284.5*	.40
COMT Learning Trial 2	7.5	1.5	4.0	2.4	F(1, 417) = 275.2*	.40
COMT Learning Trial 3	8.1	1.4	4.5	2.4	F(1, 418) = 326.7*	.44
COMT 3-5 min. Recall	7.6	1.8	2.5	2.7	F(1, 422) = 442.9*	.51
COMT 30 min. Recall	7.6	1.8	2.1	2.5	F(1, 420) = 571.6*	.58
COMT 5 min. Recognition	19.7	1.1	16.3	3.6	F(1, 422) = 219.7*	.34
COMT 30 min. Recognition	19.7	1.1	15.8	4.4	F(1, 420) = 221.2*	.34
Language						
Body Part Naming	9.9	0.4	9.4	1.8	F(1, 422) = 23.7*	.05
CERAD Animal Fluency	15.3	4.8	9.1	4.9	F(1, 411) = 110.8*	.21
Auditory Comprehension	23.7	1.8	21.1	5.0	F(1, 419) = 60.3*	.12
Visual-Spatial						
Read & Set Time	12.7	2.8	8.3	4.5	F(1, 412) = 122.5*	.23
CERAD Drawing	9.3	1.9	7.6	2.9	F(1, 417) = 39.9*	.09
WAIS-R Block Design	18.8	9.3	6.8	7.6	F(1, 412) = 119.5*	.22
Attention						
WAIS-R Digit Span	12.6	4.4	9.4	4.0	F(1, 412) = 36.7*	.08
Reasoning						
Mod. Picture Completion	7.5	2.2	5.5	2.8	F(1, 414) = 49.6*	.11
Psychomotor Speed						
Trails Making Test, Part A	73.7	50.6	122.6	77.0	F(1, 375) = 40.0*	.09

* Indicates significance at $p \leq .001$.

groups. Table 7 reports the percentage of cognitively impaired and healthy older adults scoring in the impaired range on each of the 11 tests. Scores falling at or below the fifth percentile (*i.e.*, two standard deviations below the mean, corrected for age, education, and ethnicity) are considered outside of the normal range. Clearly, the majority of healthy older adults in each of the five ethnic groups scored above the cutoff separating normal from impaired levels of performance. In contrast, many of the cognitively impaired participants scored below the cutoff, with the highest percentage showing deficits on tests of mental status (*i.e.*, CASI) and recent memory (*i.e.*, COMT).

Using the results of the earlier factor analysis, composite scores were calculated for each of the four factors by summing scores on the individual tests. These composite scores were then entered into a logistic regression equation with the CASI total score and CASI-derived MMSE score (CASI-MMSE). The Recall factor, with an Odds Ratio (*OR*) of .80 and 95% Confidence

Table 7. Percentage of healthy older adults and AD patients scoring in the impaired range on the CCNB.

CCNB Test	AD Patients (90)	Healthy Older Adults					
		Afric. Amer. (54)	Cauc. (70)	Chinese (71)	Hispan. (80)	Viet. (61)	Total (336)
Mental Status							
CASI	64.6	3.8	2.9	2.9	7.6	5.3	5.8
Recent Memory (COMT)							
Learning Trials 1-3	68.3	3.7	4.3	5.6	7.6	5.0	3.0
3-5 min. Recall	77.5	3.7	4.3	2.8	3.8	4.9	3.9
30 min. Recall	80.9	1.9	5.8	2.8	6.4	4.9	5.4
5 min. Recognition	53.9	3.7	4.3	2.8	2.5	6.6	2.4
30 min. Recognition	49.5	1.9	5.7	4.2	3.6	5.0	1.8
Language							
Body Part Naming	21.3	1.9	2.9	5.6	6.3	1.6	11.0
Animal Fluency	28.9	1.9	1.4	2.9	0.7	1.7	1.5
Aud. Comprehension	22.5	1.9	5.7	7.0	7.8	3.3	5.4
Visual-Spatial							
Read & Set Test	42.4	5.6	1.4	2.9	8.0	6.6	4.9
CERAD Drawing	10.2	3.7	4.3	4.3	1.3	3.3	1.2
WAIS-R Block Design	37.9	1.9	1.4	2.9	2.7	1.6	1.5
Attention							
WAIS-R Digit Span	9.5	0.0	0.0	1.5	1.3	3.3	1.8
Reasoning							
Mod. Pict. Completion	30.9	5.6	4.3	4.2	5.1	4.9	6.3
Psychomotor Speed							
Trails Making, Part A	17.7	3.7	2.9	3.0	4.0	4.0	6.0

Interval (*CI*) of .72 to .89, (*p* <.001), and CASI-MMSE (*OR* = .80, 95% *CI* =.68-.95, *p* < .01) produced the best overall model based on the Hosmer and Lemeshow Goodness of Fit test (1989) with a Chi-Square of 8.80, *p* = .36, and 8 degrees of freedom.

Although the complete CCNB can be administered to a cognitively impaired individual in about an hour-and-a-half, some clinicians may choose to use a shorter, less time consuming version of the battery. Logistic regression was used to identify the tests that most effectively differentiated healthy from cognitively impaired individuals. Measures that best separated the two groups included the 30-minute recall, 5-minute recognition, CASI-MMSE, WAIS-R Block Design, and Auditory Comprehension tests. The 30-minute recall was the most important of the tests (*OR* = .76, 95% *CI* = .67-.87, *p* < .001), followed by the CASI-MMSE (*OR* = .89, 95% *CI* = .82 -.96, *p* < .005), WAIS-R Block Design (*OR* = .92, 95% *CI* = .87-.97, *p* < .01), and 5-minute recognition (*OR* = .73, 95% *CI* = .56 -.95, *p* < .05). Together these four tests created a good fit to the model based on the Hosmer and Lemeshow test with a Chi-Square of 7.76, *p* = .45, and 18 degrees of freedom.

Table 8. Mean and standard deviation scores for the Hispanic controls and AD patients on the CCNB tests.

CCNB Test	Healthy Controls		AD Patients		ANOVA	Adjusted R-Square
	M	SD	M	SD		
Mental Status						
CASI	84.4	10.7	54.9	18.7	F(1, 114) = 115.8*	.50
Recent Memory						
COMT Learning Trial 1	5.8	1.5	2.7	2.0	F(1, 114) = 87.3*	.43
COMT Learning Trial 2	7.5	1.6	3.8	2.3	F(1, 114) = 97.6*	.46
COMT Learning Trial 3	8.2	1.6	4.5	2.2	F(1, 114) = 107.1*	.48
COMT 3-5 min. Recall	7.5	1.9	2.4	2.1	F(1, 114) = 165.0*	.59
COMT 30 min. Recall	7.7	1.8	1.8	2.1	F(1, 114) = 231.*	.67
COMT 5 min. Recognition	19.7	1.2	16.1	3.2	F(1, 114) = 73.7*	.39
COMT 30 min. Recognition	19.6	1.4	15.3	3.7	F(1, 114) = 78.0*	.40
Language						
Body Part Naming	9.7	0.6	9.4	1.7	F(1, 114) = 1.44 NS	.04
CERAD Animal Fluency	12.8	3.9	8.9	4.2	F(1, 114) = 23.9*	.17
Auditory Comprehension	23.7	1.7	21.3	4.7	F(1, 113) = 14.8*	.11
Visual-Spatial						
Read & Set Time	12.5	3.6	6.7	4.1	F(1, 108) = 50.8*	.31
CERAD Drawing	9.2	1.9	7.2	2.9	F(1, 113) = 18.8*	.14
WAIS-R Block Design	17.2	9.9	4.8	6.4	F(1, 107) = 45.6*	.39
Attention						
WAIS-R Digit Span	8.6	3.0	7.5	3.6	F(1, 114) = 2.9 NS	.02
Reasoning						
Mod. Picture Completion	7.5	2.2	5.1	2.5	F(1, 114) = 28.4*	.20
Psychomotor Speed						
Trails Making Test, Part A	90.0	57.3	114.5	62.9	F(1, 99) = 3.3 NS	.02

* Indicates significance at $p \leq .001$; NS indicates 'nonsignificant'.

Of the four minority groups, only the Hispanic was large enough to warrant separate analyses. When compared with the 80 Spanish-speaking healthy controls, the 39 Hispanic patients were highly similar in age and education, but differed significantly on almost all of the tests comprising the CCNB. As shown in Table 8, the Hispanic patients performed significantly worse than their healthy peers on all of the CCNB tests except Body Part Naming, WAIS-R Digit Span, and Part A of the Trail Making Tests.

A subsequent factor analysis using Varimax rotation was performed on the data from the Hispanic sample and revealed a very similar model to that seen in the entire sample. When logistic regression was performed on the data from the Hispanic subsample, scores on the 30-minute recall ($OR = .39$, $CI = .24 - .65$, $p \leq .001$), 5-minute recognition ($OR = .31$, $CI = .12 - .84$, $p \leq .05$), and Auditory Comprehension ($OR = .65$, $CI = .45-.94$, $p < .05$) best predicted AD. The model involving these three tests was a fairly good fit with a Chi-square of 1.59 and 8 degrees of freedom ($p = .99$).

Discussion

Through a comprehensive process the authors developed a set of relatively culture fair measures that assess the cognitive abilities commonly impaired in AD. When normative data from 336 healthy older adults in five ethnic groups were analyzed, the results indicated that education had the greatest effect on performance. Subsequently, the CCNB was administered to 90 cognitively impaired older adults from the same five ethnic groups. Analyses revealed that the CCNB can distinguish cognitively impaired from healthy older adults, with certain tests being more effective than others in differentiating these two groups.

Despite the best efforts of the authors to design a battery of culture fair tests, both education and ethnicity significantly affected performance on several of the instruments. Of these two factors, education had the greater influence, accounting, on average, for 15% of the variance in scores. The fact that less education was associated with lower test scores is not surprising as few tests of higher cognitive functioning are not influenced by education (Rosselli et al., 1990). Other investigators have also been unable to eliminate the impact of education on test scores (Ardila et al., 1989, 1994; Escobar et al., 1986; Ganguli et al., 1991; O'Connor et al., 1989; Taussig et al., 1992). Given the inescapable effects of education, researchers should follow the example of the present authors (Dick et al., in preparation; Kempler et al., 1998) and provide separate norms for different age, educational, and cultural groups as needed.

While ethnicity impacted performance less than education on most tests, it accounted for as much or more of the variance than education on Animal Fluency, the CERAD Drawing task, and the WAIS-R Digit Span tests. Interpretation of these results should be based on (a) a clear differentiation between statistical group effects and the range of individual differences that occur within a group, and (b) an understanding of factors such as language that may contribute to ethnic differences in test performance. First, researchers should compare the size of group effects (*i.e.*, average differences between groups) to the range of variations that occur within groups. In the CCNB normative sample, more variation occurred within the ethnic groups than between them. For any given test in the CCNB, the group effects were modest relative to the range of individual differences within the groups. As a great deal of overlap in individual performance existed between groups, it is inappropriate to interpret group effects as suggesting that everyone in a particular group (*e.g.*, Caucasians) performed better on a given test than practically everyone from another group (*e.g.*, Hispanics).

Secondly, researchers should consider the influence that a variety of factors besides cognitive ability may have on test performance. For example, the finding that Hispanics obtained significantly lower scores on the WAIS-R Digit Span tests and the Animal Fluency task than the other groups could be interpreted in light of linguistic differences. Scores on both tests may have been related to the complexity of a given language. For example, the Digit Span tests may have been more difficult for Hispanics than other participants as seven of the numbers from 1-9 are multisyllabic in Spanish. In comparison, all of the digits are monosyllabic in Chinese and Vietnamese, and only the number 7 has two syllables in English. Kempler et al. (1998) attributed the results of the Animal Fluency task to a comparable linguistic hypothesis. Interestingly, Hispanics, who scored the lowest of all the groups on this task, generated only multisyllabic words. In comparison, the Vietnamese scored the highest, with a majority of the words (80%) being monosyllabic. Word length may have reduced the scores of Hispanic participants as it is well known that multisyllabic terms take longer to articulate and retrieve from semantic memory (*e.g.*, Le Dorze, 1992), and are less successfully stored and manipulated in working memory (Baddeley, 1990; Caplan, Rochon, & Waters, 1992).

Norms are useful to the extent that they accurately represent the characteristics of a particular population. To determine the representativeness of participants in this study, the authors compared their demographic characteristics to those of the 5,262 individuals assessed at California's nine ADDTCs (now known as Alzheimer's Research Centers of California) from 1986 to 1993 (Yeo, Gallagher-Thompson, & Lieberman, 1996). Ethnic identification data indicated that 76% of the patients were Caucasian, 10% were Hispanic, 8% were African-American, 4% were Asian/Pacific Islanders, and the remainder were from other groups. This distribution mirrored the ethnic breakdown of California's older adult population at that time, with the exception of the Asian/Pacific Islanders, who were underrepresented. Upon comparing age, education, and gender data for the four groups of ADDTC patients with that of the Caucasian, Hispanic, African-American, and Asian (*i.e.*, Chinese and Vietnamese) participants in this study, the authors found a high level of similarity. In terms of age, Asians were the youngest in both the ADDTC population (*M* = 72.4) and the CCNB sample (*M* = 72.0), while Caucasians were the oldest, averaging 77 years in both the ADDTC population and our normative sample. Gender breakdown was also comparable in the ADDTC population and the CCNB sample, with the percentage of males falling at 33% and 36%, respectively. Finally, the mean number of years of schooling in the ADDTC population and CCNB sample were similar for the Hispanic (7.7 ADDTC vs. 8.3 CCNB), African-American (10.0 ADDTC vs. 11.6 CCNB), and Caucasian (12.7 ADDTC vs. 11.4 CCNB) groups. The CCNB Chinese and Vietnamese participants had attended school for an average of 11.2 and 8.6 years, respectively, while the more diverse ADDTC Asian patient group had a mean of 12.4 years of education. Overall, the comparison of CCNB participants to ADDTC patients indicates that the normative sample in this study was representative of the minority population in California.

While our sample was representative, the ethnic groups were not equivalent in years of education. The authors purposely included participants whose educational levels varied greatly as equating education would have limited the generalizability of the results. To clarify, the average educational level for Caucasians was approximately 12th grade. If participants in the other four ethnic groups were matched at this educational level, the results would not be widely applicable, for example, to Hispanics, who on average completed eight years of schooling. In addition, matching groups based on years of schooling can be relatively meaningless. Within any culture, persons who have attended school for the same number of years may differ in educational attainment due to factors (*e.g.*, rural vs. urban, public vs. private schools) that affect the quality of education. Equating education across cultures in terms of years of schooling is even more problematic, as, for example, the curriculum covered in the first six years of schooling in Vietnam may vary greatly from that taught in the United States or mainland China.

In conclusion, this multi-year project has produced a well-normed battery of cognitive tests for professionals, who are increasingly evaluating older individuals from a variety of ethnic groups for dementia. The CCNB, which is easy to administer and relatively short, can be used with several minority groups. The data reported here and elsewhere (Dick et al., in preparation; Kempler et al., 1998) delineate the range of normal functioning within five ethnic groups and report the relative influence of education, age, and ethnicity/language on performance. Further refinements, however, are necessary if the battery is to achieve widespread adoption by researchers and clinicians. In the current health care environment, patients are unlikely to receive neuropsychological testing due to the cost and time involved. Application of the CCNB in clinical settings may be limited by the 90-minute administration time. The results from the logical regression analyses suggest that certain of the tests can be eliminated, thereby shortening the battery considerably while maintaining it's diagnostic accuracy. For instance, as scores on tests such as Body Part Naming, WAIS-R Digit Span, and Part A of the Trail Making Tests do not accurately distinguish healthy from cognitively impaired Hispanic elders, these tests would not need to be included in a diagnostic evaluation. In fact, the results of the logical regression analyses performed on all of the data suggest that a much shorter "core" battery could be developed which would include just five tests namely the CASI, COMT, CERAD Drawing, Auditory Comprehension, and WAIS-R Block Design. Hopefully, by shortening the battery to include only the most essential tests this will lead to greater utilization of the CCNB in applied settings. The authors encourage interested individuals to try out this battery and hope that pooling of data in the future will allow for updated and more refined norms.

Acknowledgements

The work reported here was supported, in part, by a grant to the first author from the California Department of Health Services, Alzheimer's Disease

Program, Contract No. 93-18635. We wish to thank the following individuals who assisted with subject recruitment and data collection: Laura Bracamonte, Kim Bui, Lydia Cano, Rocco Cheng, Chen-Chen Chen, Marian Chow, Jacqueline Conyers, Fred Dewey, Marian Hsieh, Patricia Madrigal, Andy Nguyen, Pauline Pham, Maria Sandoval, Libbia Taylor, Nghia Tran, Sylvia Upchurch, and Holly Warriner.

References

Anderson, E. S. (1978). Lexical universals of body-part terminology. In J. H. Greenberg & C. A. Fergson (Eds.), *Universals of human language* (pp. 335-368). Palo Alto, CA: Stanford University Press.

Ardila, A. (1995). Directions of research in cross-cultural neuropsychology. *Journal of Clinical and Experimental Neuropsychology, 17*, 143-150.

Ardila, A. , Rosselli, M., & Puente, A. E. (1994). *Neuropsychological evaluation of the Spanish speaker.* New York: Plenum Press.

Ardila, A., Rosselli, M., & Rosas, P. (1989). Neuropsychological assessment of illiterates: Visuospatial and memory abilities. *Brain and Cognition, 11*, 147-166.

Baddeley, A. D. (1990). *Human memory: Theory and practice.* Needham Heights, MA: Allyn and Bacon.

Bird, H. R., Canino, G., Stipec, R. M., & Shrout, P. (1987). Use of the Mini-Mental State Examination in a probability sample of a Hispanic population. *The Journal of Nervous and Mental Disorders, 175*, 731-737.

Brislin, R. W., Lanner, W. J., & Thorndike, R. M. (1973). *Cross-cultural research methods.* New York: Wiley.

Caplan, D., Rochon, E., & Waters, G. S. (1992). Articulatory and phonological determinants of word length effects in span tasks. *Quarterly Journal of Experimental Psychology: Human Experimental Psychology, 45*, 177-192.

Demers, P., Robillard, A., Lafleche, G., Nash, F., Heyman, A. &, Fillenbaum, G. (1994). Translation of clinical and neuropsychological instruments into French: The CERAD experience. *Age and Aging, 23*, 449-451.

Dick, M. D., Teng, E. L., Kempler, D., Davis, D., & Taussig, I. M. (in preparation). The Cross-Cultural Neuropsychological Test Battery (CCNB): Effects of age, education, and ethnicity on performance of healthy older adults.

Elliot, K. S., Di Minno, M., Lam, D., & Tu, A. M. (1996). Working with Chinese families in the context of dementia. In G. Yeo & D. Gallagher-Thompson (Eds.), *Ethnicity and the dementias* (pp. 89-108). Washington, D.C.: Taylor & Francis.

Escobar, J. I., Burnam, A., Karno, M., Forsythe, A., Landsverk, J., & Golding, J. M. (1986). Use of the Mini-Mental State Examination in a community population of mixed ethnicity. *The Journal of Nervous and Mental Disease, 174*, 607-614.

Evans, D. A., Funkenstein, H. H., Albert, M. S., Scherr, P. A., Cook, N. R., Chown, M. J., Hebert, L. E., Hennekens, C. H., & Taylor, J. O. (1989). Prevalence of Alzheimer's disease in a community population of older persons. *Journal of the American Medical Association, 262*, 2551-2556.

Feldman, H., Anand, R., Blesa, R., Dubois, B., Gray, J., Homma, A., Mohr, E., Morris, J. C., Parys, W., Raschig, A., & Robillard, A. (1997). Translation issues in clinical trials of dementia drugs. *Alzheimer's Disease and Associated Disorders, 11*, 61-64.

Fillenbaum, G. G., Huber, M., & Taussig, I. M. (1997). Performance of elderly white and African-American community residents on the abbreviated CERAD Boston Naming Test. *Journal of Clinical and Experimental Neuropsychology, 19*, 204-210.

Folstein, M. F., Folstein, S. E., & McHugh, P. R. (1975). "Mini-Mental State": A practical method for grading the cognitive state of patients for the clinician. *Journal of Psychiatric Research, 12*, 189-198.

Fuh, J. L., Teng, E. L., Lin, K. N., Larson, E. B., Wang, S. J., Liu, C. Y., Chou, P., Kuo, B. I. T., & Liu, H. C. (1995). The Informant Questionnaire on Cognitive Decline in the Elderly (IQCODE) as a screening tool for dementia for a predominantly illiterate Chinese population. *Neurology, 45*, 92-96.

Ganguli, M., Ratcliff, G., Belle, S., Huff, F. J., & Kancel, M. J. (1991). Effects of age, gender, and education on cognitive tests in an elderly rural community sample: Norms from the Monongahela Valley Independent Elders Survey (MoVIES). *Neuroepidemiology, 10*, 42-52.

Glosser, G., Wolfe, N., Albert, M. L., Lavine, l., Steele, J. C., Calne, D. B., & Schoenberg, B. S. (1993). Cross-Cultural Cognitive Examination: Validation of a dementia screening instrument for neuroepidemiological research. *Journal of the American Geriatrics Society, 41*, 931-939.

Green, R. F., & Martinez, J. N. (1968). *Manual para la Escala de Inteligencia Wechsler para Adultos.* New York: The Psychological Corporation.

Gurland, B. J., Wilder, D. E., Cross, P., Teresi, J., & Barrett, V. W. (1992). Screening scales for dementia: Toward reconciliation of conflicting cross-cultural findings. *International Journal of Geriatric Psychiatry, 7*, 105-113.

Hasegawa, K. (1983). The clinical assessment of dementia in the aged: A dementia screening scale for psychogeriatric patients. In M. Bergener, U. Lehr, E. Lang, & R. Schmitz-Scherzer (Eds.), *Aging in the eighties and beyond* (pp. 207-218). New York: Springer.

Hosmer, D. W., & Lemeshow, S. (1989). *Applied logistic regression.* New York: Wiley & Sons.

Hughes, C. P., Berg, L., Danziger, W. L., Coben, L. A., & Martin, R. L. (1982). A new clinical scale for the staging of dementia. *British Journal of Psychiatry, 140*, 566-572.

Jacobs, D. M., Sano, M., Albert, S., Schofield, P., Dooneief, G., & Stern, Y. (1997). Cross-cultural neuropsychological assessment; A comparison of randomly selected demographically matched cohorts of English- and Spanish-speaking older adults. *Journal of Clinical and Experimental Neuropsychology, 19*, 331-339.

Jensen, A. R. (1980). *Bias in mental testing.* New York: Free Press.

Jorm, A. F., & Jacomb, P. A. (1989). The Informant Questionnaire on Cognitive Decline in the Elderly (IQCODE): Socio-demographic correlates, reliability, validity and some norms. *Psychological Medicine, 19*, 1015-1022.

Jorm, A. F., Scott, R., Cullen, J. S., & Mackinnon, A. J. (1991). Performance of the Informant Questionnaire on Cognitive Decline in the Elderly (IQCODE) as a screening test for dementia. *Psychological Medicine, 21*, 785-790.

Katzman, R., Zhang, M., Qu, O.-Y., Wang, Z., Liu, W. T., Yu, E., Wong, S. C., Salmon, D. P., & Grant, I. (1988). A Chinese version of the Mini-Mental State Examination: Impact of illiteracy in a Shanghai dementia survey. *Journal of Clinical Epidemiology, 41*, 971-978.

Kempler, D., Teng, E. L., Dick, M. B., Taussig, I. M., & Davis, D. S. (1998). The effects of age, education, and ethnicity on verbal fluency. *Journal of the International Neuropsychological Society, 4*, 531-538.

Kuo, W. (1984). Prevalence of depression among Asian-Americans. *Journal of Nervous and Mental Disease, 172*, 449-457.

Le Dorze, G. (1992). The effects of age, educational level, and stimulus length on naming in normal subjects. *Journal of Speech-Language Pathology & Audiology, 16*, 21-29.

Loewenstein, D. A., Arguelles, T., Arguelles, S., & Linn-Fuentes, P. (1994). Potential cultural bias in the neuropsychological assessment of the older adult. *Journal of Clinical and Experimental Psychology, 16,* 623-629.

Loewenstein, D. A., & Rubert, M. P. (1992). The NINCDS-ADRDA neuropsychological criteria for the assessment of dementia: Limitations of current diagnostic guidelines. *Behavior, Health, and Aging, 2,* 113-121.

López, S., & Romero, A. (1988). Assessing the intellectual functioning of Spanish-speaking adults: Comparison of the EIWA and WAIS. *Professional Psychology: Research and Practice, 19,* 263-270.

López, S. R., & Taussig, I. M. (1991). Cognitive-intellectual functioning of Spanish-speaking impaired and nonimpaired elderly: Implications for psychological assessments. *Journal of Consulting and Clinical Psychology, 3,* 448-454.

Marcos, L. R. (1979). Effects of interpreters on the evaluation of psychopathology in non-English speaking patients. *American Journal of Psychiatry, 136,* 171-174.

McKhann, G., Drachman, D., Folstein, M., Katzman, R., Price, D., & Stadlan, E. M. (1984). Clinical diagnosis of Alzheimer's disease: Report of the NINCDS-ADRDA work group under the auspices of Department of Health and Human Services Task Force on Alzheimer's disease. *Neurology, 34,* 939-944.

Morales, J-M., Gonzales-Montalvo, J-I., Bermejo, F., & Del-Ser, T. (1995). The screening of mild dementia with a shortened Spanish version of the Informant Questionnaire on Cognitive decline in the Elderly. *Alzheimer's Disease and Associated Disorders, 9,* 105-111.

Morris, J. C., Heyman, A., Mohs, R. C., Hughes, J. P., van Belle, G., Fillenbaum, G., Mellits, E. D., & Clark, C. (1989). The Consortium to Establish a Registry for Alzheimer's Disease (CERAD). Part 1. Clinical and neuropsychological assessment of Alzheimer's disease. *Neurology, 39,* 1159-1165.

National Institutes of Health (1987). Consensus Development Conference Statement. Differential Diagnosis of Dementing Disorders, *6,* 11.

O'Connor, D. W., Pollitt, P. A., & Treasure, F. P. (1989). The influence of education, social class, and sex on Mini-Mental State scores. *Psychological Medicine, 19,* 771-776.

Pontón, M. O., Satz, P., Herrera, L., Urrutia, C. P., Ortiz, F., Young, R., D'Elia, L., Furst, C., & Namerow, N. (1996). Normative data stratified by age and education for the Neuropsychological Screening Battery for Hispanics (NesSB-HIS): A standardization report. *Journal of the International Neuropsychological Society, 2,* 96-104.

Richards, M., & Brayne, C. (1996). Cross-cultural research into cognitive impairment and dementia: Some practical experiences. *International Journal of Geriatric Psychiatry, 11,* 383-388.

Ripich, D. N., Carpenter, B., & Ziol, E. (1997). Comparison of African-American and white persons with Alzheimer's disease on language measures. *Neurology, 48,* 781-783.

Roberts, R. E. (1980). Reliability of the CES-D in different ethnic contexts. *Psychological Research, 2,* 125-134.

Roberts, R. E. (1981). Prevalence of depressive symptoms among Mexican Americans. *Journal of Nervous and Mental Disease, 169,* 213-219.

Rosen , W. G., Terry, R. D., Fuld, P. A., Katzman, R., & Peck, A. (1980). Pathological verification of ischemic score in differentiation of dementia. *Annals of Neurology, 7,* 486-488.

Ross, T. P., Lichtenberg, P. A., & Christensen, B. K. (1995). Normative data on the Boston Naming test for elderly adults in a demographically diverse medical sample. *Clinical Neuropsychologist, 9,* 321-325.

Rosselli, M., Ardila, A., & Rosas, P. (1990). Neuropsychological assessment in illiterates: Language and praxis abilities. *Brain and Cognition, 12,* 281-296.

Sabin, J. E. (1975). Translation despair. *American Journal of Psychiatry, 132,* 197-199.

Taussig, I. M., Henderson, V. W., & Mack, W. (1992). Spanish translation and validation of a neuropsychological battery: Performance of Spanish- and English-speaking Alzheimer's disease patients and normal comparison subjects. *Clinical Gerontologist, 11,* 95-108.

Taussig, I. M., & Pontón, M. (1996). Issues in neuropsychological assessment for Hispanic older adults: Cultural and linguistic factors. In G. Yeo & D. Gallagher-Thompson (Eds.), *Ethnicity and the dementias* (pp. 47-58). Washington, D.C.: Taylor & Francis.

Teng, E. L. (1996). Cross-cultural testing and the Cognitive Abilities Screening Instrument. In G. Yeo & D. Gallagher-Thompson (Eds.), *Ethnicity and the dementias* (pp. 77-85). Washington, D.C.: Taylor & Francis.

Teng, E. L., Hasegawa, K., Homma, A. Imai, Y., Larson, E., Graves, A., Sugimoto, K., Yamaguchi, T., Sasaki, H., Chiu, D., & White, L. R. (1994). The Cognitive Abilities Screening Instrument (CASI): A practical test for cross-cultural epidemiological studies of dementia. *International Psychogeriatrics, 6,* 45-58.

U. S. Congress, Office of Technology Assessment (1987). *Losing a million minds: Confronting the tragedy of Alzheimer's disease and other dementias* (Publication OTABA-323). Washington, D.C.: Government Publishing Office.

U. S. Bureau of the Census & National Institute on Aging (1993). Racial and ethnic diversity of America's elderly population. *Profiles of America's Elderly, 3,* 1.

Valle, R., Hough, R., Cook-Gait, H., Lui, K. J., & Labovitiz, E. (1991). *Hispanic neuropsychological study (HNS).* California Department of Health Services: Alzheimer's Disease Program, Sacramento, CA.

Yeo, G., Gallegher-Thompson, D., & Lieberman, M. (1996). Variations in dementia characteristics by ethnic category. In G. Yeo & D. Gallagher-Thompson (Eds.), *Ethnicity and the dementias* (pp. 21-30). Washington, D.C.: Taylor & Francis.

Ying, Y-W. (1988). Depressive symptomatology among Chinese-Americans as measured by the CES-D. *Journal of Clinical Psychology, 44,* 739-746.

Yu, E. S. H., Liu, W. T., Levy, P., Zhang, M., Katzman, R., Lung, C.-T., Wong, S., Wang, Z., & Qu, O.-Y. (1989). Cognitive impairment among elderly adults in Shanghai, China. *Journal of Gerontology, 44,* 97-106.

PART II

AFRICAN /
BLACK AMERICANS

Chapter 3

THE CERAD NEUROPSYCHOLOGICAL BATTERY:

PERFORMANCE OF REPRESENTATIVE COMMUNITY AND TERTIARY CARE SAMPLES OF AFRICAN-AMERICAN AND EUROPEAN-AMERICAN ELDERLY

Gerda G. Fillenbaum, Ph.D.
Center for the Study of Aging and Human Development, Duke University Medical Center, Durham, North Carolina

Frederick W. Unverzagt, Ph.D.
Department of Psychiatry, Indiana University School of Medicine, Indianapolis, Indiana

Mary Ganguli, M.D., M.P.H.
Department of Psychiatry, School of Medicine, and Department of Epidemiology, Graduate School of Public Health, University of Pittsburgh, Pittsburgh, Pennsylvania

Kathleen A. Welsh-Bohmer, Ph.D.
Department of Psychiatry and Behavioral Sciences and Bryan Alzheimer's Disease Research Center, Duke University Medical Center, Durham, North Carolina

Albert Heyman, M.D.
Division of Neurology, Department of Medicine, Duke University Medical Center, Durham, North Carolina

Abstract

The Consortium to Establish a Registry for Alzheimer's Disease (CERAD) has developed a brief neuropsychology battery to assess performance in Alzheimer's disease (AD). In addition to use in tertiary care clinic settings, where it has been found to distinguish the cognitively normal from those with early AD, this battery has been used in three epidemiological surveys of the elderly, which were designed to identify dementia. Results from these surveys, in the Monongahela Valley of Pennsylvania; Indianapolis, Indiana; and the Piedmont area of North Carolina, are compared. Overall, the Black elderly tend to perform more poorly than White, and residents of Indianapolis and North Carolina perform more poorly than those in the Monongahela Valley. The reasons for these differences are explored.

Introduction

The Consortium to Establish a Registry for Alzheimer's Disease (CERAD) was developed in 1986 in response to a mandate from the National Institute on Aging to develop standardized assessments for Alzheimer's disease (AD). Such evaluations were intended to encourage uniform collection of data, facilitate aggregation of information, permit the development of a substantial database, and allow identification of rare variants of AD, should they exist. For this purpose CERAD developed a structured clinical evaluation for AD, and related dementias, and also for possible dementia prodromes. Additional assessments included neuropsychological, behavioral, and neuropathology instruments. The Neuropathology Assessment, in particular, has set an international standard for postmortem diagnosis of Alzheimer's disease, as well as for related dementias such as Lewy body variants and Parkinson's disease. Current guidelines from the consensus group on neuropathological standards for AD diagnosis (NIA-Reagan Institute criteria) endorse the CERAD method and expand on it with Braak staging (Anonymous, 1997).

The CERAD Neuropsychological Battery, the focus of this chapter, was originally designed to be a set of standardized measures of cognitive function relevant to patients clinically identified as having Alzheimer's disease (Morris et al., 1989). To this end, it included brief measures of memory, language impairment, apraxia, and general intellectual deterioration (Welsh et al., 1991). Eventually this battery of neuropsychological tests was found to be valuable in distinguishing persons in the early stages of AD from those who were not demented (Welsh et al., 1991). For this reason this battery was selected for use in several epidemiological surveys designed to measure the prevalence and incidence of dementia (e.g., Ganguli et al., 1993; Hendrie et al., 1995). It has also been used as a screen of cognitive functioning since it includes familiar instruments and the administration time is comparatively brief, averaging twenty minutes (Fillenbaum et al., 1998a; Ganguli et al., 1991; Hendrie et al., 1995).

This battery has been translated into many European and Asian languages and used in a wide variety of settings, e.g., clinical, academic, and population studies. This chapter describes the individual measures included in the battery and their psychometric status. We will report on the performance of African-American and European-American community resident elderly, 65 years of age and older, the majority of whom are representative of community residents their age, comparing the performance of the two racial groups. We will also examine the performance of patients with AD, and indicate whether racial differences persist in disease, and as severity of disease increases.

Certain attitudes underly our thinking in this area. Measures that are used should be valid and reliable. That is, they should measure what they claim to measure and, given the same circumstance, the response they evoke should be consistent. Comparison across studies is greatly improved (indeed, may really only be feasible) when the same measures are administered, scored, and interpreted in a uniform manner. At best, comparison can only be tenuous when criteria, as say for dementia, are operationalized in different ways (e.g., by using different tests) even when alternative tests may appropriately address the criteria agreed on. Operationalizing criteria uniformly across all settings facilitates comparison and communication which is not otherwise feasible. It permits differences to become manifest which might not otherwise be evident.

CERAD Neuropsychological Battery

The CERAD Neuropsychological Battery includes seven brief measures, each of which identify disturbances of cognitive functioning noted particularly in patients with Alzheimer's disease. In order of administration they are as follows:

Verbal Fluency. Naming as many animals as possible in 60 seconds (derived from the Set test, (Isaacs & Akhtar, 1972)). This test measures verbal production, semantic memory, and language.

Modified Boston Naming Test (Kaplan et al., 1983). Includes outline drawings of 15 of the original test's 60 items, selected so that the names of the items vary with respect to high, medium, and low frequency in the English language (i.e., five in each of the three categories). Score is the total number of items named correctly, established local variant terms are acceptable. Maximum score is 15.

Mini-Mental State Examination (MMSE) (Folstein et al., 1975). The CERAD neuropsychological battery includes the version of the MMSE developed for the Epidemiological Catchment Area study (Eaton & Kessler, 1985), modified so that the concentration section includes only spelling WORLD backwards. Serial subtraction of 7 from 100 is not included, to reduce administration time and improve accuracy of scoring. Scoring range is 0-30.

There is no prescribed way of scoring nonresponse on the MMSE. In studies reported here, refusals were scored as errors (Fillenbaum et al., 1988). However, when nonresponse was due to a physical or educational handicap (e.g., illiteracy such that the subject cannot read or write a sentence, or a disability preventing handling paper or drawing), the score on the MMSE was prorated.

Word List Memory. This is a ten-item word list learning task, similar to that in the Alzheimer's Disease Assessment Scale (Rosen et al., 1984), but specially developed for CERAD. Each of ten common nouns is shown at two second intervals. The subject reads them aloud (if unable to read, the words are read to the subject, who repeats them). The list is presented in random order on three successive occasions. After each occasion the subject reports all the words that can be recalled. Scoring range on each trial is 0-10, and number of intrusions is noted. Data on the sum of the three trials is presented here.

Constructional Praxis (Rosen et al., 1984). This task measures visuospatial and constructional abilities. The subject is shown line drawings of four figures of increasing complexity, each on a separate sheet of paper. These include a circle, diamond, intersecting rectangles and a cube. The subject is then asked to draw a copy immediately beneath each item. Scoring range is 0-11. Detailed scoring guidelines have been developed by Woods (1995).

Word List Recall. The subject is asked to recall the items of the 10-item Word List Memory task. Scoring range is 0-10.

Word List Recognition. The ten original words of the Word List Memory Task in which 10 new words are interspersed, are presented to the subject, who is then asked to distinguish the original words from the new ones. If the subject is unable to read, the words are read aloud and the subject is asked to repeat them. Scoring range is 0-20. In analysis, adjustment should be made for response set (e.g., saying "yes" or "no" to all items). Such responses should be scored as zero, so that credit is not given inappropriately.

Constructional Praxis Recall. This is a more recent addition to the battery, permitting assessment of recall of praxis items (i.e., spatial recall), as contrasted to recall of verbal material. Because of personal lack of experience with it, information on it is not provided here. It does, however, enjoy increasing use (e.g., Spangenberg et al., 1997).

Comparison with the Alzheimer's Disease Assessment Scale and other structured assessments of dementia

The CERAD neuropsychological battery was developed by one of the neuropsychologists instrumental in developing the Alzheimer's Disease Assessment Scale (ADAS) (Rosen et al., 1984). While there is overlap in inquiry between the cognitive portion of ADAS and the CERAD battery, there are also notable differences. The ADAS includes 12 measures. Constructional

Praxis is identical in the two assessments, while the ADAS Word Recall is comparable to the CERAD Word List Memory Task. The ADAS Word List Recognition Task, however, differs from that in CERAD as do the measures of language, comprehension, following commands and naming. The ADAS orientation items largely overlap those included in the MMSE. ADAS also includes inquiry not present in CERAD, such as into ideational praxis (preparing a letter for mailing). ADAS has a long and successful history of use in drug intervention trials. Since its inception, more strictly standardized administration and scoring procedures have been developed (Standish et al., 1996). The cognitive portion of ADAS and the CERAD Neuropsychological Battery are not equivalent, and cannot be substituted for each other.

The other primary structured assessments for dementia used in English-speaking countries are GMS-AGECAT (Copeland et al., 1986) and CAM-DEX (Roth et al., 1986). GMS-AGECAT contains no neuropsychology measures. CAMDEX includes a neuropsychological battery called CAMCOG. Included in CAMCOG, in addition to the MMSE and its components, are measures of language, memory for familiar events, recognition of familiar people and common items, praxis, calculation, abstract thinking and perception. Thus, the areas of cognitive function examined are not identical to those included in the CERAD Neuropsychological Battery. The equivalence of the CERAD and CAMCOG batteries for identifying dementia does not appear to have been assessed.

Limitations of the CERAD Neuropsychological Battery

The CERAD Neuropsychological Battery has certain limitations. As stated above, selection of measures for the test battery focused on those that characterize the primary cognitive manifestations of AD. Measures considered to be related specifically to nonAD dementias (e.g., frontal lobe dementia, vascular dementia) may be inadequate or absent. The original battery is therefore not recommended for differential diagnosis of dementing disorders. CERAD has identified sets of measures to be added to the battery to make it appropriate for evaluating alternative dementias and possible dementia prodrome or mild cognitive impairment (i.e., patients whose cognitive impairment suggests, but is not yet sufficiently severe, to warrant a diagnosis of dementia). In its present state, however, the battery should be adequate to identify the presence of a dementing disorder.

In common with other measures, administration of the CERAD battery is difficult in subjects with hearing loss, visual difficulty, physical impairment, or poor education. While problems related to hearing loss can, at times, be handled by the use of hearing amplification devices or by asking the test-taker to read the directions, this approach is not feasible where the test-taker is required to repeat a spoken phrase (as in the MMSE). Visual difficulty may hinder administration of the modified Boston Naming test, the constructional praxis test, and the constructional praxis item of the MMSE. Illiteracy prevents administration of two items of the MMSE, and requires an alternate administration of two of the Word List tests. For those who are unable to read because of literacy or visual problems, the items of the Word List Memory test and the Word List Recognition test are read aloud, with the subject or patient repeating them, so maintaining two input modalities. Physical impairment which prevents handling paper or pencil means that certain parts of the MMSE and the constructional praxis test cannot be administered. Such problems, however, are inherent in nearly all neuropsychology measures.

The measures are not designed for persons with limited education or with non-mainstream cultural backgrounds. Such persons may perform more poorly because of lack of familiarity with the tasks and activities involved. Minimal accommodation in scoring is made for such difficulty; no adjustments for race, culture, or environmental circumstances have, as yet, been proposed. In part this is becaue such adjustments inhibit examination of these issues. But in part it also reflects a need for additional experience with such groups, in order to determine how best to handle the problems that arise.

Psychometric Characteristics of the CERAD Neuropsychological Battery

Reliability

Considerable attention has been paid to ensuring the reliability of this battery. Reliability is encouraged through careful training of the test administrators. A videotape for this purpose is available. In addition, directions for administration are printed with the test, and specific guidelines for scoring are typically placed on the page facing the test.

One month test–test reliability has been established by CERAD (unpublished data) for carefully evaluated patients with AD who were at the mild or moderate level of disease as assessed by the Clinical Dementia Rating (CDR) scale (Morris, 1993), and for control subjects. Details are given in Table 1 for both African-American and European-American AD cases and control subjects. The lower correlations found for some of the measures reflect restriction in range of scores – a floor effect for cases (e.g., African-American cases on Word List Recall) and a ceiling effect for control subjects (e.g., for both African-American and European-American control subjects on Word List Recognition).

The intraclass correlation coefficients for inter-rater scoring reliability range from a low of 0.92 for Constructional Praxis to 1.00 for Word List Recall for raters in the CERAD study (Morris et al., 1989). For subjects evaluated in an epidemiological study of the incidence and prevalence of dementia, the intraclass correlation coefficients ranged from 0.71-1.00, and were typically 0.90 or higher (Fillenbaum et al., 1998a).

Table 1. One month test-retest correlations of CERAD neuropsychology measures based on CERAD registry data.

	African American		European American	
	Cases (N=88)	Controls (N=20)	Cases (N=525)	Controls (N=372)
Verbal Fluency	.82	.72**	.79	.69
Modified Boston Naming test	.90	.75	.90	.68
Mini-Mental State	.92	.86	.85	.48
Word List Learning	.84	.86	.78	.62
Constructional Praxis	.77	.86	.80	.58
Word List Recall	.44	.61*	.59	.65
Word List Recognition				
Original items	.60	.33[NS]	.51	.36
Foils	.71	−.08[NS]	.57	.16***

All correlations statistically significant at $p < .0001$, except when indicated by *** ($p < .001$), ** ($p < .01$), * ($p < .05$) or NS (nonsignificant).

Validity

The original purpose of the CERAD Neuropsychological Battery was to assess level of severity of AD. In that regard the battery has content validity, since the measures selected were those which identify the neuropsychological losses most likely to occur in that disorder (Morris et al., 1989; Welsh et al., 1991).

Important for epidemiological purposes, the measures in the battery show discriminative validity in distinguishing older community residents with dementia from those without such cognitive impairment. Studies by Welsh et al. (1991, 1992) found that the ability to recall two words or less on the Word List Recall measure distinguished mild cases of AD from cognitively intact control subjects. Ganguli et al. (1993), using an expanded CERAD Neuropsychological Battery, found that combined use of several measures resulted in better sensitivity for dementia than did the MMSE score alone. She operationalized dementia based on DSM-III-R and NINCDS-ADRDA criteria (McKhann et al., 1984) and identified the status of community residents whose scores on a measure of memory and on a minimum of two other areas of cognitive function fell at the 5th and 10th percentiles.

Sensitivity to change

The measures of the CERAD Neuropsychological Battery are also sensitive to progression of AD, and possibly to aging. Examined over a period of one year, the average level of performance of patients with AD declined on each measure, whereas the average performance of control subjects remained stable, or improved (perhaps due to a learning effect) (Morris et al., 1989). Examined over a period of two years (n=300) and three years (n=285) average scores of these control subjects continued to remain stable. Patients with AD, however, showed notable declines on all measures except Word List Recall, which had initially been close to the floor. For control subjects, standard deviations were stable (or increased slightly through the second year), but with the exception of the MMSE there was no further increase in variability three years after initial evaluation. Similarly, over a period of two years, in a representative community sample not demented at the start of the study, average level of performance remained stable, or declined slightly (Ganguli et al., 1996). The decline found in that study may reflect the effects of aging in a more diverse community sample, or the development of cognitive impairment, perhaps heralding dementia.

Factorial Structure

Factor analysis of data from the first 354 AD cases in CERAD, the vast majority of whom were European-American (Morris et al., 1989), indicated that the seven measures fell on three factors, which together explained 73% of the variance. The three Word List measures fell on the first factor, which appears to measure memory. Verbal Fluency and the modified Boston Naming test fell on the second factor (measuring language), and the MMSE and Constructional Praxis fell on the third factor, which appears to measure praxis. The MMSE has slightly lower, but notable loadings on factors 1 and 2, supporting a view that it is a general measure of cognitive functioning in those with impaired cognitive status.

Data from cognitively normal African-Americans indicated that the measures fell on two factors and explained 67% of the variance. One appeared to be a global nonmemory factor (including Verbal Fluency, modified Boston Naming, MMSE and Constructional Praxis), while the other was considered to be a memory factor (consisting of the three Word List tasks) (Unverzagt et al., 1996).

Further studies are needed to determine whether the factorial structure varies as a function of race or dementia status.

Normative Data for Community-Representative Subjects

Because of cost, norms for the CERAD Neuropsychological Battery are not available from a nationally representative sample. However, norms for community-representative subjects are available from studies in the South, Northeast, and Midwest. The first is a study of a stratified random sample of African-American and European-American community residents 68 years of age and over when initially sampled for a study of the prevalence and incidence of dementia (Fillenbaum et al., 1998a). They lived in five adjacent counties (one urban, four rural) in the Piedmont area of North Carolina. Person weights are available, which permit data from this group to be made representative of persons their age living in this area. Thirty five percent of the elderly in this area are African-American.

The second study was carried out in the Monongahela Valley of Pennsylvania, a rural non-farm rust-belt area, 25 miles south of Pittsburgh. The study subjects were an age-stratified random sample of community residents, 65 years of age and older, fluent in English, and (with the exception of those 85 years of age or older) with a minimum of a sixth grade education. Almost all (97%) were European-American (Ganguli et al., 1991).

The third study, carried out in Indianapolis, Indiana, provided normative data for a study of the prevalence and incidence of dementia in African-American elderly living in that area. The subjects consist of a purposive group of 83 healthy African-American community residents, 65 years of age and older, without a history of stroke, dementing, psychiatric or neurological disorders (Unverzagt et al., 1996). These three studies provide a means to examine the generalizability of norms for representative community residents. There are some minor differences in the administration of the battery in the different studies. In particular in the Indianapolis study, repeating the days of the week backwards was substituted for backwards spelling of WORLD in the MMSE. This task also requires concentraton, but was considered more feasible for persons who might have minimal literacy. For similar reasons, the items of the Word List Learning task were read to the subject, who did not see or repeat them. Such differences in administration could result in differences in performance.

Table 2 shows basic comparative demographic information for the Indianapolis (African-American) and Monongahela Valley (European-American) samples, in addition to mean scores on each of the CERAD Neuropsychology measures for each of these groups. The scores reported in Table 2 for the Piedmont, North Carolina group were derived from regression equations using data adjusted for oversampling of people likely to be demented. They reflect the scores predicted for persons of the same race, gender distribution, mean age and mean education as the comparison Indianapolis (African-American) and Monongahela Valley (European-American) groups. Although the North Carolina study is designed to provide gender specific norms, such norms have not been published by the two other community studies.

Comparison of the two studies with information on the performance of African-Americans indicates that in the Piedmont area this racial group performs more poorly than those in Indianapolis on all measures. With the exception of Verbal Fluency, the European-Americans of the Piedmont, NC study perform more poorly than the members of the same racial group in the Monongahela Valley.

Although the better performance of the African-Americans in Indianapolis may reflect their better health, such an explanation does not account for the differences in scores of the two European-American groups, since both are designed to be community representative. However, with the exception of those 85 years of age and older, the European-Americans in the Monongahela Valley had a minimum of a sixth grade education. No minimum educational level was required by the Piedmont, NC study, indeed the median level of

Table 2. Comparison of mean scores in the Indianapolis; Piedmont, North Carolina[1], and Monongahela Valley studies on the measures of the CERAD Neuropsychological Battery[3].

	Indianapolis	Piedmont, North Carolina		Monongahela Valley
	African-American	African-American	European-American	European-American
Men (%)	29.0			45.0
Age: Mean	74.6			73.1
Education: Mean	10.2			12.0
Verbal Fluency	14.4	13.0	14.6	14.2
Modified Boston Naming	12.2	10.9	12.1	14.0
Mini-Mental State	26.1	23.9	26.1	27.2
Word List Learning[2]	14.8	13.2	14.5	18.7
Constructional Praxis	9.0	7.6	8.5	10.5
Word List Recall	4.0	3.4	4.6	7.0
Word List Recognition	18.3	16.1	18.0	19.1

[1] The Piedmont, NC data are regression-derived scores for a sample matching the race, age, education and gender distribution of the African Americans in Indianapolis and the European Americans in the Monongahela Valley.

[2] In Indianapolis, the items of the Word List Learning test were read aloud by the examiner, but not seen or repeated by the subject.

[3] Reproduced in modified form with permission of the Journal of the International Psychological Society.

education in this community was 8 years, notably less than the mean of 12 years in the Monongahela Valley.

Effect of demographic characteristics on score

This raises the question of the extent to which level of performance on the CERAD neuropsychology measures is affected by health status and demographic characteristics. The effects of physical health status have not been examined. Each of the three studies, however, has explored the impact of gender, age and education. In addition, racial differences (between African-Americans and European-Americans) have been examined in the Piedmont, NC study. Table 3 provides information from the Piedmont, NC study. The rightmost column indicates the extent to which demographic characteristics (race, sex, age, education) explain variance in score on each of the measures. Asterisks in the body of the table indicate which demographic characteristics explain each score. The rows labeled with the name of a particular measure can be treated as regression equations. Given a particular individual, that person's unique demographic characteristics can be weighted by the parameter estimates supplied, and summed to provide the score that a person of that particular race, sex, age and education who is at the 50th percentile can be expected to make. This score can then be compared with that actually made by the individual. Hence it is possible to determine whether score is within selected normal bounds, or not.

Table 3. Regression-based parameter estimates for CERAD neuropsychology measures. Data from Piedmont, NC.

	Intercept	Race	Gender	Age	Education	R^2
Verbal Fluency	20.63	-0.17	-1.00	-0.16**	0.51****	.24
95% CI	10.70,30.55	-1.60,1.26	-2.37,0.36	-0.29,-0.04	0.34,0.68	
Modified Boston						
Naming	26.32	-0.43	-1.29*	-0.21****	0.15*	.18
95% CI	18.46,34.19	-1.56,0.70	-2.37,-0.21	-0.31,-0.11	0.02,0.29	
Mini-Mental State	38.48	-0.82	-1.38	-0.23***	0.43****	.27
95% CI	28.63,48.33	-2.24,0.59	-2.74,-0.02	-0.35,-0.11	0.27,0.60	
Word List Learning	24.46	-0.39	1.44*	-0.22**	0.44****	.22
95% CI	14.03,34.90	-1.89,1.12	0.00,2.88	-0.35,-0.09	0.26,0.61	
Constructional Praxis	19.66	-0.20	-0.54	-0.18****	0.19**	.19
95% CI	12.99,26.33	-1.16,0.76	-1.46,0.38	-0.27,-0.10	0.08,0.30	
Word List Recall	12.28	-0.51	0.54	-0.13****	0.09*	.17
95% CI	7.61,16.94	-1.18,0.16	0.10,1.19	-0.18,-0.07	0.01,0.17	
Word List Recognition	26.34	-1.05	0.72	-0.18*	0.37***	.13
95% CI	14.32,38.36	-2.78,0.68	-0.94,2.38	-0.33,-0.03	0.17,0.57	

Race: 0 = European-American, 1 = African-American; Gender: 0 = male, 1 = female; Age and education in years. * $p < 0.05$; ** $p < 0.01$; *** $p < 0.001$; **** $p < 0.0001$.

The present data indicate that the demographic characteristics considered explain between 13% and 27% of the variance in score depending on the measure examined. With the exception of Constructional Praxis, the Indiana-polis study found an even stronger association between demographic charac-teristics and score (Unverzagt et al., 1996). While the Piedmont NC study is the only one in which direct controlled comparison of African-Americans and European-Americans is possible (no statistically significant racial differences were found), all three studies considered here have compared the effects of sex, age and education in controlled analyses (Table 4).

For all measures, with the exception of Word List Recognition which was not examined in all three studies, in controlled analyses increased education predicted a better score. On the other hand, with increased age, scores tended to be lower in two of the studies (Piedmont, NC and Monongahela Valley), but in Indianapolis this finding only held for Word List Learning and Word List Recall. Absence of an age effect on the other measures, particularly on the MMSE, is unexpected, since such an effect has otherwise been consist-ently found (e.g., Tombaugh & McIntyre, 1992; Crum et al., 1993). A gender effect was found for some measures, but was only consistent across the three studies for Word List Learning. When a gender effect was present, women typically performed better than men.

All three community samples found that education was a significant pre-dictor of performance on the Word List Recall test. The ability of score on the Word List Recall task to distinguish early AD cases, and the original findings from clinical control subjects that score on this measure was not affected

Table 4. Comparison of significant demographic characteristics identified in three community-based studies[1].

	Piedmont, NC	Indianapolis	Monongahela Valley
Verbal Fluency			
Sex			
Age	X**		X+
Education	X***	X***	X+
Modified Boston naming			
Sex	-W*		+W+
Age	X****		X+
Education	X*	X***	X+
Mini-Mental State			
Sex			+W+
Age	X**		X+
Education	X****	X***	X+
Word List Learning			
Sex	+W*	+W**	+W+
Age	X**	X***	X+
Education	X****	X***	X+
Constructional Praxis			
Sex			
Age	X****		X+
Education	X**	X**	X+
Word List Recall			
Sex			+W+
Age	X****	X**	X+
Education	X*	X***	X+

X = statistically significant determinant in multivariable analysis including sex, age and education. When significant, younger age and increased education are related to better performance.

W = significant gender effect, +W = women perform better than men, -W = significant gender effect, women perform worse than men.

* $p < .05$; ** $p < .01$; *** $p < .001$; **** $p < .0001$; $+p < .003$ or better.

[1] Reproduced in modified form with permission of the Journal of the International Psychological Society.

by education (Welsh et al., 1994) were highly attractive for epidemiologists looking for a brief, valid tool to identify likely cases of dementia in surveys. It is possible that, as cognitive impairment increases the protective effects of education decline. The Word List Recall task does appear to be a satisfactory screen.

Normative Data for African-Americans and European-Americans with Dementia and for Control Subjects

The CERAD Neuropsychological Battery was developed for use in tertiary care medical centers to determine the status of patients with AD. In this section we will describe the performance of African-American and European-

American patients with AD who were entered into the CERAD program and compare it with that of African-American and European-American subjects with dementia identified in the epidemiological surveys in Indianapolis and the Monongahela Valley. We will also present data for European-American control subjects who were enrolled in CERAD. These persons underwent clinical and neuropsychological testing comparable to that developed for the patients with AD enrolled in CERAD, but were determined neither to be demented nor to have an illness associated with dementia.

CERAD has made publicly available on CD-ROM, information on 196 African-Americans and 858 European-Americans at the mild, moderate, and severe stages of AD as determined by the Clinical Dementia Rating scale (CDR) (Morris, 1993). Entry scores on these patients, adjusted in terms of gender, age and education, is shown in Table 5. Information on Word List Recognition is not provided because of the skew of these data. In general, the European-Americans perform somewhat better on the neuropsychology measures of the CERAD battery than do the African-Americans, but, with the exception of the modified Boston Naming measure, the differences are

Table 5. CERAD AD entrants: adjusted score on CERAD neuropsychology measures by race and CDR[a].

	African-American cases CDR stage			European-American cases CDR stage		
	1 (n=101)	2 (n=76)	3 (n=19)	1 (n=463)	2 (n=349)	3 (n=46)
Verbal Fluency						
Mean	5.3	3.4	1.9	5.8	4.0	2.4
S.E.	0.3	0.3	0.5	0.1	0.1	0.3
Modified Boston Naming						
Mean	10.2	7.6	4.8	11.5	9.5	6.0
S.E.	0.3	0.4	0.8	0.1	0.2	0.5
Mini-Mental State						
Mean	19.6	12.5[b]	8.3	19.7	14.8	7.6
S.E.	0.4	0.6	1.1	0.2	0.3	0.7
Word List Learning						
Mean	9.2	4.9[c]	3.4	8.8	5.5	1.6
S.E.	0.4	0.5	0.6	0.2	0.2	0.4
Constructional Praxis						
Mean	7.2	4.9	4.1	7.7	6.0	3.9
S.E.	0.3	0.3	0.7	0.1	0.2	0.4
Word List Recall						
Mean	1.0	0.3	0.2	0.9	0.4	0.1
S.E.	0.1	0.1	0.1	0.1	0.1	0.1

CDR = Clinical Dementia Rating Scale (Morris, 1993).
[a] Score adjusted in terms of gender, age and education.
[b] Race difference for MMSE at CDR = 2 is $p < .0008$.
[c] Race difference for Word List Learning at CDR = 2 is $p < .02$.

not substantial. They reach statistical significance for the MMSE at CDR = 2 ($p < .0008$) and for Word List Learning at the same stage ($p < .02$). On the modified Boston Naming task there is a difference of greater than one point at each level of the CDR. This may reflect bias in the items, since some (e.g., tongs) are less familiar to African-Americans. It is important to note that, in each racial group, and for each measure, score declines with increasing severity of disease. Floor effects are found sooner for certain measures, in particular Word List Recall.

Welsh et al. (1995) analyzed data from a subsample of the AD patients mentioned above. After controlling for age, education, estimated duration of illness, ability to perform activities of daily living as assessed by the Blessed Dementia Rating Scale (Blessed et al., 1968), and CDR score (gender was not included since it had not been found to be related to race), a significant race effect was found overall for the five measures examined (Verbal Fluency, modified Boston Naming, MMSE, Word List Learning and Constructional Praxis). While African-Americans performed more poorly than European-Americans on all measures, univariate analyses indicated statistically significant differences for the modified Boston Naming, MMSE and Constructional Praxis. Because of the skew of the data, two measures, Word List Recall and Word List Recognition, could not be examined.

Thus, while race did not appear to influence score on the CERAD neuropsychology measures in a community-based sample (with gender, age and education controlled), race does affect scores in patients with carefully identified AD. In fact, Welsh et al. (1995) recommend that cultural or experiential differences, as well as age and education be taken into account when interpreting the performance on neuropsychological measures of African-American patients with dementia.

While there may be racial differences in performance at entry into CERAD, a follow-up study, which examined progression of AD over the period of a year in a subgroup of the same patients (Fillenbaum et al., 1998b), found that race effects were mild ($p < .047$) after age, education, initial level of performance and stage of disease at entry had been controlled. Indeed, African-American patients had significantly less decline on the Boston Naming and Word List Learning tests. While suggesting that the two groups do not differ markedly in progression of disease, this study cannot be considered definitive. The duration is brief because the dropout rate of the African-American patients was high, a not unusual finding. While 82% of the European-American patients were still in the study a year after entry, this was true for only 66% of the African-American patients. Constraints such as lack of transportation or financial difficulties, and greater acceptance of diseases related to aging, may help to explain the higher attrition rate (Ballard et al., 1993).

We are not able to determine whether race also influences performance of subjects identified as demented in epidemiological surveys, but data in Table 6 does permit some comparison. It should be noted that for the Monongahela Valley (Ganguli et al., 1997), data for all cases with dementia at a mild or greater level have been combined. In Indianapolis, the numbers at CDR stages 2 and 3 are small, but the same held for the CERAD data for this racial group. First, it should be noted that, even with all stages of dementia combined, the European-Americans of the Monongahela Valley perform at a notably higher level than do the African-Americans at a mild stage of disease in Indianapolis. We have not taken into account here differences in age, gender distribution, or education, each of which may contribute to the difference found. Further, those with dementia in the Monongahela Valley also appear to have, for two measures (modified Boston Naming, MMSE) the same, and for four measures a better level of performance than the European-American patients with AD enrolled in CERAD. While the median age of the CERAD European-Americans was 1.3 years greater than for the total Monongahela Valley sample (which would reduce their level of performance), their average level of

Table 6. Score on CERAD neuropsychology measures by race and CDR stage for epidemiologically identified cases with dementia.

	Indianapolis African-American CDR stage			Monongahela Valley European-American CDR stage
	1 (n=89)	2 (n=23)	3 (n=20)	≥ 1 (n=82)
Verbal Fluency				
Mean	7.8	3.9	2.1	8.2
S.D.	4.0	3.3	2.6	3.9
Modified Boston Naming				
Mean	9.1	5.3	3.5	11.3
S.D.	2.7	2.7	1.6	3.0
Mini-Mental State[1]				
Mean	17.8	10.1	5.3	20.0
S.D.	4.2	3.3	4.9	5.9
Word List Learning[2]				
Mean	6.9	3.5	2.0	10.1
S.D.	3.5	2.7	3.3	4.7
Constructional Praxis[3]				
Mean				8.5
S.D.				2.1
Word List Recall				
Mean	0.6	<0.1	0.1	1.8
S.D.	1.0	0.3	0.4	2.0
Word List Recognition				
Mean	13.2	10.4	10.2	16.4
S.D.	3.0	2.3	2.5	2.2

[1] In Indianapolis, saying the days of the week backwards was used instead of spelling WORLD backwards.

[2] In Indianapolis, the items of the Word List Learning test were read aloud by the examiner, but not seen or repeated by the subject.

[3] Full Constructional Praxis not routinely administered in Indianapolis.

education was slightly higher and their gender distribution was comparable. The effect of these demographic differences between the samples can be
expected to cancel each other out.

The African-Americans with dementia in Indianapolis came from two representative samples, one of community residents, the other of residents of
nursing homes. Here data for these two groups have been combined. On
verbal fluency these community and nursing home residents perform better
than the carefully selected African-American CERAD patients with AD, on
all other measures their performance is poorer. This may reflect differences
in assignment of CDR score. The scores at each CDR level are, however,
compatible.

Thus, while for African-Americans with dementia, performance on the
CERAD Neuropsychological Battery reflects stage of disease rather than location where identified, this situation is not clear for European-Americans with
dementia. Confusing the issue further is the fact that the data from CERAD
on the performance of those with dementia are based solely on patients with
AD. The community and nursing home samples include persons with all types
of dementia. For these people the present measures may vary in the extent to
which they are sensitive indicators of stage of disease. So, while these measures
can distinguish different levels of severity of dementia, more information is
needed on how those with different types of dementia perform on these tests.

Conclusions

The CERAD Neuropsychological Battery is reliable and valid. It can be used
to distinguish, both in the tertiary care and in the community setting, those
who are cognitively normal from those who are demented. Although in the
community no race bias was identified statistically, nevertheless, the performance of African-Americans was at a lower level than that of European-
Americans, and significant differences were found in controlled analyses for
some measures in the tertiary care setting. Cultural bias may be present,
particularly for the modified Boston Naming test (Fillenbaum et al., 1997).
The effects of age and education may, however, be more serious than the
effects of race. As with all measures, performance should be interpreted cautiously, and individual circumstances should be taken into account.

Acknowledgements

Work on this chapter was supported by the following grants: NIA grant
no. AG08937 (GGF), NIA grant No. AG06790 (GGF, A.H. & KW-B), NIA
grants No. AG09997, AG05128 (KW-B), NIA grants no. AG06782 and
AG07562 (MG), NIA grants no. AG09956 and AG10133 and Alzheimer
Association grant no. IIRG-95-084 (FU).

References

Anonymous (1997). Consensus recommendations for the postmortem diagnosis of Alzheimer's disease. The NIA and Reagan Institute Working Group on Diagnostic Criteria for the Neuropathological Assessment of AD. *Neurobiology of Aging, 18,* S1-2.

Ballard, E., Nash, F., Raiford, K. & Harrell, L. (1993). Recruitment of black elderly for clinical research studies of dementia: The CERAD experience. *Gerontologist, 33,* 561-565.

Blessed, G., Tomlinson, B.E., & Roth, M. (1968). The association between quantitative measures of dementia and of senile change in the cerebral grey mater of elderly subjects. *British Journal of Psychiatry, 114,* 797-811.

Copeland, J.R., Dewey, M.E. & Griffiths-Jones, H.M. (1986). A computerized psychiatric diagnostic system and case nomenclature for elderly subjects: GMS and AGECAT. *Psychological Medicine, 16,* 89-99.

Crum, R.M., Anthony, J.C., Bassett, S.S., & Folstein, M.F. (1993). Population-based norms of the Mini-Mental State Examination by age and education level. *Journal of the American Medical Association, 269,* 2386-2391.

Eaton, W.W. & Kessler, L.G. (Eds.) (1985). *Epidemiologic field methods in psychiatry: The NIMH Epidemiologic Catchment Area program.* New York: Academic Press.

Fillenbaum, G.G., George, L.K., & Blazer, D.G. (1988). Scoring nonresponse on the Mini-Mental State examination. *Psychological Medicine, 18,* 1021-1025.

Fillenbaum, G.G., Huber, M., & Taussig, I.M. (1997). Performance of elderly white and African-American community residents on the abbreviated CERAD Boston Naming Test. *Journal of Clinical and Experimental Neuropsychology, 19,* 204-210.

Fillenbaum, G.G., Heyman, A., Huber, M.S., Woodbury, M.A., Leiss, J., Schmader, K.E., Bohannon, A., & Trapp-Moen, B. (1998a). The prevalence and 3-year incidence of dementia in older Black and White community residents. *Journal of Clinical Epidemiology, 51,* 587-595.

Fillenbaum, G.G., Peterson, B., Welsh-Bohmer, K.A., Kukull, W.A., & Heyman, A. (1998b). Progression of Alzheimer's disease in black and white patients. The CERAD experience, Part XVI. *Neurology, 51,* 154-158.

Folstein, M.F., Folstein, S.E., & McHugh, P.R. (1975). Mini-mental state: A practical method for grading the cognitive state of patients for the clinician. *Journal of Psychiatric Research, 12,* 189-198.

Ganguli, M., Ratcliff, G., Huff, F.J., Belle, S., Kancel, M.J., Fischer, L., Seaberg, E.C., & Kuller, L.H. (1991). Effects of age, gender, and education on cognitive tests in a rural elderly community sample: Norms from the Monongahela Valley Independent Elders Survey. *Neuroepidemiology, 10,* 42-52.

Ganguli, M., Belle, S., & Ratcliff, G. (1993). Sensitivity and specificity for dementia of population-based criteria for cognitive impairment: the MoVIES project. *Journal of Gerontology: Medical Sciences, 48,* M152-M161.

Ganguli, M., Seaberg, E.C., Ratcliff, G.G., Belle, S.H., & DeKosky, S.T. (1996). Cognitive stability over two years in a rural elderly population: The MoVIES project. *Neuroepidemiology, 15,* 42-50.

Ganguli, M., Ratcliff, G., & DeKosky, S.T. (1997). Cognitive test scores in community-based older adults with and without dementia. *Aging and Mental Health, 1,* 176-180.

Hendrie, H.C., Osuntokun, B.O., Hall, K.S., Ogunniyi, A. O., Hui, S. L., Unverzagt, F. W., Gureje, O., Rodenberg, C. A., Baiyewu, O., Musick, B. S., Adeyinka, A., Farlow, M. R., Oluwole, S. O., Class, A. C., Komolafe, O., Brashear, A., & Burdine, V. (1995). Prevalence of Alzheimer's disease and dementia in two communities: Nigerian Africans and African-Americans. *American Journal of Psychiatry*, *152*, 1485-1492.

Isaacs, B., & Akhtar, A.J. (1972). The Set Test. *Age and Ageing*, *1*, 222-226.

Kaplan, E.F., Goodglass, H., & Weintraub, S. (1983). *The Boston Naming Test*. Philadelphia, PA: Lea & Febiger.

McKhann, G., Drachman, D., Folstein, M., Katzman, R., Price, D., & Stadlan, E.M. (1984). Clinical diagnosis of Alzheimer's disease: Report of the NINCDS-ADRDA Work Group under the auspices of Department of Health and Human Services Task Force on Alzheimer's disease. *Neurology*, *34*, 939-944.

Morris, J.C. (1993). The Clinical Dementia Rating (CDR): Current version and scoring rules. *Neurology*, *43*, 2412-2414.

Morris, J.C., Heyman, A., Mohs, R.C., Hughes, J. P., van Belle, G., Fillenbaum, G., Mellits, E. P., Clark, C., and the CERAD investigators (1989). The Consortium to Establish a Registry for Alzheimer's Disease (CERAD). Part I: Clinical and neuropsychological assessment of Alzheimer's disease. *Neurology*, *39*, 1159-1165.

Rosen, W.G., Mohs, R.C., & Davis, K.L. (1984). A new rating scale for Alzheimer's disease. *American Journal of Psychiatry*, *141*, 1356-1364.

Roth, M., Tym, E., Mountjoy, C.Q., Huppert, F.A., Hendrie, H., Verma, S. & Goddard, H. CAMDEX. (1986). A standardized instrument for the diagnosis of mental disorder in the elderly with special reference to early detection of dementia. *British Journal of Psychiatry*, *149*, 698-709.

Spangenberg, K.B., Henderson, S. & Wagner, M.T. (1997). Validity of a recall and recognition condition to assess visual memory in the CERAD battery. *Applied Neuropsychology*, *4*, 154-159.

Standish, T.I., Molloy, D.W., Bedard, M., Layne, E.C., Murray E.A., & Strang, D. (1996). Improved reliability of the standardized Alzheimer's Disease Assessment Scale (SADAS) compared with the Alzheimer's Disease Assessment Scale (ADAS). *Journal of the American Geriatrics Society*, *44*, 712-716.

Tombaugh, T.N., & McIntyre, N.J. (1992). The Mini-Mental State Examination: A comprehensive review. *Journal of the American Geriatrics Society*, *40*, 922-935.

Unverzagt, F.W., Hall, K.S., Torke, A.M., Rediger, J.D., Mercado, N., Gureje, O., Osuntokun, B.O., & Hendrie, H.C. (1996). Effects of age, education, and gender on CERAD neuropsychological test performance in an African-American sample. *Clinical Neuropsychologist*, *10*, 180-190.

Welsh, K., Butters, N., Hughes, J.P., Mohs, R.C., & Heyman, A. (1991). Detection of abnormal memory decline in mild cases of Alzheimer's disease using CERAD neuropsychology measures. *Archives of Neurology*, *48*, 278-281.

Welsh, K., Butters, N., Hughes, J.P., Mohs, R.C., & Heyman, A. (1992). Detection and staging of dementia in Alzheimer's disease - use of the neuropsychology measures developed for the Consortium to Establish a Registry for Alzheimer's Disease. *Archives of Neurology*, *49*, 448-452.

Welsh, K., Butters, N., & Mohs, R.C., et al. (1994). The Consortium to Establish a Registry for Alzheimer's Disease (CERAD) Part V: a normative study of the neuropsychological battery. *Neurology*, *44*, 609-614.

Welsh, K.A., Fillenbaum, G., & Wilkinson, W., et al. (1995). Neuropsychological test performance in African-American and white patients with Alzheimer's disease. *Neurology*, *45*, 2207-2211.

Woods, D.C. (1995). CERAD Constructional Praxis scoring rules. Ms., Alzheimer Center, Case Western Reserve University and University Hospitals of Cleveland, April 27.

Chapter 4

NEUROPSYCHOLOGICAL ASSESSMENT OF AFRICAN AMERICANS

Gary T. Miles, Ph.D.
Department of Veterans Affairs, Palo Alto Health Care System, Palo Alto, California

Abstract

Accurate assessment of African-American patients involves a consideration of a complex interaction of variables. Much debate has occurred regarding the relevance of many of these variables and the impact that they may or may not exert on the level of performance in this population. These variables are identified and their implications discussed.

Introduction

An aspect of conducting neuropsychological evaluation and interpretation with African Americans involves an understanding of the patient/client with respect to cultural background, educational history, academic achievement, issues surrounding acculturation/assimilation, as well as level of motivation for undergoing an evaluation. Oftentimes, the purpose of the evaluation and how this process may be useful has not been fully explained, which may set up an atmosphere of mistrust, anger and resentment for what appears to be an unnecessary procedure.

In the United States, there have been several instances in which test data have been misused to incorrectly diagnose and/or classify African Americans, ultimately establishing a culture of mistrust of these processes. In the 1970s, a class action suit was filed by a group of African-American parents against the San Francisco Unified School District. In the suit, the parents alleged that test scores were being utilized to incorrectly label their children, resulting in placement in Developmentally Delayed (DD) classes. The parents alleged that the civil rights of the children, guaranteed by the Fourteenth Amendment of the Constitution, had been violated and they had been denied equal opportunity to education guaranteed by the Civil Rights Act of 1964 and the California Education Code. The plaintiffs alleged that their children had been inappropriately classified and placed in DD classes; that their children represented a class of "all black children in the state wrongly labelled and retained in DD classes." That the plaintiffs' children, and the class they represented, had never been mentally retarded, but had been wrongfully placed in DD classes through the use of standardized IQ tests in the State of California, which failed to account for their (plaintiff's children) cultural background and home experiences. That use of culturally biased IQ tests resulted in a disproportionately large number of black children being wrongly labelled mentally retarded and inappropriately placed in DD classes (Dent, 1986).

On June 21, 1972, Judge Robert F. Peckham issued a preliminary injunction against the San Francisco Unified School District to enjoin the district from requiring the use of IQ tests that do not account for the cultural and experiential background of black children. On December 14, 1974, Judge Peckham extended the class of children to include all black children in the State of California and enjoined the state from requiring the use of culturally biased IQ tests for the purpose of placing black children in DD classes (Dent, 1986).

Even though these parents were successful in over-turning the requirement that their children be tested, the damage had been done. Intelligence testing, psychological testing, and ultimately neuropsychological testing, are often viewed with mistrust and apprehension by African Americans due in large measure to the historical adverse use of test data in ways that did not appear to have the best interest of the examinee at heart.

Culture-Free, Culture-Fair Testing

For several decades, the argument for culture-free, culture- fair tests has been waged. Test developers scrutinize the content of the test questions, as well as the way in which questions are phrased. Both psychological and neuropsychological tests are developed with a broad perspective as to who will be taking the test, with emphasis on how the test data will be used.

Research on ethnic differences has been accumulating since the mid 1960s, with the majority of the research focusing on African Americans. Typically, researchers appear interested in answering questions pertaining to bias in test construction and interpretation (Anastasi, 1988). Anastasi (1988) indicated that the focus of research has begun to shift somewhat, from the evaluation of test bias, to the design of selection strategies for fair test use with cultural minorities.

Anastasi (1988) suggested that the issue of cross-cultural testing had been a problem at least since 1910. She reported that the waves of immigrants entering the United States were often culturally isolated and had had very little contact with Western culture. As a result, most of the instruments that had been developed for a more technologically advanced culture were not appropriate for this newly arrived population.

Anastasi (1988) posited that education, language and performance speed are prominent variables on which cultures vary. When educational background is poor, the issue of illiteracy may be prevalent. Issues of language must be considered, largely due to regional variations in dialect and nomenclature. Performance speed is yet another parameter detailed by Anastasi (1988) on which the dominant culture may differ from a sub-culture. She indicates that there is often a different tempo of life, adding that the value of hurrying through a task (rapid performance) may not be clearly recognizable within certain cultural sub-groups. As an example, consider the general differences between rural and urban subcultures. Life in many major metropolitan centers in the U.S. is a fast-paced, dog-eat-dog, hustle/bustle, 24-hour culture. In contrast, life in a rural environment conjures up images of a much slower existence; an existence where porch swings prevail and people appear less concerned with the passage of time and more concerned with experiencing their lives.

Approaches to Cross-Cultural Testing

Briefly, Anastasi (1988) suggested that there were three basic approaches for developing tests appropriate for cross-cultural use. The first approach involved selecting items common to many different cultures which are then followed by validation of the test items against local criteria among several different cultures. A second approach involved the development of test items within one culture which is then followed by subsequent administration to individuals with divergent cultural backgrounds. A third, and final approach, involves the development of different tests for each culture, utilizing the test only on the population for which it was developed. Each of the aforementioned strategies has its pros and cons. Regarding any test developed for a given culture as the yardstick against which all cultures are measured puts one at risk for overgeneralizing from the test results. Or, assuming that a low score obtained by a patient/client from a different culture on which the test was normed as equivalent to a low score obtained by someone from the normative population creates the tendency to over-pathologize the individual when that individual is from a different cultural subgroup. Overall, however, in the development of culture-fair tests, the objective seems largely to have been to select test items from a broadly defined area, which are reflective of several cultures followed by the validation of the test against local criteria in many different cultures (Anastasi, 1988; Berry, 1983; Segal, 1983; Whiting, 1976).

The Black Intelligence Test of Cultural Homogeneity (BITCH) was developed to examine and quantify knowledge comprehension of urban slang used by African Americans. Test items were selected from a fairly narrow area of African-American culture, based on empirical differences in black-white performance. What the test developer found was that most Caucasian examinees and some African-American examinees, who hadn't been familiar with African-American culture, performed poorly (Williams, 1972a, 1972b). The BITCH test is a fair example of what occurs when a test is developed for a relatively small segment of the population, the utility of the test in the general population becomes limited.

Problems in Cross-Cultural Testing

Cross-cultural testing, in general, is not a simple issue. The issue becomes increasingly complex when considering how cultural differences impact group differences in behavior. Certain test items may have no impact when presented to certain members of a group, which may result in lowering the validity of the test for the entire population. Let us consider briefly, Scale 8 of the Minnesota Multiphasic Personality Inventory 2. A clinical score elevation $T > 65$ in a Caucasian sample would likely be interpreted as suggestive of psychotic, or disorganized thought processes. The same scale elevation in an African-American population would likely be interpreted more cautiously, secondary to considering questions about the respondent's religious and spiritual beliefs. As noted earlier, the responses of the subgroup can alter both the validity and reliability of the test for the entire group.

Anastasi (1988) proposed that there is a continuum of cultural differentials with the effects being superficial, or temporary, ranging to far-reaching, or permanent, disabilities. Language was cited as one of the more superficial cultural differentials in that language ability can be improved with training. She cites factors that are environmentally determined as being longer-term and not necessarily remediable. Intellectual or emotional damage may be created by persistent, negative, adverse environmental factors.

Knobloch and Pasamanick (1966) and Pasamanick and Knobloch (1966) found that prenatal and perinatal disorders were significantly related to behavioral disorders and mental retardation. Low socio-economic-scale (SES) was shown to be related to deficiencies in maternal nutrition. There was also a concomitant increase in other medical complications in mothers with a lower SES, and the frequency of these complications was higher in African Americans when compared to Caucasians. Anastasi (1988) further suggested that these cultural differentials are directly linked with behavioral deficiencies. Furthermore, the effects of these deficiencies persist, resisting extinction for generations. The authors emphasized the fact that these issues are not mediated by genetic factors, adding that environmental conditions need to change in order for improvement to occur.

Cultural Differences and Cultural Handicap

Environment also plays a role in influencing behavior. Individuals reared within a distinct cultural milieu evince behaviors consonant with that milieu. These cultural influences are reflected in the behavioral patterns of the inhabitants of the milieu and should therefore be reflected in test performance. For example, consider the common violin. For a certain segment of the population, when asked to identify the object, the respondents will reply that it is a "violin." The same object, taken, perhaps to a more rural population, will be called a "fiddle." Regional differences, or cultural milieu, affect nomenclature, but they are also responsible for affecting behavior. Consider again the violin/fiddle. That same instrument, played in New York City is likely to yield a distinct, stylistically different sound when compared with someone playing that same instrument in a style that originated and was nurtured in that rural setting.

The goal of cross-cultural testing becomes to construct tests that examine common characteristics between varying cultural groups. It is probably unlikely that any one test will be universally fair across all cultural groups. It is equally unlikely that any single test will be equally fair to more than one cultural group. Each cultural reference group possesses unique qualities and ways of behaving which cause them to stand out as distinct, whether it be performance speed, problem solving ability, motivation to succeed, mathematical ability, or high academic expectation, to name but a few. If a cultural subgroup does not value academic success, then test performance will be negatively affected. Eells and Davis (1951) examined a group of children who came from a reference group of lower socioeconomic status families. These children tended to rush through the test, marking answers to questions in a random fashion. The authors concluded that the poor performance on the part of the students was due to less value being placed on academic success by the culture in which they were raised. These results have been replicated by several researchers (Anastasi & Cordova, 1953; Smith, 1942). While this behavior may be rewarded within the culture from which it emanates, it quickly becomes a liability when the individual changes subgroups and tries to compete within a new group (Anastasi, 1988).

Acculturation

Webster's Dictionary defines acculturation as "the process of adapting to a new, or different culture with more or less advanced patterns." As subgroups begin to integrate with the dominant culture, it becomes increasingly important to acquire those skills and abilities which will allow them to compete successfully within the dominant culture. When the process of acculturation is incomplete, the individual not only experiences a greater likelihood of failure, but he/she has an increasing likelihood of coming to the attention of psychologists, neuropsychologists or social workers who are then called upon to assess, quantify, and/or rehabilitate the identified deficits in order that the individual becomes more successful.

Cultural Deprivation

In addition to an individual being handicapped by his or her inability to adapt to a new cultural subgroup, they can also be handicapped by the family culture in which they develop. Feuerstein (1979) hypothesized that individuals teach behaviors to their children that are not flexible, or adaptive when the need arises to compete within another cultural subgroup. He labelled this cultural deprivation and describes it as a state of reduced cognitive modifiability which is produced by a lack of mediated learning experience. Feuerstein (1979) states that the transmission of accumulated knowledge is an experience common only to humans, with the caregiver acting as the mediating agent. Because the caregiver acts as the mediating agent, they are the gate-keepers charged with selecting and organizing stimulus material presented to the child. Such mediated learning is thought to be necessary for cognitive development because it establishes patterns of learning necessary for successful cognition. If a child does not experience sufficient mediated learning, they will lack the building blocks for higher-order cognitive functioning. Those who have been exposed to mediated learning experiences are then prepared to adapt to the demands of new subcultures with only relative difficulty.

Test Performance

Turning to an examination of the cross-cultural literature as it relates to neuropsychology, it appears clear that significant differences between racial groups have been inconsistently demonstrated in the score patterns of tests of cognitive functioning (Faulstitch, McAnulty, Carey, & Gresham, 1987; Kaufman, McLean, & Reynolds, 1988; Vernon, 1979). In an examination of neuropsychological test performance in African-American and Caucasian patients with Alzheimer's disease, Welsh, Fillenbaum, Wilkinson, Heyman, Mohs, Stern, Harrell, Edland, and Beekly (1995) suggested that performance on specific neuropsychological tests may be modified by cultural and experiential differences. They also suggested that it may be important to examine broader variables such as age and educational background when interpreting neuropsychological test performance in elderly African-American patients with dementia.

Racial differences as an issue affecting test performance continues to be controversial and unsettled. Generally, Caucasians tend to outperform African Americans on many tests of cognitive ability (Kaufman et al., 1988). Amante et al. (1977) suggested that this performance differential can be explained by the increased economic advantage that Caucasians have when compared to African Americans, and are not mediated by racial factors. If this economic advantage is solely responsible for this performance differential, then the argument becomes circular when you consider that, on the average, African Americans earn less money per capita when compared to Caucasians, which may be partially explained by education, and/or lack of opportunity. Further, if African Americans, overall, are less well educated, it seems likely that opportunities for increased financial gain also become limited. It seems likely therefore, that race affects not only economic advantage, but educational opportunity as well, which should be sufficient to indicate that race is indeed a mediating variable, and that race may also mediate this performance differential. Others (Kaufman et al., 1988), through factor-analytic examination, have suggested that the underlying cognitive abilities are identical for Caucasians and African Americans, while Helms (1992) found that cultural differences between the races accounted for the differential performance on standardized tests.

Norman, Evans, Miller, and Heaton (2000) examined whether there were performance differences on the California Verbal Learning Test in a sample of Caucasians and African Americans. They found significant differences based on the demographic characteristics of age, education, ethnicity, and gender.

In a study of HIV positive African-American males, Richardson, Satz, Myers, Miller, Bing, Fawzy, and Maj (1999) found that standard cut-scores for self-report inventories appear to over-estimate psychiatric morbidity.

Akpaffiong, Kunik, Hale, Molinari, and Orengo (1999) examined the phenomenological and treatment differences between Caucasian and African-American patients presented to a geropsychiatric unit for treatment of behavioral problems associated with dementia. Using the Mini-Mental State Examination, the Cohen-Mansfield Agitation Inventory, Brief Psychiatric Rating Scale and the Positive and Negative Syndrome Scale for Schizophrenia, the test results and treatment outcomes between the two groups were the same. The authors felt this was because standardized tests (and standard cut-scores) were used.

In support of seeking appropriate normative data, Gladsjo, Schuman, Evans, Peavy, Miller, and Heaton (1999) used multiple regression analysis to develop demographically corrected norms for letter and category fluency in a sample of Caucasian and African-American adults. Participants ranged in age from 20 to 101 years, with 0-20 years education. Age, education, and ethnicity were significant predictors of letter and category fluency performance, accounting for 15% and 25% of variance, respectively.

Manly, Miller, Heaton, Byrd, Reilly, Velasquez, Saccuzzo, and Grant (1998) suggested that accounting for acculturation might improve the diagnostic accuracy of certain neuropsychological tests. They examined the relationship of neuropsychological test performance in a group of medically healthy, non-impaired African Americans compared with a group of HIV-positive subgroups of African Americans and Caucasians matched for age, education, sex, and HIV disease status. The examiners measured acculturation through self-report. They also measured "Black English" use in a subset of medically healthy subjects. They determined that Black English use was correlated with performance deficits on the Trail Making Test, part B, and the Information subtest on the WAIS-R. After accounting for acculturation, they determined that ethnic group differences on all measures, with the exception of Story Learning, became nonsignificant.

A group of African Americans with unilateral brain damage and non-brain-damaged controls was compared using the Hooper Visual Organization Test (VOT). The VOT is a measure of hemisphere-specific, region-specific, or non-specific brain damage. The examiners demonstrated that VOT performance is differentially sensitive to regional cerebral pathology. They question, however, the claim that the test is appropriate for use with patients with right posterior cerebral damage. The normative data for this test were not different for African Americans (Lewis et al., 1997).

In an examination of performance differences between African-American and Caucasian subjects on six abilities from Horn's Gf-Gc theory for five age groups between 15-19, and 55-93 years, Caucasian respondents scored significantly higher on all six abilities. Differences in fluid reasoning and short-term apprehension and retrieval were less than .5 SD. Interactions of age x race were non-significant, indicating that the discrepancies between scores of African-American and Caucasian subjects did not vary as a function of age (Chen, Kaufman, & Kaufman, 1994).

Examining differences in reaction times in African-American and Caucasian alcoholics, York and Biederman (1991) found that the effects of alcohol use remained statistically significant. The obtained values for African Americans were 5% slower than were the values for Caucasians; values for alcoholics were approximately 4.6% slower than those for controls.

In an example of how cultural or experiential differences may mediate neuropsychological test performance, Welsh, Fillenbaum, Wilkinson, Heyman, Mohs, Stern, Harrell, Edland, and Beekly (1995) examined a group of African-American and Caucasian patients with Alzheimer's disease. The authors concluded that it is useful to consider cultural and experiential differences, along with age and education, when interpreting the neuropsychological test performance of elderly African-American patients with dementia.

In many ways, racial differences appear to have a significant impact on the quantitative differences in cognition. Researchers have presented evidence suggesting that race and formal education impact cognitive performance. In addition, there are several disease processes that contribute to neuropsychological impairment. In most group comparisons, Caucasians appear to outperform African Americans on cognitive tests (Kaufman, McLean, &

Reynolds, 1988). Amante et al. (1977) feet that many of these differences are mediated by the socioeconomic advantages of Caucasians. Other researchers suggested that the underlying abilities for these groups are identical (Faulstich et al., 1987; Kaufman, Mc Lean, & Reynolds, 1991).

Turning briefly to the Wechsler Adult Intelligence Scales, Kaufman, McLean and Reynolds (1988) found that Caucasians performed consistently better on the Vocabulary subtest, compared to African Americans. Educational differences were not examined, however. Vernon (1979) and Anastasi (1988) believed that the Vocabulary scaled score performance was probably more representative of the patient's socioeconomic level and cultural development rather than educational level.

Scaled scores on the Information subtest were 1.5 to 2 points lower for African-American elderly patients, compared to similar Caucasians. The authors reported that the scaled score differences were also apparent in African Americans over the age of 55 residing in rural versus urban environments. These differences were not apparent in younger patients. It was suggested that the effects of mass-media exposure erased this performance difference in younger people (Kaufman, McLean & Reynolds, 1988). Using a modified 200-item version of the Paced Auditory Serial Addition Task, Diehr, Heaton, Miller, and Grant (1998) found that age, education, and ethnicity were significant predictors, accounting for nearly 23% of the variance in test performance.

Although the literature appears somewhat mixed relative to the acceptance of race as a mediating variable in neuropsychological performance (Gould, 1981; Loehlin et al., 1975), test examiners probably owe it to their examinees to consider the possibility that race is indeed a factor, and to consider the degree to which performance deficits may be accounted for by this factor. In general, Caucasians tend to outperform African Americans on many tests (Kaufman, McLean & Reynolds, 1988). Caucasians also tend to be more advantaged relative to socioeconomic status (Amante et al., 1977). Kaufman et al. (1991) and Faulstich et al. (1987) report that the underlying abilities were identical across racial groups as demonstrated by congruent factor structures. Helms (1992), however, suggested that cultural differences between the races may explain the differential performance on standardized tests. Overall, it appears more likely that any combination of variables, i.e., race, culture or socioeconomic status, may account for the observed differences in level of performance, rather than those differences being attributed to any one variable.

Disease Processes

Historically, African Americans have had poorer access to health care in the United States. As a result, disease processes often go undetected, untreated, under-treated, or mistreated. There are several disease processes that are more common in African Americans, many of them having implications for neuropsychological impairment, i.e., hypertension, diabetes, cerebro-vascular disease and early-onset dementia.

The incidence of hypertension in African Americans is greater than that of the dominant culture in our society. Similarly, the incidence of alcoholism and substance abuse in the African-American community is also likely to make a contribution to neuropsychological impairment. Neurological disorders tend to be more common in African-American patients. Those who acquired the diseases through intravenous drug use rather than sexual contact appear to show higher rates of impairment (Kaemingk & Kasniak, 1989).

In a field investigation of stroke survivors, males had a higher age adjusted stroke prevalence ratio regardless of race when compared to women. African-American subjects of either sex had a higher age-adjusted prevalence ratio than did Caucasians. For all groups the prevalence ratios increased with age (Schoenberg, 1986).

The literature on cerebrovascular disease appears more consistent than is true for the coronary heart disease (CHD) literature. In a group of 164 African-American elderly living in central Harlem, Teresi, Albert, Holmes, and Mayeux (1999) utilized cognitive screening instruments in an effort to examine signs of CVA and symptoms of Parkinson's disease. These researchers found that 2-3% of the sample were communication-disordered; 5% had significant ambulation disorders.

Greater cognitive decline has also been associated with less formal education, with greater decline observed in African-American patients with fewer than eight years formal education. Having more than eight years formal education was associated with less decline. Formal education beyond nine years was not associated with further reduction in cognitive decline (Lyketsos, Chen, & Anthony, 1999).

Diabetes is raised as an issue in neuropsychological impairment because of its profile of complications. Individuals who are diagnosed as diabetic tend to have higher incidences of heart disease, stroke, kidney failure, blindness and peripheral vascular disease. African Americans have experienced a tremendous increase in the prevalence and mortality of this disease. Roseman (1985) reported that in the period from 1961 to 1983 alone, the prevalence of diabetes increased 175% in African Americans and 106% in Caucasians, with African Americans experiencing greater risk for the aforementioned complications (Office of Minority Health Resource Center, 1988).

The third leading cause of death in the African-American population is cerebrovascular disease. When compared to Caucasians, African Americans, between the ages of 35 and 74, are more likely to die from CVAs. African-American women have greater incidences of stroke until the age of 75, when compared with African-American men (Gillum, 1988). Geographical differences have been observed in the incidence of cerebrovascular accidents, with a higher incidence observed in the Southeastern United States (Report of the Secretary's Task Force on Black and Minority Health, 1986).

Regardless of age, education, acculturation, or race, the basic patho-physiology in organic brain disorders is generally assumed to have the same biophysical manifestations (Valle, 1981). Heyman, Fillengaum, Prosnitz, Willians, Burchett, Clark, and Woodbury (1988) however, suggest that there are differences in the rates at which elder African Americans experience dementia, compared to their Caucasian counterparts. One-hundred-forty-four patients with clinically documented dementia were autopsied at Johns Hopkins Hospital between 1973 and 1986. De la Monte, Hutchins, and Moore (1989) reported that there were racial differences in the etiology of the dementing illness. Caucasians demonstrated 2.6 times greater frequency of dementia than African Americans and 3.86 times greater risk for developing Alzheimer's disease. African Americans had 5.56 times greater frequencies of multi-infarct dementia while the risk of Parkinson's was higher in Caucasians. African Americans demonstrated an 8.44 times greater likelihood of dementia associated with chronic EtOH abuse. The authors stated that additional study is required as their results may not be generalizable beyond the community served by Johns Hopkins. Heyman et al. (1988) also found that African Americans demonstrated a higher prevalence for dementia when compared with Caucasians. African Americans were more likely to report heart attacks, CVAs, HTN, and diabetes when compared to Caucasians.

Roca and co-workers (1984) reported that the diagnosis of dementia is often missed or inappropriately diagnosed (Roca, Klein, Kirby, McArthur, Vogelsang, Folstein, & Smith, 1984). Diagnoses of dementia are often overlooked in patients who are younger or incorrectly diagnosed in those with less formal education (Roca et al., 1984). If the observed differences in prevalence is due to formal education, these differences are hypothesized to disappear as African Americans overall achieve greater formal education (Macken, 1986).

In a survey of 20,000 rural African Americans and Caucasians, the prevalence of dementia increased with age, and did not appear affected by race or gender (Kramer, German, Anthony, Von Korff, & Skinner, 1985). Females had a higher percentage of primary progressive dementia while African Americans had a marginally higher percentage of cases diagnosed. Non-white males had a significantly higher rate of cognitive impairment compared to white males in the 65 to 74 and 75+ age range. No differences were seen in the women in the same age ranges. The authors concluded that the differences in prevalence may be attributed to diet, environment, heredity, or several of these factors in combination. A similar conclusion was reached by Breitbach, Alexander, Daltroy, Liang, Boll, Karlson, Partridge, Roberts, Stern, Wacholtz, & Straaton (1998). In an examination of patients with SLE, the authors report no significant interaction between race and disease. They suggested that increased frequency of cognitive impairment in African Americans with SLE is due to the additive effects of psychosocial variables.

Conclusions

In assessing African Americans, it becomes incumbent upon the examiner to take into account the interaction of several variables when selecting, scoring, and interpreting neuropsychological tests. Age and level of education are routinely considered to be significant variables; however, level of acculturation and assimilation of the patient with the dominant culture is often overlooked. Those who demonstrate disparities with the dominant culture can be expected to perform less well on standardized tests and are likely to be over-pathologized.

In selecting tests, those tests that rely less on written language are more likely to be "culture-fair" compared to those which rely more heavily on language skill. Particular attention should be paid to dialect and regional differences in nomenclature as these differences may result in performance deficits.

Age was also mentioned earlier as a significant mediating variable. Older African-American patients tend to perform less well due to greater incidences of health problems which have been shown to have consequences for neuropsychological impairment.

It is imperative that the examiner explain why the patient is being tested and to discuss how those results are to be utilized. Try to make the patient an ally in the assessment process by gaining his/her trust in the utility of the procedures.

Overall, the differences in assessing African Americans may appear subtle; however, the effects of ignoring these differences can be enormous. Lezak (1995) wrote "it should be emphasized that the statistical adjustment in test scores, cutoffs, and prediction formulas hold little promise as a means of correcting social inequities. More constructive approaches are suggested...one is illustrated by multiple aptitude testing and classification strategies, which permit the fullest utilization of the diverse aptitude patterns fostered by different cultural backgrounds. Another approach is through adaptive treatments, such as individualized training programs in order to maximize the fit of such programs as accurately as possible to the person's present level of development..." By altering our approach relative to the assessment of African Americans, we can increase the utility and the effectiveness of our interventions with this special population.

References

Akpaffiong, M., Kunik, M.E., Hale, D., Molinari, V., & Orengo, C. (1999). Cross-cultural differences in demented geropsychiatric inpatients with behavioral disturbances. *International Journal of Geriatric Psychiatry, 14* (10), 845-850.

Amante, D., VanHouten, V. W., Grieve, J. H., Bader, C. A., & Marquez, P. H. (1977). Neuropsychological deficit, ethnicity, and socioeconomic status. *Journal of Consulting and Clinical Psychology, 45*, 524-535.

Anastasi, A. (1988). *Psychological testing*, 6 ed., New York: McMillan.

Anastasi, A., & Cordova, F. A. (1953). Some effects of bilingualism upon the intelligence test performance of Puerto Rican children in New York City. *Journal of Educational Psychology, 44*, 1-19.

Berry, J. W. (1983). Textured contexts: Systems and situations in cross-cultural psychology. In S. H. Irvine & J. W. Berry (Eds.), *Human assessment and cultural factors* (pp. 117-125). New York: Plenum Press.

Breitbach, S. A., Alexander, R. W., Daltroy, L. H., Liang, M. H., Boll, T. J., Karlson, E. W., Partridge, A. J., Roberts, W. N., Stern, S. H., Wacholtz, M. C., & Straaton, K. V. (1998). Determinants of cognitive performance in systemic lupus erythematosus. *Journal of Clinical Experimental Neuropsychology, 20* (2), 157-166.

Chen, T. H., Kaufman, A. S., & Kaufman, J. C. (1994). Examining the interaction of age x race pertaining to black-white differences at ages 15 to 93 on six Horn abilities assessed by K-FAST, K-SNAP, and KAIT subtests. *Perceptual and Motor Skills, 79* (3, pt 2), 1693-1690.

De la Monte, S. M., Hutchins, G.M., & Moore, G. W. (1989). Racial differences in the etiology and frequency of Alzheimer's lesions in the brain. *Journal of the National Medical Association, 81* (6), 644-652.

Dent, H. (1986). Presentation on "The Larry P. Case" presented to the Bay Area Association of Black Psychologists, September 1986.

Diehr, M.C., Heaton, R. K., Miller, W., & Grant, I. (1998). The Paced Auditory Serial Addition Task (PASAT): norms for age, education and ethnicity. *Assessment, 5* (4), 375-387.

Eells, K., & Davis, A. (1951). *Intelligence and cultural differences.* Chicago: University of Chicago Press.

Faulstich, M.E., McAnulty, D.A., Carey, M.P., & Gresham, F. M. (1987). Topography of human intelligence across race: Factorial comparison of black-white WAIS-R profiles for criminal offenders. *International Journal of Neuroscience, 35*, 181-187.

Feuerstein, R. (1979). *The dynamic assessment of retarded performers: The Learning Potential Assessment Device, theory, instruments, and techniques.* Baltimore: University Park Press.

Gillum, R.F. (1988). Stroke in blacks. *Stroke, 19*, 1-9.

Gladsjo, J. A., Schuman, C. C., Evans, J. D., Peavy, G. M., Miller, S. W., & Heaton, R. K. (1999) Norms for letter and category fluency: demographic corrections for age, education, and ethnicity. *Assessment, 6* (2), 147-178.

Gould, S. J. (1981). *The mismeasure of man.* New York: W.W. Norton.

Helms, J. E. (1992). Why is there no study of cultural equivalence in standardized cognitive ability testing? *American Psychologist, 47*, 1083-1101.

Heyman, A., Fillenbaum, G.G., Prosnitz, B., Williams, K., Burchett, B., Clark, C., & Woodbury, M. (1988). Estimated prevalence of dementia among elderly black and white community residents. Paper presented at the 41st Annual Scientific Meeting of the Gerontological Society of America, San Francisco, CA.

Kaemingk, K.L., & Kasniak, A.W. (1989). Neuropsychological aspects of human immunodeficiency virus infection. *The Clinical Neuropsychologist, 3*, 309-326.

Kaufman, A.S., McLean, J.E., & Reynolds, C.R. (1988). Sex, race, residence, region, and education differences on the 11 WAIS-R subtests. *Journal of Clinical Psychology, 44*, 231-248.

Knobloch, H., & Pasamanick, B. (1966). Prospective studies on the epidemiology of reproductive casualty: Methods, findings, and some implications. *Merrill-Palmer Quarterly, 12*, 27-43.

Kramer, M., German, P.S., Anthony, J. C., Von Korff, M., & Skinner, E. A. (1985). Patterns of mental disorders among the elderly residents of Eastern Baltimore. *Journal of the American Geriatrics Society, 33* (4), 236-245.

Lewis, L., Campbell, A., Takushi-Chinen, R., Brown, A., Dennis, G., Wood, D., & Weir, R. (1997). Visual organization test performance in an African-American population with acute unilateral cerebral lesions. *International Journal of Neuroscience, 91* (3-4), 295-302.

Lezak, M. D. (1995). *Neuropsychological assessment* (3rd ed.). New York: Oxford University Press.

Loehlin, J. C., Lindzey, G., & Spuhler, J.N. (1975). *Race differences in intelligence.* San Francisco: W. H. Freeman.

Lyketsos, C. G., Chen, L. S., & Anthony, J. C. (1999). Cognitive decline in adulthood: an 11.5-year follow-up of the Baltimore Epidemiologic Catchment Area Study. *American Journal of Psychiatry, 156* (1), 58-65.

Macken, C.L. (1986). A profile of functionally impaired elderly persons living in the community. *Health Care Financing Review, 7* (4), 33-49.

Manly, J. J., Miller, S. W., Heaton, R. K., Byrd, D., Reilly, J., Velasquez, R. J., Saccuzzo, D. P., & Grant, I. (1998). The effect of African-American acculturation on neuropsychological test performance in normal and HIV-positive individuals. The HIV Neurobehavioral Research Center (HNRC) Group. *Journal of the International Neuropsychological Society, 4* (3), 291-302.

Norman, M.A., Evans, J.D., Miller, W. S., & Heaton, R. K. (2000). Demographically corrected norms for the California Verbal Learning Test. *Journal of Clinical Experimental Neuropsychology, 22* (1), 80-94.

Office of Minority Health Resource Center (1988). *Closing the gap: Diabetes and minorities.* (pp. 1-4). Washington, D.C.: Office of Minority Health, Public Health Service, U.S. Department of Health and Human Services.

Pasamanick, B., & Knobloch, H. (1966). Retrospective studies on the epidemiology of reproductive casualty: Old and new. *Merrill-Palmer Quarterly, 12,* 7-26.

Report of the Secretary's Task Force on Black & Minority Health (1986). *Cardiovascular and cerebrovascular disease (Vol. IV, Part I).* Washington, D.C.: Department of Health and Human Services, U. S. Government Printing Office.

Richardson, M. A., Satz, P.F., Myers, H.F., Miller, E.N., Bing, E.G., Fawzy, F.I., & Maj, M. (1999). Effects of depressed mood versus clinical depression on neuropsychological test performance among African-American men impacted by HIV/AIDS. *Journal of Clinical Experimental Neuropsychology, 21* (6), 769-783.

Roca, R. P., Klein, L., Kirby, S., McArthur, J., Vogelsang, G., Folstein., M., & Smith, C. (1984). Recognition of dementia among medical patients. *Archives of Internal Medicine, 144,* 73-75.

Roseman, J.M. (1985). Diabetes in black Americans. In National Diabetes Data Group (Eds.), *Diabetes in America* (NIH Publication No. 85-1468, pp. 1-24).Washington, D.C.: U.S. Government Printing Office.

Schoenberg, B.S. (1986). Racial differentials in the prevalence of stroke: Copia County Mississippi. *Archives of Neurology, 43,* 565-568.

Segal, M. H. (1983). On the search for the independent variable in cross-cultural psychology. In S. H. Irvine & J. W. Berry (Eds.), *Human assessment and cultural factors* (pp. 127-137). New York: Plenum Press.

Smith, S. (1942). Language and non-verbal test performance of racial groups in Honolulu before and after a 14-year interval. *Journal of General Psychology, 26,* 51-93.

Teresi, J. A., Albert, S. M., Holmes, D., & Mayeux, R. (1999). Use of latent class analyses for the estimation of prevalence of cognitive impairment, and signs of stroke and Parkinson's disease among African-American elderly of central Harlem: results of the Harlem Aging Project. New York: Columbia University Center for Geriatrics and New York State Psychiatric Institute.

Valle, R. (1981). Natural support systems, minority groups, and the late life dementias: Implications for service delivery, research, and policy. In N.E. Miller & G.D. Cohen (Eds.), *Clinical aspects of alzheimer's disease and senile dementia,* [*Aging* special issue], *15*, 277-299.

Vernon, P. E. (1979). *Intelligence: Heredity and environment.* San Francisco: W. H. Freeman.

Welsh, K. A., Fillenbaum, G., Wilkinson, W., Heyman, A., Mohs, R.C., Stern, Y., Harrell, L., Edland, S. D., & Beekly, D. (1995). Neuropsychological test performance in African-American and white patients with Alzheimer's disease. *Neurology, 45* (12), 2207-2211.

Whiting, B. B. (1976). The problem of the packaged variable. In K. Riegel and J. Meacham (Eds.). *The developing individual in a changing world, Vol. 1* (pp. 303-309). The Hague: Mouton.

Williams, Robert (1972a). *BITCH 100: A culture-specific test.* Paper presented to the American Psychological Association Convention, Honolulu, September 1972.

Williams, Robert (1972b). *BITCH 100: A culture-specific test.* Williams and Associates, Inc., 6374 Delmar Blvd. St. Louis, MO 63130.

York, J. L., & Biederman, I. (1991). Hand movement speed and accuracy in detoxified alcoholics. *Alcohol and Clinical Experimental Research, 15* (6), 982-990.

Chapter 5

FUTURE DIRECTIONS IN NEUROPSYCHOLOGICAL ASSESSMENT WITH AFRICAN AMERICANS

Jennifer J. Manly & Diane M. Jacobs
Cognitive Neuroscience Division, Taub Institute for Research on Alzheimer's Disease and the Aging Brain, Department of Neurology and the G.H. Sergievsky Center, Columbia University College of Physicians and Surgeons, New York, New York

Abstract

Most previous research on cognitive test performance of African Americans has compared African Americans to non-Hispanic Whites on intelligence tests, screening measures, and to some extent, neuropsychological tests. These comparisons have generally shown that despite equivalence on demographic variables such as years of education and socioeconomic status, African Americans obtain lower scores on both verbal and non-verbal cognitive tasks and therefore, the specificity of many neuropsychological measures is inadequate when used among African Americans. Establishing separate neuropsychological test norms for African Americans may be an important first step to avoid misdiagnosis of cognitive impairment; however, many problems with this approach remain. First, because "Black" and "African American" are political classifications instead of culturally or scientifically-based categories, it is unclear who should be included in these normative studies and to whom these norms should be applied. This chapter challenges neuropsychologists investigating cognitive test performance of African Americans to clarify the independent influences of race, culture, educational experience, and socioeconomic status on neuropsychological test performance. The authors clarify definitions and research operationalizations of race, ethnicity, and education, and explore how each of these variables might play a part in African-American neuropsychological test performance. Recent research regarding the influence of stereotype threat, acculturation, educational setting, and literacy on neuropsychological test performance in African Americans is reviewed. Finally, the authors discuss how investigation of specific cognitive processes related to racial, cultural, and educational differences (such as familiarity with items, effect of timing, emphasis of holistic aspects versus details of stimuli, and categorization of items using pragmatic versus abstract classifications) will help clarify previous research findings and shed light on the relationship of culture to cognition.

Introduction

Few cognitive ability measures have been properly validated for use among ethnic minorities in the United States. Lack of such validation may account for the fact that, based on neuropsychological test performance, African Americans are judged to be cognitively impaired more often than non-Hispanic White persons. Many investigators have concluded that separate neuropsychological test norms for Black Americans are the solution to this problem. Race-specific norms may improve the specificity of neuropsychological measures when used among African Americans; however, this approach avoids the extraordinary diversity within those who identify as Black, and fails to illuminate the underlying reasons for performance discrepancies between African Americans and Whites. This chapter will argue that future studies of neuropsychological assessment among African Americans should focus investigation on cultural factors which influence cognitive test performance and which can explain ethnic group differences in test scores. We believe this effort should begin with the clarification of the independent influences of race, culture, educational experience, and socioeconomic status on neuropsychological test performance.

In this chapter, we will first discuss previous research on neuropsychological test performance of African Americans. Collection of race-specific norms is currently the most popular direction of research, and we will discuss the advantages and disadvantages of this approach. Along with definitions and research operationalizations of race, ethnicity, and culture, recent research regarding the influence of cultural experience, quality of education, and stereotype threat on neuropsychological test performance of African Americans will be reviewed. As the effect of cultural experience on cognitive processes is emphasized, the importance of racial classifications is reduced, and the distinctiveness and depth of African-American culture is highlighted. We will therefore end with a brief exploration of the possibility of creating measures that are sensitive to those cognitive abilities salient within African-American culture.

Previous Research

Previous research on cognitive test performance of African Americans has compared African Americans to Whites on intelligence tests (Chen, Kaufman, & Kaufman, 1994; Heaton, Ryan, Grant, & Matthews, 1996; Kaufman, McLean & Reynolds, 1988; Kush & Watkins, 1997; Overall & Levin, 1978; Reynolds, Kaufman, & McLean, 1987; Vincent, 1991) and screening measures (Bohnstedt, Fox, & Kohatsu, 1994; Fillenbaum, Heyman, Williams, Prosnitz, & Burchett, 1990; Fillenbaum, Hughes, Heyman, George, & Blazer, 1988; Ford, Haley, Thrower, West, & Harrel, 1996; Kuller et al., 1998; Murden, McRae, Kaner, & Bucknam, 1991; Teresi et al., 1995; Unverzagt, Hall, Torke, & Rediger, 1996; Welsh et al., 1995). Prior research has also investigated performance of African Americans on neuropsychological tests of naming (Lichtenberg, Ross, & Christensen, 1994; Roberts & Hamsher, 1984; Ross, Lichtenberg, & Christensen, 1995), reading (Boekamp, Straus, & Adams, Boake, Crain, 1995), non-verbal abilities (Adams et al., 1982; Anger et al., 1997; Bernard, 1989; Brown et al., 1991; Campbell et al., 1996; Heverly, Isaac, & Hynd, 1986; Miller, Bing, Selnes, Wesch, & Becker, 1993), and dementia batteries (Carlson, Brandt, Carson, & Kawas, 1998; Inouye, Albert, Mohs, Sun, & Berkman, 1993; Manly et al., 1998b; Marcopulos, McLain, & Giuliano, 1997; Ripich, Carpenter, & Ziol, 1997; Unverzagt, Hal, Torke, & Rediger, 1996; Welsh et al., 1995). These ethnic comparisons have generally shown that despite equivalence on demographic variables such as years of education and socioeconomic status, African Americans obtain lower scores on both verbal and non-verbal cognitive tasks and therefore, the specificity of many neuropsychological measures is inadequate when used among African Americans.

A number of studies, however, have reported no discrepancies in test performance after matching African Americans and Whites on years of education (Carlson, Brandt, Carson, & Kawas, 1998; Ford, Haley, Thrower, West, & Harrel, 1996), after statistically adjusting for education (Marcopulos, McLain, & Giuliano, 1997), or after cut-scores were adjusted for those with low education(Murden, McRae, Kaner, & Bucknam, 1991). However, the statistical power to detect a significant difference in some of these studies was severely limited by their small sample sizes of African-American participants. For example, a recent publication (Ripich, Carpenter, & Ziol, 1997) described a small number of African Americans ($n = 11$) and Whites ($n = 32$) with Alzheimer's disease and reported that there were no significant ethnic differences on measures of naming, picture vocabulary, verbal abstraction, verbal list learning, and pragmatic language use after controlling for MMSE score and years of education. Another study found that among 18 Black and 114 White participants who met NINCDS-ADRDA criteria (McKhann et al., 1984) for AD, there were no significant differences by race on decline in MMSE score over an average 2.5-year period, whereas left-handedness, more years of education, and family history of dementia were associated with more rapid decline (Rasmusson, Carson, Brookmeyer, Kawas, & Brandt, 1996).

Taken together, most previous studies of ethnic group differences in performance on intelligence, screening, and neuropsychological measures have shown that discrepancies between scores of African Americans and Whites persist, despite equating groups on other demographics such as age, education, sex, and socioeconomic background. These discrepancies result in attenuated specificity of verbal and non-verbal neuropsychological tests, such that cognitively normal African Americans are more likely to be misdiagnosed as impaired as compared to Whites (Ford-Booker et al., 1993; Klusman, Moulton, Hornbostle, Picano, & Beattie, 1991; Manly et al., 1998c; Stern et al., 1992; Welsh et al., 1995).

Possible Solutions

Persisting test score discrepancies between African Americans and Whites suggest that many neuropsychological tasks are not functionally equivalent between the two ethnic groups (Helms, 1992; van de Vijver, 1997). That is, measures developed in White, Western, middle class culture may not assess the same cognitive ability in the same way if applied to African Americans. As an example, a traditional African-American cultural background may dictate that relating primarily to the perceptual aspects of an object is more important than the object's taxonomic category. If responses to a classification task were graded according to White, Western, middle-class norms, however, the perceptual response would receive less credit than the taxonomic one. Both responses are correct, but vary according to cultural differences in categorization style. This classification task is therefore not functionally equivalent among African Americans and Whites, since categorization skills operate differently in each culture.

There are several possible ways to improve the accuracy of neuropsychological tests when used among African Americans. These approaches acknowledge the fact that cognition is always embedded in culturally meaningful contexts, and that sociocultural factors determine which cognitive processes come into play in a particular situation. One approach to improving the accuracy of neuropsychological assessment in African Americans is to create new tests that are culturally specific and specialized for detecting impairment among African Americans. This approach avoids the fallacy of using definitions of optimal performance that are bound to White-American culture. By using an "emic" approach to assessment, cognitive skills that are salient within a culture are measured using methodology that is familiar to members of that culture. A major weakness of this approach, however, is that eventually it will lead to an unwieldy number of tests.

Instead of developing multiple, culturally specific measures, another solution is to develop new measures that are as culturally neutral as possible and thus can be used among all ethnic groups – the "etic" approach. Whether it is possible to develop a truly "culture-free" test has been challenged both theoretically and empirically; nevertheless, a major concern for neuropsychologists is that the cost of the "culture-free" approach may be that the measures are less sensitive to subtle cognitive impairment. A final approach is to improve the sensitivity and specificity of existing measures by collecting separate normative data for African Americans. To date, this approach has received the most attention.

Available norms for African Americans

Development of separate norms for African Americans attempts to address the fact that most traditional neuropsychological tests use primarily middle-class White normative and validation samples. Several investigators have commented on the potential for misdiagnosis of cognitive impairment when these inappropriate normative samples are used among ethnic minorities in general (Ardila, 1995; Loewenstein, Arguelles, Arguelles, & Linn-Fuentes, 1994) and African Americans in particular (Campbell et al., 1996; Manly et al., 1998d). In response, several researchers have begun to establish separate test norms for African Americans (Miller, Kirson, & Grant, 1997) or regression-based corrections that include ethnicity (i.e., African-American or White) as a factor. Three studies have been published thus far using data from the San Diego African American Neuropsychological Norms Project: Evans et al. (1999) evaluated the CVLT; Gladsjo et al. (1999) analyzed letter and category fluency, and Diehr et al. (1998) evaluated the PASAT. Lichtenberg and his colleagues in Detroit have developed a Normative Studies Research Project Battery for use among African Americans (Lichtenberg, Ross, Youngblade, & Vangel, 1998). A number of studies have provided normative data for mental status examinations and domain-specific tests designed to detect dementia. These data come from the CERAD study (Fillenbaum, Huber, & Taussig, 1997; Welsh et al., 1995); North Carolina (Fillenbaum, Heyman, Williams, Prosnitz, & Burchett, 1990); Indianapolis (Unverzagt, Hall, Torke, & Rediger, 1996), New York City (Manly et al., 1998b), and rural Virginia (Marcopulos, McLain, & Giuliano, 1997).

Forthcoming normative data include complete information from the San Diego African American Neuropsychological Norms Project, which utilized an expanded Halstead-Reitan Battery; the Mayo Older American Norms Study in Jacksonville, FL; as well as information about African Americans who participated in the WAIS and WMS-III normative sample.

African-American Neuropsychological Test Norms – Issues

Despite the likely reduction of misdiagnosis of cognitive impairment associated with using separate ethnic group norms, there are significant disadvantages of this approach. Primarily, use of separate norms leaves ethnic differences in test performance unexplained, unexamined, and thus not understood. Many authors (Helms, 1992; Neisser et al., 1996) have described how genetic or biological factors are often invoked to account for these unexplained differences. What we have only begun to explore are the underlying cultural factors that might account for ethnic group differences in test performance; some of these investigations are described below.

The fallacy underlying all comparisons of test performance between African Americans and Whites is the assumption imbedded in racial and ethnic classifications: that they are biological or genetic categories. Use of norms separated on the basis of race or ethnicity also assumes that ethnic classifications are scientifically rigorous. In the following section, we discuss racial and ethnic classifications in more detail.

Use of Race and Ethnicity as Scientific Variables

One of the most important directions for future research of neuropsychological test performance among African Americans will be to challenge the basic notions of race, ethnicity, and culture. These terms are often confused and used interchangeably (Wilkinson & King, 1987). Part of the confusion stems from the tremendous heterogeneity within the traditional, "federally" defined ethnic group classifications in the United States that are typically used in studies of ethnicity and cognitive test performance. These classifications, based on the protocol used by the US Census (United States Bureau of the Census, 1991), are actually a combination of racial self-categorization (White, Black, Asian, Pacific Islander, American-Indian, other) and ethnicity (Hispanic/non-Hispanic). Hispanics can be of any race using this classification method. This protocol confuses issues of heritage and immigration status; for example, in some studies, "African Americans" include only non-Hispanic Black individuals who were born in the United States (African Americans), whereas other studies may also include Black immigrants from the West Indies or Africa. Race, nationality, place of birth, and immigration status are not the only sources of heterogeneity within these traditional ethnic group classifications; the level at which the culture of origin is maintained also varies among individuals within one ethnic group. Therefore, the "federally" defined ethnic groups not only confuse racial and ethnic classifications, but also obscures cultural heterogeneity within ethnicity to reflect a homogeneous culture.

Race. Race is generally defined as any relatively large division of persons that can be distinguished from others on the basis of inherited physical characteristics. Racial classifications as they are currently used in the United

States were constructed during the 18th century to refer to those populations brought together in colonial America: American Indians, Europeans, and African slaves, and have served as the basis for "scientific" theories of racial and genetic inferiority.

Many researchers view race as reflecting an underlying genetic homogeneity. It is common practice, however, to assign race on socially defined classification of phenotypic traits such as skin color and hair features (Wilkinson & King, 1987). Because of this incongruity between theory and research practice, race is a construct that lacks scientific basis (Zuckerman, 1990). There is more genotypic variation within races than between them (Lewontin, Rose, & Kamin, 1984; Wilkinson & King, 1987), therefore, it is difficult to classify humans into discrete biological categories with rigid boundaries. Racial classifications, although untenable as biological or genetic categories, are certainly related to experiences of and reactions to racism and institutionalized segregation (Helms, 1997). Therefore, the influence of racial identity and experiences of racism on cognitive testing must be considered in future studies of African-American test performance.

Ethnicity. Unlike race, ethnicity is universally accepted as a socially defined variable. Psychologically, ethnicity can be used to describe the behaviors, attitudes, and values which define ethnic groups, ethnic identity, as well as experiential aspects of minority status (Phinney, 1996). Ethnicity is not only how people identify themselves, but is also the result of labeling by other groups in a multicultural society. As such, ethnic classifications are as inconstant as racial categories, and can also change depending on societal forces. In general, the stronger the ethnic identity, the more traditional ethnic cultural values and behavior are retained (i.e., the less acculturated the individual is likely to be). When defined behaviorally and experientially, this concept of acculturation and ethnic identity can have substantial implications for research on African-American test performance, as described in detail below.

In conclusion, the interchangeable use of race and ethnicity can be a serious barrier to understanding neuropsychological test performance among African Americans. This discussion highlights that a person's racial classification reveals nothing about their cultural, socioeconomic, educational, or racial experiences. Race and ethnicity may be surrogates for or be confounded by other relevant variables, such as socioeconomic status; therefore, information on these other variables must be considered. Because the concepts of race and ethnicity are fluid, those who identify themselves as African American will change depending on the population under study and over time. Researchers must contend with the fact that their results may rapidly become outdated or will be geographically specific. However, if we explicitly measure behavioral, attitudinal, experiential, and psychological variables of interest that may underlie ethnic classifications, we can take advantage of this variability and improve our understanding of the role of race and culture on cognitive test performance.

Influence of Within-Group Variables on Test Performance

As suggested by Helms (1992), specification of experiential, attitudinal, or behavioral variables which distinguish those belonging to different ethnic groups, and which also vary among individuals within an ethnic group, may allow investigators to understand better the underlying reasons for the relationship between ethnic background and cognitive test performance. There is tremendous diversity in geographic, economic, and educational experiences, as well as level of exposure to White-American culture among African Americans. Current racial and ethnic classifications ignore this diversity. Yet it is these cultural and experiential factors that may account for the differences between ethnic groups on cognitive tests. Why not define and measure cultural experience instead of using classifications that ignore it? The following sections will describe investigations of within-group cultural and educational factors on neuropsychological test performance among African Americans. This investigational approach may illuminate factors which can explain not only ethnic group differences on cognitive tests, but can inform us in future development of measures designed to measure cognitive abilities salient within African-American culture. In addition, the effect of these cultural and educational factors on cognitive test performance must be well understood before we attempt to develop "culture fair" measures.

Cultural Experience

Level of acculturation is one way in which social scientists have operationalized within-group cultural variability. Acculturation has been defined as the level at which an individual shares the values, language, and cognitive style of their own ethnic community versus those of the dominant culture. Previous studies have identified ideologies, beliefs, expectations, and attitudes as important components of acculturation, as well as cognitive and behavioral characteristics such as language and customs (Berry, 1976; Moyerman & Forman, 1992; Negy & Woods, 1992; Padilla, 1980). Acculturation has traditionally been measured among immigrant groups such as Hispanics and Asian Americans. Landrine and Klonoff (1994, 1995) recently reported the development of a reliable and valid measure of African-American acculturation. This scale has been found to assess key dimensions in African-American cultural experience, including traditional childhood experiences, religious beliefs and practices, preferences for African-American music, media, and people, and preparation and consumption of traditional foods. By measuring acculturation, regardless of race, the association of cultural experience with cognitive test performance can be assessed, and we can test the hypothesis that individuals with lifestyles that are very dissimilar to White-American culture will also obtain lower scores on traditional neuropsychological tests.

Few studies have examined the relationship of cognitive test performance to within-group ethnic or cultural factors independent of those associated with socioeconomic status. Arnold and his colleagues (Arnold et al., 1994) found a relationship between Hispanic acculturation and performance on selected tests of the Halstead-Reitan Battery among college students. Artiola and her colleagues (Artiola i Fortuny, Heaton, & Hermosillo, 1998) reported that among Mexican and Mexican-American residents of a US-border region, percentage of life in which individuals lived in the US was significantly and negatively related to number of words generated on a Spanish oral fluency measure, especially among those with fewer than eight years of education. In addition, those who spent a greater percentage of their life in the US made fewer perseverative errors on the Wisconsin Card Sorting Test, and bilingualism was significantly and positively associated with performance on a Spanish Verbal Learning Test.

Three studies have explored the relationship of African-American cultural experience (as measured by the African American Acculturation Scale (Landrine & Klonoff, 1994, 1995) to cognitive test performance. We found that among neurologically intact African Americans between the ages of 20 and 65, those who were less acculturated (more traditional) obtained lower scores on measures of general information and naming than more acculturated African Americans (Manly et al., 1998d). Among elderly residents of Northern Manhattan (Manly et al., 1998a), acculturation accounted for a significant amount of variance in several neuropsychological measures assessing verbal and non-verbal abilities after accounting for age, education, and sex. Among elderly African Americans living in Jacksonville, FL, acculturation accounted for a significant amount of variance in Verbal IQ (as measured by the Wechsler Adult Intelligence Scale), Boston Naming Test, and delayed recall of stories from the Wechsler Memory Scale – Revised (Lucas, 1998).

Taken together, investigations of acculturation level suggest that there are cultural differences within those of the same ethnicity that relate to neuropsychological measures of verbal and non-verbal skills, and that accounting for cultural experience may help to improve the accuracy of certain neuropsychological tests. Acculturation level probably reflects other cognitive and non-cognitive factors that have a direct influence on test performance. For example, acculturation level may reflect the salience that a particular task has in everyday life. Specifically, those with ethnically traditional lifestyles may engage in fewer activities that are similar to those required for successful neuropsychological test performance. Acculturation may also reflect the emphasis that was placed on a particular task during development. Traditional African Americans may not be as "testwise" or as proficient in the implicit and explicit requirements of cognitive measures. Acculturation may also reflect motivation or attitude toward testing. If individuals are suspicious as to the value of a task, they may not deliver their maximum performance. We assume that internalized competition will cause everyone to try their hardest, but competition on formal cognitive tests may be more valued in White-American culture, and thus vary with level of acculturation.

Years of Education/Quality of Education/Literacy

Extreme differences in educational level are often found between African Americans and Whites. Cross-cultural researchers are therefore challenged to find measures that are sensitive to cognitive impairment across these broad educational backgrounds (Ratcliff et al., 1998). In addition, it is common for investigators to use covariance or matching procedures in order to equate ethnic groups on years of education before comparing neuropsychological test performance. However, matching on quantity of formal education does not necessarily mean that the quality of education received by each ethnic group is comparable (Whitfield, 1996).

In the United States there is a great deal of discordance between years of education and quality of education; this is true especially among African Americans. Previous studies revealed that elderly African Americans have reading skills which were significantly below their self-reported education level (Albert & Teresi, 1999; Baker, Johnson, Velli, & Wiley, 1996; Manly et al., 1999). African Americans educated in the South before the Supreme Court's 1954 *Brown v. Board of Education* decision attended segregated schools, which received inferior funding as compared to White Southern schools and most integrated Northern schools (Anderson, 1988). Since the Coleman report (Coleman, 1966) was released, the source of this discordance between years of education and achievement has been investigated through studies of school characteristics, such as pupil expenditures, teacher quality, pupil/teacher ratios, presence of special facilities such as science laboratories, length of school year/days attended, and peer characteristics such as the educational background and aspirations of other children in the school. These school variables have been shown to account for much of the difference in achievement and other outcomes (e.g., wage earnings), between African Americans and Whites (Hanushek, 1989; Hedges. Laine, & Greenwald, 1994; O'Neill, 1990). The unequal distribution of funds to segregated African-American schools in the South in the first half of this century, and the subsequent lower quality of education, was related to lower earnings among African Americans in a number of studies (Margo, 1985, 1990; Smith, 1984; Smith & Welch, 1977; Welch, 1966, 1973). Margo (1985) also found that the opportunity gaps resulting from African American children being employed rather than attending school played a role in reducing attendance during the year, and therefore quality of schooling and literacy levels.

Therefore, disparate school experiences, and resulting different bases of problem-solving strategies, knowledge, familiarity, and practice could explain why some African Americans obtain lower scores on cognitive measures even after controlling for years of education. Statistical control of years of education may be inadequate or inappropriate since different scales of measurement may be used among (and within) each ethnic group (Loewenstein, Arguelles, Arguelles, & Linn-Fuentes, 1994).

Presence of poor literacy skills is a particularly relevant issue for neuropsychologists attempting to accurately detect cognitive impairment. Reading level, as measured by a bilingual measure of reading comprehension, was found to be more related to Mini-Mental State Exam (MMSE) score than were years of education, age, or ethnicity (Weiss, Reed, Kligman, & Abyad, 1995). These results suggest that interpretation of cognitive test performance is more dependent on knowledge of literacy or reading skills than years of education. Nevertheless, only a few studies have been conducted to identify ways to accurately assess literacy and reading level among African Americans (Baker, Johnson, Velli, & Wiley, 1996; Boekamp et al., 1995)

Our first attempts to assess the effect of quality of education have focused on reading level (Manly et al., 1999, 2000). We hypothesized that reading achievement, as assessed by the WRAT-III reading subtest, would reflect educational experience. We sought to determine whether reading level had a significant relationship to cognitive test performance even after accounting for the effects of years of education. Among community-dwelling elders, we found that 1) African Americans were over-represented within the group for which self-reported years of education was an overestimate of actual reading level (47% among African Americans versus 18% among Whites; 2) although demographics (age, sex, and years of education) explained a significant amount of variance on most cognitive measures, WRAT-III reading level had a significant, independent effect on measures of verbal and non-verbal learning and memory, orientation, verbal and non-verbal abstraction, language, and construction; and 3) significant discrepancies in neuropsychological test performance between education-matched African-American and White elders become non-significant when WRAT-III reading score was used as a covariate.

These results suggest that reading level is sensitive to aspects of educational experience important for successful performance on measures across several cognitive domains that are not captured by years of education. Future work must clarify whether reading level is an accurate measure of quality of education, and whether reading level-based norms provide more accurate detection of cognitive deficit than ethnicity- or education-based norms.

Stereotype Threat

Level of comfort and confidence during the testing session may also vary among African Americans. The concept of stereotype threat has been described as a factor that may attenuate the performance of African Americans on cognitive tests. Stereotype threat describes the effect of attention diverted from the task at hand to the concern that one's performance will confirm a negative stereotype about one's group. Steele and his colleagues (Steele, 1997; Steele & Aronson, 1995) demonstrated that when a test consisting of difficult verbal GRE exam items was described as measuring intellectual ability, Black undergraduates at Stanford University performed worse than SAT score-matched Whites. However, when the same test was described as a "laboratory problem-solving task" or a "challenging test" which was unrelated to intellectual ability, scores of African Americans matched those of White students. Researchers have also shown that when sex differences in math ability were invoked, stereotype threat undermined performance of women on math tests (Spencer, Steele, & Quinn, 1999), and among White males (when comparisons to Asians were invoked) (Aronson et al., 1999). The role of stereotype threat in neuropsychological test performance of African Americans has not been investigated to date. In addition, it is likely that the salience of negative stereotypes differs among African Americans, and therefore, stereotype threat will likely affect some test takers more than others. Investigation of the experiential, social, and cultural variables that affect vulnerability to stereotype threat should be examined.

African American Cognition

Traditional neuropsychological assessment is based on skills that are considered important within White, Western, middle-class culture, but which may not be salient or valued within African-American culture (Helms, 1992; Helms, 1997). Therefore, differences in salience of cognitive skills, exposure to items, and familiarity with certain problem-solving strategies could attenuate performance of African Americans on neuropsychological measures. Cultural variability in response set, participant/examiner interactions, test-taking attitudes, and motivation during the testing session may also account for ethnic group differences found on tests of verbal and non-verbal ability.

Prior research shows that African Americans categorize information, such as word lists, pictures, and situations differently than Whites (Shade, 1991). Therefore, culturally influenced variability in organization and information analysis (e.g., holistic vs. detail-oriented, functional vs. descriptive) may explain the observed ethnic group differences on several measures.

Cognitive skills and strategies of ethnic minorities are not adequately tapped by standard cognitive tasks – existing tests simply do not elicit the full potential of African Americans. Assessment of these yet unmeasured strengths could be the best way to detect subtle neurocognitive dysfunction among ethnic minorities. When test stimuli are more culturally pertinent to the experiences of African Americans, performance improves (Hayles, 1991). Prior research indicates that African Americans obtain higher scores on measures of divergent thinking or creativity (Price-Williams & Ramirez, 1977; Torrance, 1971). In addition, some research shows that African Americans obtain higher scores on measures of facial recognition (both White and Black faces) as compared to Whites (Barkowitz & Brigham, 1982). These studies point to several ways in which neuropsychological measures can be used to assess cognitive abilities that are salient within African-American culture.

Conclusions

While no one educational or cultural factor can completely explain cognitive test performance of African Americans or differences between Whites and African Americans, continued evaluation of the independent and combined predictive power of these factors on test performance will allow us to improve the specificity of existing neuropsychological measures. Studies of the effect of within-group cultural and educational factors on test performance can serve as hypothesis generators for in-depth study of the effect of these variables on specific cognitive functions.

Thus far, the most emphasis has been placed on developing separate norms for existing neuropsychological tests. We hope that this chapter has demonstrated that new normative data is not the only solution. Once we understand the nature of the relationship between cultural and educational variables and test performance, we may be able to more successfully develop tests that are specific and sensitive to neurocognitive impairment among African Americans.

References

Adams, R. L., Boake, C., & Crain, C. (1982). Bias in a neuropsychological test classification related to age, education and ethnicity. *Journal of Consulting and Clinical Psychology, 50*, 143-145.

Albert, S. M. & Teresi, J. A. (1999). Reading ability, education, and cognitive status assessment among older adults in Harlem, New York City. *American Journal of Public Health, 89*, 95-97.

Anderson, J. D. (1988). *The education of blacks in the South, 1860-1935.* Chapel Hill: University of North Carolina Press.

Anger, W. K., Sizemore, O. J., Grossman, S. J., Glasser, J. A., Letz, R., & Bowler, R. (1997). Human neurobehavioral research methods: Impact of dubject variables. *Environmental Research, 73*, 18-41.

Ardila, A. (1995). Directions of research in cross-cultural neuropsychology. *Journal of Clinical and Experimental Neuropsychology, 17*, 143-150.

Arnold, B. R., Montgomery, G. T., Castaneda, I., & Longoria, R. (1994). Acculturation and performance of Hispanics on selected Halstead-Reitan neuropsychological tests. *Assessment, 1*, 239-248.

Aronson, J., Lustina, M. J., Good, C., Keough, K., Steele, C. M., & Brown, J. (1999). When White men can't do math: Necessary and sufficient factors in stereotype threat. *Journal of Experimental and Social Psychology, 35*, 29-46.

Artiola i Fortuny, L., Heaton, R. K., & Hermosillo, D. (1998). Neuropsychological comparisons of Spanish-speaking participants from the U.S.-Mexico border region versus Spain. *Journal of the International Neuropsychological Society, 4*, 363-379.

Baker, F. M., Johnson, J. T., Velli, S. A., & Wiley, C. (1996). Congruence between education and reading levels of older persons. *Psychiatric Services, 47*, 194-196.

Barkowitz, P. & Brigham, J. C. (1982). Recognition of faces: own-race, incentive, and time-delay. *Journal of Applied Social Psychology, 12*, 225-268.

Bernard, L. (1989). Halstead-Reitan neuropsychological test performance of Black, Hispanic, and White young adult males from poor academic backgrounds. *Archives of Clinical Neuropsychology, 4,* 267-274.

Berry, J. W. (1976). *Human ecology and cognitive style.* New York: Sage-Halstead.

Boekamp, J. R., Strauss, M. E., & Adams, N. (1995). Estimating premorbid intelligence in African-American and White elderly veterans using the American version of the National Adult Reading Test. *Journal of Clinical and Experimental Neuropsychology, 17,* 645-653.

Bohnstedt, M., Fox, P. J., & Kohatsu, N. D. (1994). Correlates of Mini-Mental Status Examination scores among elderly demented patients: the influence of race-ethnicity. *Journal of Clinical Epidemiology, 47,* 1381-1387.

Brown, A., Campbell, A., Wood, D., Hastings, A., Lewis-Jack, O., Dennis, G., Ford-Booker, P., Hicks, L., Adeshoye, A., Weir, R., & Davis, T. (1991). Neuropsychological studies of Blacks with cerebrovascular disorders: A preliminary investigation. *Journal of the National Medical Association, 83,* 3-217.

Campbell, A., Rorie, K., Dennis, G., Wood, D., Combs, S., Hearn, L., Davis, H., Brown, A., & Weir, R. (1996). Neuropsychological assessment of African Americans: Conceptual and methodological considerations. In R. Jones (Ed.), *Handbook of tests and measurement for black populations, Vol. 2* (pp. 75-84). Berkeley: Cobb and Henry.

Carlson, M. C., Brandt, J., Carson, K. A., & Kawas, C. H. (1998). Lack of relation between race and cognitive test performance in Alzheimer's disease. *Neurology, 50,* 1499-1501.

Chen, T.-H., Kaufman, A. S., & Kaufman, J. C. (1994). Examining the interaction of age x race pertaining to black-white differences at ages 15 to 93 on six Horn abilities assessed by K-FAST, K-SNAP, and KAIT subtests. *Perceptual and Motor Skills, 79,* 1683-1690.

Coleman, J. (1966). *Equality of educational opportunity.* Washington, D.C.: Government Printing Office.

Diehr, M. C., Heaton, R. K., Miller, S. W., & Grant, I. (1998). The Paced Auditory Serial Addition Task (PASAT): Norms for age, education, and ethnicity. *Assessment, 5,* 375-387.

Evans, J. D., Norman, M. A., Miller, S. W., Kramer, J. H., Delis, D. C., & Heaton, R. K. (1999). Age-, education-, gender- and race-corrected norms for the California Verbal Learning Test (CVLT). *Journal of the International Neuropsychological Society, 5,* 110.

Fillenbaum, G., Heyman, A., Williams, K., Prosnitz, B., & Burchett, B. (1990). Sensitivity and specificity of standardized screens of cognitive impairment and dementia among elderly black and white community residents. *Journal of Clinical Epidemiology, 43,* 651-660.

Fillenbaum, G. G., Huber, M., & Taussig, I. M. (1997). Performance of elderly White and African American community residents on the abbreviated CERAD Boston Naming Test. *Journal of Clinical and Experimental Neuropsychology, 19,* 204-210.

Fillenbaum, G. G., Hughes, D. C., Heyman, A., George, L. K., & Blazer, D. G. (1988). Relationship of health and demographic characteristics to Mini-Mental State examination score among community residents. *Psychological Medicine, 18,* 719-726.

Ford, G. R., Haley, W. E., Thrower, S. L., West, C. A. C., & Harrell, L. E. (1996). Utility of Mini-Mental State Exam scores in predicting functional impairment among White and African American dementia patients. *Journals of Gerontology. Series A, Biological Sciences and Medical Sciences, 51,* 185-188.

Ford-Booker, P., Campbell, A., Combs, S., Lewis, S., Ocampo, C., Brown, A., Lewis-Jack, O., & Rorie, K. (1993). The predictive accuracy of neuropsychological tests in a normal population of African Americans. *Journal of Clinical and Experimental Neuropsychology, 15*, 64.

Gladsjo, J. A., Evans, J. D., Schuman, C. C., Peavy, G. M., Miller, S. W., & Heaton, R. K. (1999). Norms for letter and category fluency: demographic corrections for age, education, and ethnicity. *Assessment, 6*, 147-178.

Hanushek, E. (1989). The impact of differential expenditures on school performance. *Educational Researcher, 18*, 45-51.

Hayles, V. R. (1991). African American strengths: a survey of empirical findings. In R.L. Jones (Ed.), *Black psychology* (3rd ed., pp. 379-400). Berkeley, CA: Cobb & Henry Publishers.

Heaton, R. K., Ryan, L., Grant, I., & Matthews, C. G. (1996). Demographic influences on neuropsychological test performance. In I. Grant & K. M. Adams (Eds.), *Neuropsychological assessment of neuropsychiatric disorders* (2nd ed., pp. 141-163). New York: Oxford University Press.

Hedges, L. V., Laine, R. D., & Greenwald, R. (1994). Does money matter? A meta-analysis of studies of the effects of differential school inputs on student outcomes. *Educational Researcher, 23*, 5-14.

Helms, J. E. (1992). Why is there no study of cultural equivalence in standardized cognitive ability testing? *American Psychologist, 47*, 1083-1101.

Helms, J. E. (1997). The triple quandry of race, culture, and social class in standardized cognitive ability testing. In D.P.Flanagan, J. L. Genshaft, & P. L. Harrison (Eds.), *Contemporary intellectual assessment: theories, tests, and issues* (pp. 517-532). New York: Guilford Press.

Heverly, L. L., Isaac, W., & Hynd, G. W. (1986). Neurodevelopmental and racial differences in tactile-visual (cross-modal) discrimination in normal black and white children. *Archives of Clinical Neuropsychology, 1*, 139-145.

Inouye, S. K., Albert, M. S., Mohs, R., Sun, K., & Berkman, L. F. (1993). Cognitive performance in a high-functioning community-dwelling elderly population. *Journals of Gerontology. Series A, Biological Sciences and Medical Sciences, 48*, 146-151.

Kaufman, A. S., McLean, J. E., & Reynolds, C. R. (1988). Sex, race, residence, region, and education differences on the 11 WAIS-R subtests. *Journal of Clinical Psychology, 44*, 231-248.

Klusman, L. E., Moulton, J. M., Hornbostle, L. K., Picano, J. J., & Beattie, M. T. (1991). Neuropsychological abnormalities in asymptomatic HIV seropositive military personnel. *Journal of Neuropsychology and Clinical Neurosciences, 3*, 422-428.

Kuller, L. H., Shemanski, L., Manolio, T., Haan, M., Fried, L., Bryan, N., Burke, G. L., Tracy, R., & Bhadelia, R. (1998). Relationship between ApoE, MRI findings, and cognitive function in the Cardiovascular Health Study. *Stroke, 29*, 388-398.

Kush, J. C. & Watkins, M. W. (1997). Construct validity of the WISC-III verbal and performance factors for Black special education students. *Assessment, 4*, 297-304.

Landrine, H. & Klonoff, E. A. (1994). The African American Acculturation Scale: Development, reliability, and validity. *Journal of Black Psychology, 20*, 104-127.

Landrine, H. & Klonoff, E. A. (1995). The African American Acculturation Scale II: Cross-validation and short form. *Journal of Black Psychology, 21*, 124-152.

Lewontin, R., Rose, S., & Kamin, G. (1984). *Not in our genes: Biology, ideology, and human nature*. New York: Pantheon.

Lichtenberg, P. A., Ross, T., & Christensen, B. (1994). Preliminary normative data on the Boston Naming Test for an older urban population. *Clinical Neuropsychologist, 8*, 109-111.

Lichtenberg, P. A., Ross, T. P., Youngblade, L., & Vangel, S. J. (1998). Normative Studies Research Project test battery: Detection of dementia in African American and European American urban elderly patients. *Clinical Neuropsychologist, 12*, 146-154.

Loewenstein, D. A., Arguelles, T., Arguelles, S., & Linn-Fuentes, P. (1994). Potential cultural bias in the neuropsychological assessment of the older adult. *Journal of Clinical and Experimental Neuropsychology, 16*, 623-629.

Lucas, J. A. (1998). Acculturation and neuropsychological test performance in elderly African Americans. *Journal of the International Neuropsychological Society 4*, 77.

Manly, J. J., Jacobs, D. M., Sano, M., Bell, K., Merchant, C. A., Small, S. A., & Stern, Y. (1998a). African American acculturation and neuropsychological test performance among nondemented community elders. *Journal of the International Neuropsychological Society, 4*, 77.

Manly, J. J., Jacobs, D. M., Sano, M., Bell, K., Merchant, C. A., Small, S. A., & Stern, Y. (1998b). Cognitive test performance among nondemented elderly African Americans and Whites. *Neurology, 50*, 1238-1245.

Manly, J. J., Jacobs, D. M., Sano, M., Bell, K., Merchant, C. A., Small, S. A., & Stern, Y. (1998c). Cross-cultural comparison of neuropsychological test performance and diagnosis of dementia. *Neurology 50*, 91.

Manly, J. J., Jacobs, D. M., Sano, M., Small, S. A., Merchant, C., Touradji, P., & Stern, Y. (1999). Quality of education and neuropsychological test performance among nondemented community-dwelling elders. *Neurology, 52*, A433.

Manly, J., Jacobs, D., Touradji, P., Small, S., Merchant, C., Bell, K., & Stern, Y. (2000). Are ethnic group differences in neuropsychological test performance explained by reading level? A preliminary analysis. *Journal of the International Neuropsychological Society, 6*, 245.

Manly, J. J., Miller, S. W., Heaton, R. K., Byrd, D., Reilly, J., Velasquez, R. J., Saccuzzo, D. P., Grant, I., & the HIV Neurobehavioral Research Center Group (1998d). The effect of African-American acculturation on neuropsychological test performance in normal and HIV positive individuals. *Journal of the International Neuropsychological Society, 4*, 291-302.

Marcopulos, B. A., McLain, C. A., & Giuliano, A. J. (1997). Cognitive impairment or inadequate norms: A study of healthy, rural, older adults with limited education. *Clinical Neuropsychologist, 11*, 111-131.

Margo, R. A. (1985). *Disenfranchisement, school finance, and the economics of segregated schools in the United States south, 1980-1910*. New York: Garland Publishing.

Margo, R. A. (1990). *Race and schooling in the South, 1880-1950: An economic history*. Chicago: University of Chicago Press.

McKhann, G., Drachman, D., Folstein, M., Katzman, R., Price, D., & Stadlan, E. (1984). Clinical diagnosis of Alzheimer's disease: report of the NINCDS-ADRDA Work Group under the auspices of the Department of Health and Human Services Task Force on Alzheimer's Disease. *Neurology, 34*, 939-944.

Miller, E. N., Bing, E. G., Selnes, O. A., Wesch, J., & Becker, J. T. (1993). The effects of sociodemographic factors on reaction time and speed of information processing. *Journal of Clinical and Experimental Neuropsychology 15*, 66.

Miller, S. W., Heaton, R. K., Kirson, D., & Grant, I. (1997). Neuropsychological (NP) Assessment of African Americans. *Journal of the International Neuropsychological Society, 3*, 49.

Moyerman, D. R. & Forman, B. D. (1992). Acculturation and adjustment - a meta-analytic study. *Hispanic Journal of Behavioral Sciences, 14*, 163-200.

Murden, R. A., McRae, T. D., Kaner, S., & Bucknam, M. E. (1991). Mini-Mental State exam scores vary with education in blacks and whites. *Journal of the American Geriatrics Society, 39*, 149-155.

Negy, C. & Woods, D. J. (1992). The importance of acculturation in understanding research with Hispanic-Americans. *Hispanic Journal of Behavioral Sciences, 14*, 224-247.

Neisser, U., Boodoo, G., Bouchard, T. J. J., Boykin, A. W., Brody, N., Ceci, S. J., Halpern, D. F., Loehlin, J. C., Perloff, R., Sternberg, R. J., & Urbina, S. (1996). Intelligence: Knowns and unknowns. *American Psychologist, 51*, 77-101.

O'Neill, J. (1990). The role of human capitol in earning differences between Black and White men. *Journal of Economic Perspectives, 4*, 25-45.

Overall, J. E. & Levin, H. S. (1978). Correcting for cultural factors in evaluating intellectual deficit on the WAIS. *Journal of Clinical Psychology, 34*, 910-915.

Padilla, A. M. (1980). *Acculturation: theory, models, and some new findings.* Boulder, CO: Westview Press for the American Association for the Advancement of Science.

Phinney, J. S. (1996). When we talk about American ethnic groups, what do we mean? *American Psychologist, 51*, 918-927.

Price-Williams, D. R. & Ramirez, M. (1977). Divergent thinking, cultural deficiencies and civilizations. *Journal of Social Psychology, 103*, 3-11.

Rasmusson, D. X., Carson, K. A., Brookmeyer, R., Kawas, C., & Brandt, J. (1996). Predicting rate of cognitive decline in probable Alzheimer's disease. *Brain and Cognition, 31*, 133-147.

Ratcliff, G., Ganguli, M., Chandra, V., Sharma, S., Belle, S., Seaberg, E., & Pandav, R. (1998). Effects of literacy and education on measures of word fluency. *Brain and Language, 61*, 115-122.

Reynolds, C. R., Chastain, R. L., Kaufman, A. S., & McLean, J. E. (1987). Demographic characteristics and IQ among adults: Analysis of the WAIS-R standardization sample as a function of the stratification variables. *Journal of School Psychology, 23*, 323-342.

Ripich, D. N., Carpenter, B., & Ziol, E. (1997). Comparison of African-American and white persons with Alzheimer's disease on language measures. *Neurology, 48*, 781-783.

Roberts, R. J. & Hamsher, K. D. (1984). Effects of minority status on facial recognition and naming performance. *Journal of Clinical Psychology, 40*, 539-545.

Ross, T. P., Lichtenberg, P. A., & Christensen, B. K. (1995). Normative data on the Boston Naming Test for elderly adults in a demographically diverse medical sample. *Clinical Neuropsychologist, 9*, 321-325.

Shade, B. J. (1991). African American patterns of cognition. In R.L.Jones (Ed.), *Black Psychology* (3rd ed., pp. 231-247). Berkeley, CA: Cobb & Henry Publishers.

Smith, J. P. (1984). Race and human capital. *American Economic Review, 4*, 685-698.

Smith, J. P. & Welch, F. (1977). Black-White male wage ratios: 1960-1970. *American Economic Review, 67*, 323-328.

Spencer, S. J., Steele, C. M., & Quinn, D. M. (1999). Stereotype threat and women's math performance. *Journal of Experimental and Social Psychology, 35*, 4-28.

Steele, C. M. (1997). A threat in the air. *American Psychologist, 52*, 613-629.

Steele, C. M. & Aronson, J. (1995). Stereotype threat and the intellectual test performance of African Americans. *Journal of Personality and Social Psychology, 69*, 797-811.

Stern, Y., Andrews, H., Pittman, J., Sano, M., Tatemichi, T., Lantigua, R., & Mayeux, R. (1992). Diagnosis of dementia in a heterogeneous population. Development of a neuropsychological paradigm-based diagnosis of dementia and quantified correction for the effects of education. *Archives of Neurology, 49*, 453-460.

Teresi, J. A., Golden, R. R., Cross, P., Gurland, B., Kleinman, M., & Wilder, D. (1995). Item bias in cognitive screening measures: comparisons of elderly white, Afro-American, Hispanic and high and low education subgroups. *Journal of Clinical Epidemiology, 48,* 473-483.

Torrance, E. P. (1971). Are the Torrance Tests of Creative Thinking biased against or in favor of "disadvantaged" groups? *Gifted Child Quarterly, 15,* 75-80.

United States Bureau of the Census (1991). *Census of Population and Housing 1990. Summary tape file 1, technical documentation prepared by the Bureau of the Census.* Washington, D.C.: Bureau of the Census.

Unverzagt, F. W., Hall, K. S., Torke, A. M., & Rediger, J. D. (1996). Effects of age, education and gender on CERAD neuropsychological test performance in an African American sample. *Clinical Neuropsychologist, 10,* 180-190.

Van de Vijver, F. (1997). Meta-analysis of cross-cultural comparisons of cognitive test performance. *Journal of Cross-Cultural Psychology, 28,* 678-709.

Vincent, K. R. (1991). Black/White IQ differences: Does age make the difference? *Journal of Clinical Psychology, 47,* 266-270.

Weiss, B. D., Reed, R., Kligman, E. W., & Abyad, A. (1995). Literacy and performance on the Mini-Mental State Examination. *Journal of the American Geriatric Society, 43,* 807-810.

Welch, F. (1966). Measurement of the quality of education. *American Economic Review, 56,* 392.

Welch, F. (1973). Black-White differences in returns to schooling. *American Economic Review, 63,* 893-907.

Welsh, K. A., Fillenbaum, G., Wilkinson, W., Heyman, A., Mohs, R. C., Stern, Y., Harrell, L., Edland, S. D., & Beekly, D. (1995). Neuropsychological test performance in African-American and white patients with Alzheimer's disease. *Neurology, 45,* 2207-2211.

Whitfield, K. E. (1996). Studying cognition in older African Americans: some conceptual considerations. *Journal of Aging and Ethnicity, 1,* 41-52.

Wilkinson, D. Y. & King, G. (1987). Conceptual and methodological issues in the use of race as a variable: policy implications. *Milbank Quarterly, 65* (suppl. 1), 56-71.

Zuckerman, M. (1990). Some dubious premises in research and theory on racial differences: Scientific, social, and ethical issues. *American Psychologist, 45,* 1297-1303.

PART III

ASIAN /
PACIFIC ISLANDERS

Chapter 6

CURRENT ISSUES IN NEUROPSYCHOLOGICAL ASSESSMENT IN JAPAN

Toshiya Murai, M.D.
Max-Planck-Institute of Cognitive Neuroscience, Leipzig, Germany

Kazuo Hadano, M.D.
Department of Psychogeriatrics, National Institute of Mental Health, Ichikawa, Japan

Toshihiko Hamanaka, M.D.
Department of Psychiatry, Nagoya City University, Nagoya, Japan

Abstract

Since the majority of neuropsychological studies have been conducted with patients whose mother tongue is one of the major European languages, neuropsychological studies of Japanese-speaking patients may provide unique insights. Among the differences between Japanese and the major European languages, those of syntax and orthography are the most prominent.

The most remarkable grammatical structure of the Japanese language is its word order (Subject-Object-Verb). This unique syntactical feature is reflected in the error patterns of Japanese aphasic patients. As to the Japanese orthography, two different types of writing systems are used in combination, i.e., the kana systems and the kanji system. Clinical syndromes such as pure alexia, surface dyslexia, or constructional agraphia provide rich examples of neuropsychological problems specific to the Japanese orthography. In this chapter, the authors propose that investigation of problems specific to the Japanese language will also lead to understanding language-independent universal neuropsychological problems.

Introduction: A Brief History and Present Status of Neuropsychology in Japan

Neuropsychology in Japan began at the end of the 19th century when the first article on aphasia was published. At the beginning of 20th century, unique characteristics of the Japanese language, namely, the dual writing systems (kanji/kana) were already mentioned in conjunction with aphasic patients (Miura, 1901: see Hamanaka, 1994). One of the earliest contributions to international neuropsychological journals by Japanese researchers dates to this decade, when Imamura (1903) reported a study investigating the roles of the corpus callosum in visual recognition. As early as 1935, the significance of the "apractoagnostic" aspects of apraxic disorders was mentioned by Akimoto (1976) who published the first monograph on neuropsychology in Japan. The original description of Gogi aphasia, a special form of transcortical sensory aphasia (see Section 3-5), was reported in 1943 by Imura (1943).

Contemporary neuropsychology began during the 1970's when the Neuropsychological Association of Japan (1977) and the Japanese Society of Aphasiology (1975) were established. Along with the translation of major European and American textbooks, the first comprehensive textbook of general neuropsychology was published as early as 1960 (Ohashi, 1960). In addition to various neuropsychological tests developed in Europe/North-America (Boston Naming Test, Token Test, etc.), several standardized tests specific to the Japanese language, such as the Standardized Language Test for Aphasia (Japanese Society of Aphasiology, 1977), the Test of Syntactical Expression and Comprehension (Fujita & Miyake, 1984), have been developed to capture unique orthographic and grammatical impairments in Japanese aphasia. Educational and training systems of neuropsychological specialists have also been established and integrated into the medical systems (Hamanaka 1994; Table 1).

Most of the neuropsychological topics studied in Europe/North America have been extensively studied in Japan in the last three decades. There are a number of pioneering contributions of Japanese researchers to international journals. Along with these studies, Japanese researchers continued to be interested in the uniqueness of their own language and its effect on the neuropsychological deficits of Japanese-speaking patients. Consequently, it became clear that neuropsychological studies of Japanese-speaking patients

Table 1. History of neuropsychology in Japan.

1893	First article on aphasia (Onishi)
1901	Comment on aphasia, referring to Kanji/Kana problem (Miura)
1935	Monograph on apraxia (Akimoto)
1943	Description of Gogi (word meaning) aphasia (Imura)
1960	The first comprehensive monograph; "Aphasia, Apraxia and Agnosia" (Ohashi)
1976	Founding of *The Japanese Society of Aphasiology*
1975	Standardized Language Test for Aphasia (Japanese Society of Aphasiology)
1977	Founding of *The Neuropsychology Association of Japan*
1979	Founding of the National Institute of Rehabilitation for the Handicapped.

would contribute substantially to the understanding of language specific clinical problems as well as neuropsychological problems in general.

Syntactic Disturbances in the Japanese Language

1. Characteristics of syntax in the Japanese language

Although it is naïve to state that Japanese is the most unique language among the whole range of world languages, it is no overstatement to say that the Japanese language is quite different from major European languages (English, French, Spanish, German, Italian etc.) in many aspects (syntax, lexicon, orthography, phonology, etc.). Since the majority of neuropsychological studies have been conducted with patients whose mother tongues are one of the major European languages, neuropsychological studies of Japanese-speaking patients should provide unique insights.

Among the differences between Japanese and the major European languages, those of syntax and orthography are the most prominent. An example of Japanese sentences is shown in Fig. 1, to demonstrate a brief outlook of the basic characteristics of Japanese. We begin with neuropsychological topics on syntactic problems in Japanese-speaking patients, and later describe topics on reading/writing impairment.

Syntactical characteristics of Japanese include highly differentiated honorific systems, topic formation with the postpositional particle 'wa', etc. However, perhaps the most unique grammatical structure of Japanese is its word orders. As opposed to major European languages with the word order SVO (Subject-Verb-Object), Japanese is an SOV (Subject-Object-Verb) language; in a given transitive sentence, both the subject and the object precede the verb. Japanese is called an "ideal" SOV language because the word-order "dependent-head" is consistently maintained in all types of constituent (Shibatani, 1990).

Also, Japanese is an agglutinating language in which the concept of a "phrase" (*bunsetsu*) is different from that in major European languages. A Japanese "phrase" often consists of a substantive word with a content

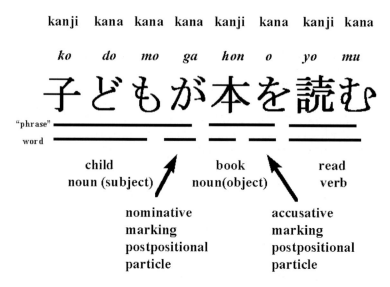

The child reads a book.

Fig. 1. A Japanese sentence is written as a mixture of kanji characters and kana characters. There is a one to one correspondence between kana-characters and their pronunciation, whereas the pronunciation of a kanji character generally depends on the word which contains that kanji character. Some Japanese words are written with a single character, whereas others consist of plural characters. No space is allocated between words in a written sentence. The most typical word order is Subject-Object-Verb (SOV), in contrast with the SVO order in English. Another grammatical characteristic of the Japanese language is the use of a variety of postpositional particles, which determine the grammatical function of preceding words. For example, case marking postpositional particles determine the case (nominative, accusative etc.) of preceding words. A combination of a single substantive word (e.g. noun, verb, adjective) and one or a few function word(s) (e.g. such as postpositional particles) following the substantive word constitutes a subunit of a sentence. This grammatical unit is called *Bunsetsu* (phrase).

meaning, including a noun, verb and adjective, and a single (or a few) grammatical function word(s) agglutinated to the former, including postpositional particles and auxiliaries. Function words indicate the relationship between phrases, and their grammatical functions are equivalent to tense, mode, case, and voice in European inflectional languages (Hadano & Hamanaka, 1997).

2. Clinical studies and assessment of syntactic impairments in Japanese aphasia

Syntactic impairments are common in patients with aphasia both in speech production and comprehension. Agrammatism, a syntactic impairment in speech production (often associated with Broca aphasia), is characterized by fragmental sentences in which function words and inflections are missing. In an extreme case, it is called telegraphic speech. Although this characterization has mostly been based on the observations of patients whose native language is one of the major European languages, several researchers have reported characteristics of Japanese agrammatism.

In the early literature, Ohashi (1960) summarized characteristics of Japanese agrammatism as follows: (1) instability of word order, (2) marked reduction in the ability of using auxiliaries (resulting in simplification of predicates) as well as various particles, and (3) impaired use of honorifics. Although the empirical data are limited to confirm this early description in detail, a unanimous observation of subsequent studies is the omission of function words, which is common with agrammatic patients speaking major European languages. Among the functional words, however, postpositional particles are most frequently omitted, which is specific to Japanese agrammatism (e.g. *kodomo* (child) – *ga* (nominative marking particle) – *hon* (book) -*o* (accusative marking particle) – *yomu* (read) ------> *kodomo – hon – yomu*). Recently, Sasanuma et al. (1990) identified a hierarchy of tendency in omitting postpositional particles; frequently omitted postpositional particles are those that participate in core sentential structures (e.g. case marking particles '*ga*', '*o*', the topic marking particle '*wa*', the quotative particle '*to*'), whereas particles which are not essential in determining the basic grammatical structures of sentences, e.g. discourse particles like '*yo*', are relatively spared.

These basic observations on syntactic impairment in Japanese aphasia could provide an insight into general theory of syntactic impairment and normal syntactic processing. Characterization of syntactic impairment in Japanese aphasics is also essential for the optimal evaluation and programming of therapy of Japanese-speaking patients. The Test of Syntactic Processing in Aphasia (Fujita & Miyake, 1984) is designed to capture typical syntactic impairments in Japanese aphasia. This test battery consists of two sections, comprehension and production. Each section is structured hierarchically; this is supported by the finding that Japanese aphasic patients show worse performance as the level of syntactic complexities increases (Fujita & Miyake, 1985).

For example, the comprehension section focuses on the frequent error of subject/object confusion by aphasic patients (Table 2). In Japanese sentences, case-marking postpositional particles determine subjects and objects of preceding nouns or pronouns (postpositional particle strategy). However, even without knowledge of the grammatical function of these particles, determining subjects and objects is often successful with alternative strategies. Since the most common word order of Japanese transitive sentence is SOV, it is

Table 2. The hierarchical structure of Japanese syntactical comprehension (Fujita et al., 1984).

Level	Available strategy to determine the subject and object	Complement clause	Example
1	word meanings word orders postpositional particles	–	*kodomo-ga doa-o osu.* (The child pushes the door.)
2	word orders postpositional particles	–	*kodomo-ga haha-o osu.* (The child pushes the mother.)
3	postpositional particles	-	*kodomo-o haha-ga osu.* (The child pushes the mother.)
4	postpositional particles	+	*kodomo-ga haha-ni boshi-o torareru.* (The child is taken the hat by the mother.)

most likely that the first noun is the subject and the second is the object (word order strategy). In some sentences, it is self-explanatory from the meaning of a pair of nouns in the sentence, which is the subject and which is the object (word meaning strategy).

Sentences presented to patients in the comprehension section of the Test of Syntactic Processing in Aphasia are classified into four groups with differing complexity regarding the available strategies to determine the subject and the object. Patients are requested to choose figures corresponding to auditorily or visually presented sentences. A test session begins with the most simple sentences showing SOV structure, in which reversal of subjects and objects makes nonsense sentences (e.g. *kodomo* (child) – *ga* (nominative marking particle) – *doa* (door) *-o* (accusative marking particle) *osu* (push); The child pushes the door). In these sentences, patients can use all three strategies (word meaning strategy, word order strategy and postpositional particle strategy) to determine the subject and the object. When the patients pass this level, they proceed to the next level. Sentences used in the second level also have SOV structure, while substitution of subjects and objects makes meaningful sentences (e.g. *kodomo* (child) – *ga* (nominative marking particle) – *haha* (mother) *-o* (accusative marking particle) *osu* (push); The child pushes the mother). The word meaning strategy is unavailable here to determine the subject and the object, while the word order strategy and the postpositional particle strategy is still available. At the third level, the word order of sentences is OSV structure, which is also possible in Japanese language though uncommon (e.g. *kodomo – o (accusative) haha – ga (nominative) osu.* The mother pushes the child.). At this level, the correct understanding of postpositional particles is essential to determine the subject and object. Finally, sentences in the last stage are more complex including complement clauses.

3. Syntactic disturbance in Japanese aphasia: linguistic approaches

Subject/object confusion, on which the comprehension section of the Test of Syntactic Processing in Aphasia focuses, is a frequent finding in aphasia regardless of languages. In English-speaking agrammatic patients, a sentence such as "it was the bear that the lion chased" is frequently confused with "it was the tiger that chased the lion". These typical errors suggest that comprehension errors in agrammatic patients have some discrete tendencies, which may shed light on the underlying mechanism of human syntactic processing. According to an early hypothesis (Grodzinsky, 1995), the first noun is likely to be taken as the *<agent>* (the performer of the action, usually corresponding to the subject in active sentences) and the second as the *<patient>* (the element which is affected by the action, usually corresponding to the object in active sentences). This theory has been revealed to explain a variety of comprehension errors by English-speaking agrammatic patients.

However, a question remains. Does the hypothesis also hold true for the Japanese language, where the canonical sequence is not SVO but SOV ? Are the error patterns of patients not language-independent but language-specific?

Hagiwara and Caplan (1990) investigated the comprehension of sentences with different category order (noun-noun-verb, noun-verb-noun), thematic role order (*<agent>* – *<patient>*, *<patient>* – *<agent>*), and voice (active, passive) in Japanese-speaking patients with aphasia. For example, the sentence "*kuma* (bear) -*o* (accusative marking particle) *ositanowa* (pushed) – *zoo* (elephant) – *da* (copula); That which pushed the bear was the elephant", is an active sentence with the word order noun – verb – noun, in the order *<patient>* – *<agent>*. Patients were requested to manipulate toy animals (a bear, an elephant) to demonstrate the situation of auditorily presented sentences. The number of correct responses was compared between different category orders, thematic role orders and voices. The findings indicated that the patients tended to understand sentences better when an immediately preverbal noun has the role of *<patient>*. For example, "*kuma* (bear) – *o* (accusative marking particle) – *ositanowa* (pushed) – *zoo* (elephant) – *da* (copula); That which pushed the bear was the elephant", is more easily understood than "*kuma-ga* (nominative marking particle) – *ositanowa-zoo-da*; What the bear pushed was the elephant".

This could not be predicted from the hypothesis of the "*<agent>*-first" rule of Grodzinsky (1995). Hagiwara and Caplan's interpretation was that it was not the order of the *<agent>* and the *<patient>*, but the position of the *<patient>* relative to the verb that was the critical factor in determining the tendency of errors. In Japanese, following the natural order of *<patient>* –

verb, aphasic patients tend to judge the immediately pre-verbal noun as the
<patient>.

These findings highlight both the language-universal and language-specific
components involved in processing syntax. A close relationship between the
verb and the *<patient>* appears to be common to English and Japanese. In
Japanese, the immediately pre-verbal *<patient>* is easy to understand, while in
English, the immediately post-verbal *<patient>* is easier; this is the language-
specific component of syntactic processing.

4. Aphasic speech output observed in Japanese language: semistereotypic speech

Another unique grammatical feature of Japanese is that it is an agglutinating
language (like Turkish, etc.) which is different from inflectional languages
such as English or German. In an inflectional language, an exact segmenta-
tion of root and derivational morphemes is not always possible. In contrast,
in Japanese, as an agglutinative language, variety of grammatical function
is expressed with function words which are easily separable from content
words (e.g. *kodomotachino* (children's) = *kodomo* (child) – *tachi* (plural) –
no (genitive);).

Hadano and Hamanaka (1997) described a Japanese patient with global
aphasia, whose speech was characterized by 'semistereotypic speech' (SSS),
which has not been reported in the European/American literature. We shall
see the relationship between these unique utterances and the grammatical
characteristics of Japanese as an agglutinative language.

[Case M.M. (Hadano & Hamanaka, 1997)]
A 63-year-old right-handed woman (M.M.) was hospitalized because of a
sudden onset of speech disturbance and motor weakness on the right side.
She was diagnosed as having had a cerebral infarction based on neurological
and neuroradiological examinations. Computed tomography (CT) performed
1.6 months after disease onset revealed a large and circumscribed lesion with
a low density in the areas of the anterior and the middle cerebral arteries in
the left hemisphere. Neuropsychiatric evaluation 3.9 months after the onset
revealed complete hemiparesis of the right side, a general loss of initiative,
severe global aphasia, orofacial apraxia, ideomotor and ideational apraxia,
and constructional disabilities. She could only utter some undifferentiated
syllables like "ee", "aha", etc. At a neuropsychological re-evaluation about
1.7 years after onset, however, it was discovered that she made the following characteristic utterances. When she spoke, different kinds of grammatical function words (postpositional particles, auxiliary verbs, conjunctions,
verbs with uncertain meanings) were almost always agglutinated to KICHI-
KICHI (KICHIKICHI-ya-naa, KICHIKICHI-dosse, KICHIKICHI-ya-sakai,
etc.) (Table 3-1). She made these utterances with natural feelings and into-
nations as though she was enjoying normal conversation. Once she began
to utter the SSS, she never ceased to do so. All her speech productions in

Table 3. Examples of MM's speech production.

3-1 During conversation:
Examiner: Onamae-o osshat-te kudasai (Please say your name)
MM: O O /kitʃikitʃi/ (Oh, Oh, KICHIKICHI)
E.: Okiraku-ni site kudasai-ne (Please make yourself at home)
MM: Iya KICHIKICHI-ya-ne KICHI (No, [something] is KICHIKICHI, KICHI)
E.: Juusho-o itte kudasai (Please tell me your home address)
MM: KICHIKICHI-ya-na ([Something] is KICHIKICHI)
E.: Y.ku ? ([Is it] District Y.?)
MM: KICHIKICHI-ya ([Something] is KICHIKICHI)
E.: Seinengappi-wa? (When is your birthday?)
MM: Un Un (Well, well)
E.: Tanjoobi (Your birthday)
MM: Un ka-na KICHIKICHI-ya-na (Well, maybe KICHIKICHI)
E.: Nangatsu-desu-ka? (In what month?)
MM: KICHIKICHI-ya-kara (because of KICHIKICHI)
E.: Ouchi-no oshigoto-wa nan-desu-ka? (What did your husband do?)
MM: Un KICHIKICHI-ya-kara (Well, because of KICHIKICHI)
E.: Kazoku-wa nannin? (How large is your family ?)
MM: KICHIKICHIKICHI
E.: Kodomo-wa? (How many children [do you have]?)
MM: KICHIKICHI-ya un ([Something] is KICHIKICHI, well)

3-2 In confrontation naming:
Fish: KICHI KICHI
Telephone: Un KICHI   (Well, KICHI)
Pencil: Ka-na demo KICHIKICHI-ya-kara (Maybe, but because of KICHI-
            KICHI)
Shoes: Demo KICHIKICHI-ya-kara (But because of KICHIKICHI)
Watch: KICHIKICHI
Umbrella: KICHIKICHI KICHIKICHI-nan-ya-kedo (KICHIKICHI, but [something]
            is KICHIKICHI)

response to formal neuropsychological testing, including confrontation naming (Table 3-2) and reading aloud, consisted of this type of utterance and its
variations except for some interjections.

Recurring utterances or speech automatism is stereotypic speech, which
is observed in some patients with global aphasia. A patient with recurring
utterances answers every question with the same (often nonsense) word or
short phrase. M.M.'s utterances "KICHIKICHI..." were not consistent with
the usual form of recurring utterances, which, as a rule, are completely stereotypic. While usually recurring utterances consist only of invariable parts and
contain no variable parts, e.g. Broca's (1861) famous description of a patient
with recurring utterance "Tan, Tan", M.M.'s utterances "KICHIKICHI..."
contain variable parts attached to the invariable part " KICHIKICHI". No
other patient with this type of speech has been reported in the literature
except for another Japanese-speaking patient (Takewaka et al., 1995). Thus,
Hadano and Hamanaka suspect that the very nature of Japanese as an agglu-

tinative language, in which functional words are attached to substantive words posteriorily, like a suffix, may be responsible for the occurrence of the SSS.

Although such utterance seems unique to the Japanese language, its occurrence provides support for the general model of speech automatisms by Blanken et al. (1988). These researchers claimed that speech automatism (recurring utterances) does not result from the general breakdown of the language-related functions, and that relatively unaffected levels of language processing exist among automatism-generating aphasics. The language production model by Blanken et al. (1987) assumes that human language is processed sequentially by three separable apparatuses, i.e. a prelinguisitic "pragmatic-conceptual apparatus", a linguistic "formulation apparatus" and a postlinguistic "articulatory apparatus" (see Blanken et al., 1987; Fig. 2).

The pragmatic conceptual apparatus builds the conceptual structure of the intended speech act. The formulation apparatus consists of three components: the lexicalization, the grammaticalization, and the prearticulatory-segmental processing components. The lexicalization component mediates access to lexical items, the grammaticalization component performs the linearization of the sentence constituents. Subsequent to interactive and parallel processing by these two components, the prearticulatory-segmental process-

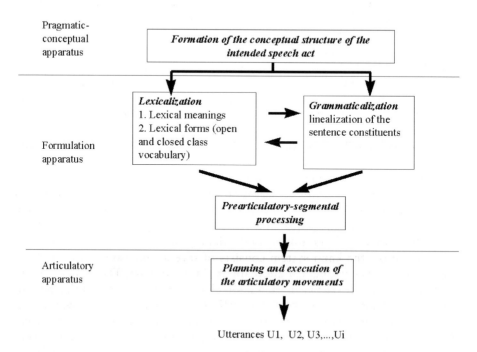

Fig. 2. A neurolinguistic working model of language production (Blanken et al., 1987, 251).

ing component is activated, which determines detailed phonological forms of words on a prearticulatory level. Finally, the articulatory apparatus plans and executes articulatory motor movements.

The fact that M.M. showed neither articulatory nor phonemic disturbances in uttering both the stereotypic and the variable functional parts suggested the existence of preserved function in the prearticulatory-segmental processing unit as well as the articulatory apparatus. The stereotypic part of the SSS is supposed to be generated from the highly impaired lexicalization component, whereas the variable part may be processed in the relatively preserved grammaticalization component.

The suspected mechanism regarding semistereotypic speech, i.e. impoverishment of lexical sources and preserved grammatical functions, could probably occur regardless of the language. However, it might only be in an agglutinative language that the dissociation between these two functional components is explicitly revealed in spontaneously produced utterances of aphasic patients.

The Writing System of the Japanese Language and its Impairments: Kanji-Kana Problems

1. The Japanese writing system and Kanji-Kana problems

In the Japanese writing system, three different systems are used in combination, namely two kana systems (hiragana and katakana) and the kanji system.

Both hiragana and katakana systems consist of 75 characters (the number can differ slightly depending on the way of counting), and each character corresponds to a certain syllable (strictly speaking, corresponds to a mora) of spoken language. There is an almost one-to-one correspondence between each kana character and its pronunciation, with only a few exceptions. For example, a hiragana character 'か' is pronounced as *ka* in any word or in any combination with other characters; 'さか' and 'かわ' are pronounced as *sa-ka, ka-wa*, respectively. There is no other hiragana pronounced '*ka*'. With only a few exceptions, each kana character has no static meaning of its own. The meaning is determined only in combination with other characters, at the level of words. 'さか' (*sa-ka*) means slope, and 'かわ' (*ka-wa*) means river or skin. This is similar to English where the letter 'p' has no static contribution of meaning to the words 'picture', 'pen', 'cup', etc. In this sense kana characters are called phonograms or syllabograms.

In contrast, the kanji system consists of several thousands of characters, among which approximately 2000 are used for daily use. There is no one-to-one correspondence between each kanji character and its pronunciation. For example, a kanji character '人', by itself, is pronounced *hito*. However, it is also used in combination with other characters. In the word '人口' (*jin-kou*), '人' is pronounced *jin*, in the word '役人' (*yaku-nin*), '人' is pronounced as *nin*. Furthermore, there are many kanji characters that are pronounced as *nin*; '認', '任', '忍', '仁', and so on. Unlike kana characters, the correspondence of each kanji character and its pronunciation is not so strict, although most kanji characters contain a relatively static meaning of their own that contributes to the meaning of words which contain those characters. The kanji character '人' adds a meaning of 'man' or 'human-being' to the words which contain this character (e.g., '人口' (*jin-kou*) means population, '役人' (*yaku-nin*) means officer, and so on). Consequently, kanji characters are often called ideograms or morphograms.

The uniqueness of Japanese orthography as a dual writing system provides an opportunity to test universal and language-specific neuropsychological theories of reading/writing. For example, *kenkyu* (research) can be alternatively written using kana 'けんきゅう' or using kanji '研究'. If certain patients can not write 'けんきゅう' but can write '研究', it might be hypothesized that the damaged brain area is specifically related to kana (phonogram) writing. Or, if certain patients can not read '研究' but can read 'けんきゅう', it seems plausible to say that the observed area of lesion is specifically related to kanji (ideogram) reading. Although such conclusions may seem reasonable, there are a number of pitfalls that one must be aware of when interpreting the neuropsychological evidence of kanji/kana dissociation. These issues will be discussed in the following section.

2. Kanji-Kana problems in neuropsychology: methodological problems

As mentioned above, because the Japanese writing system is a dual system of kanji and kana, many words can be written alternatively using either kanji or kana. However, some words are customarily written using kanji, and other words are customarily or exclusively written in kana. For example, while *kenkyu* (research) can be written as '研究' using kanji or alternatively as 'けんきゅう' using kana, kana is very rarely used to spell this word in daily writing. There are several conventions regarding the use of kanji or kana; most of the abstract nouns are written using kanji; most words of foreign origin are written using katakana; postpositional particles are exclusively written using hiragana, and so on. Thus, simple comparison of reading abilities of the same words written alternatively using kana or kanji makes little sense, because the familiarity of each orthography is different. When comparing the number of errors in kanji or kana in writings of aphasic patients, one may also be comparing the difference among several grammatical categories (nouns and particles etc.) rather than ideogram/phonogram differences (Hamanaka et al., 1980).

Another problem is that although kanji characters are often called ideograms, strictly speaking, they are not 'ideal' ideograms. It is true that a kanji character can be pronounced more than one way, but this does not mean that any pronunciation is legal for a given kanji character. The possible pronunciation is usually restricted to a few ways, which is in contrast with ideal ideograms, such as the footprint ideograms invented by Varney (1984) which have no phonological decoding rule. In addition, while correspondence to a certain meaning often exists in certain kanji characters, the meaning of each kanji character sometimes plays a minor role in words. For example, a kanji character ' 仏 ', pronounced as *hotoke* or *butu*, usually adds the meaning of Buddha to words which contain this character. However, in the word ' 仏国 ', *futsu-koku*, France, ' 仏 ' has semantically nothing to do with France. ' 仏 ' is used only due to its acousitic similarity with *france*. We can only say that kanji characters are relatively closer to 'ideal' ideograms than kana characters. Thus, evidence of dissociation between kanji and kana reading/writing performance in aphasic patients does not automatically mean a dissociation between ideogram and phonogram reading/writing.

When interpreting findings of kanji/kana dissociation in aphasic, alexic, agraphic patients, or normal healthy subjects, it is important to consider several attributes other than ideogram/phonogram differences, which may affect the apparent difference of kanji/kana dissociation. Hamanaka et al. (1980) described those attributes as follows:

1) *Psychophysiological (visuo-spatial, audiophonological, kinaesthetico-graphic, articulo-phonetic) qualities of each character.* For example, the structural complexity of Japanese characters is highly variable from a very simple character '一' to very complex '鬱'. Thus, if this factor is not controlled, findings of apparent dissociation in kanji/kana reading/writing might be due to disturbance of processing complex characters regardless of kanji/kana difference.

2) *Frequency, familiarity, and learnedness.* The Japanese characters, especially kanji characters, are highly variable regarding these factors. Thus, findings of apparent dissociation in kanji/kana reading/writing performance might only be due to the disturbance of processing less frequent or less familiar characters.

3) *Grammatical category.* Conventionally, some words belonging to certain grammatical categories are written in kana, whereas some others are written in kanji. Thus, findings of apparent kanji/kana dissociation might be due to selective disturbance of processing words which belong to a certain grammatical category.

4) *Semantic category (concrete-/abstractness, picturability, operability/figurability, special categories such as number or color).* Some words belonging to certain semantic categories are preferentially written in kana, whereas others are written in kanji. Findings of apparent kanji/kana dissociation might be due to the selective disturbance of processing words which belong to a certain semantic category.

3. Kanji-Kana problems in pure alexia

Various factors mentioned above would limit one's ability to interpret data concerning the patients' performance of reading and writing. In early Japanese literature of aphasia or alexia, one would frequently encounter descriptions such as "In this patient, the impairment is more severe in kanji than in kana", or "In this subtype of aphasia, impairment in kana is more prominent than in kanji". However, a close examination of these studies reveals that only a small number of characters was used (Sugishita et al., 1992), or only the verbal description of physicians without concrete data were reported (Hadano et al., 1985).

Hadano et al. (1985, 1986) investigated how those factors affect the conclusion of kanji/kana discrepancy. Hadano et al. (1985) administered a single letter reading task to eight patients with pure alexia. Simple comparison between the performance of kanji reading and kana reading revealed significant differences in seven of the eight patients (six patients were better in kana reading, one patient was better in kanji reading). However, after the complexity, frequency and the school grade at which each character was taught were matched between kanji and kana, only two patients showed a significant difference between kanji and kana reading. Using a multivariate analysis (Hayashi's quantification method of the second type), they also investigated the effect of ten attributes of each character on the reading performance of the same eight patients (Hadano et al., 1986). They were, 1) kanji/kana difference, 2) complexity, 3) school grade at which each character is taught, 4) frequency, 5) right-left separability (some characters such as '任' are composed of separable right and left parts, while others such as '国' are not), 6) ideographic nature, 7) visual associability (in their study, characters provoking more visual images were defined as those with high visual associability), 8) auditory associability, 9) somatosensory associability, and 10) adjectivity (characters, by which derivative adjectives can be made, are defined as those with adjectivity; e.g. '赤' aka -->'赤い' aka-i, red). Among the six patients who matched the mathematical model of this statistical analysis, the kanji/kana differences had the greatest influence upon reading performance in two patients, whereas the school grade at which each character is taught had the greatest influence in three patients, and the ideographic nature of the letters (pictograph or simple ideograph) had the greatest influence in one patient. These findings suggest that not only kanji/kana differences, but also other attributes of each character affected the performance of the patients. The Japanese characters, especially kanji, include so many variables that it might be difficult to attribute patients' performance solely to kanji/kana differences.

4. Kanji-Kana problems and hemispheric asymmetries of their processing

Early studies with tachistoscopic presentation revealed a left hemisphere (right visual field) advantage for the identification of alphabets or kana. In contrast, several studies using the same design by Japanese or Chinese speakers demonstrated that single kanji characters are processed preferentially with the right hemisphere (Hatta, 1977, Tzeng et al., 1979). These surprising findings, suggesting that kanji is a unique verbal material processed in the brain differently from other verbal materials such as kana or alphabet, stimulated a series of studies using similar experimental paradigms.

Hatta (1983) performed a study in which they asked subjects to perform semantic comparative judgments (Fig. 3). In experiment 1, a pair of Arabic numerals of different physical size were displayed either on the right visual field or on the left, and subjects were asked to judge whether the physical size of the stimulus and the numerical magnitude were congruent or not. In experiment 2, a pair of physically different-sized kanji characters representing concrete objects were displayed and subjects were required to judge whether the physical size of the kanji character was congruent or not with the relative real life object size. In experiment 3, a pair of physically different-sized kanji characters representing numerical magnitude were displayed and subjects judged whether the physical size of the kanji character and the numerical magnitude were congruent or not. Results showed that the reaction time was faster using a right-visual-field presentation in experiments 1 and 3, whereas in experiment 2, the reaction time was faster using a left-visual-field presentation. These findings indicated that in semantic comparative judgment tasks kanji characters representing concrete objects are preferentially processed by the right hemisphere. The author's interpretation is that there are two types of semantic processing of verbal materials one relying on the verbal code and the other relying on the use of imagery; the former is more strongly engaged by the left hemisphere while the latter is more strongly engaged by the right hemisphere.

As described earlier, Japanese characters include varieties of attributes other than the kanji/kana dichotomy. Thus, to reveal the underlying mechanism of preferential right-hemispheric processing of kanji characters, it is essential to examine the effect of each attribute separately. The effects of

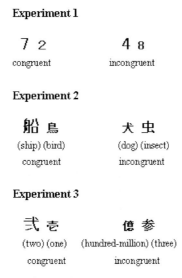

Figure 3. Samples of the paired stimuli in Hatta (1983)'s experiments.

various attributes, such as complexity, familiarity, or imaginability have been examined (Hatta, 1992). Since kanji characters are generally more complex than kana characters, the greater complexity of kanji characters may be responsible for the apparent right hemispheric advantage in kanji recognition. To date, it still remains controversial whether the reported right-hemispheric (left visual field) advantage of kanji is due to the greater structural complexity of kanji (Coney, 1998; Hartje et al., 1986).

5. Dual route model of reading and Kanji-Kana problems

In 1973, Marshall and Newcombe (1973) identified different types of dyslexic patients, and proposed the so-called 'dual route model of reading' to explain the difference (Fig. 4). The first type is surface dyslexia, and the second type is deep dyslexia[1]. The essential feature of surface dyslexia is the marked difficulty in reading irregular words (e.g. pint, yacht, colonel, listen) and frequent regularization errors (e.g. pint with short i, disease as decease). Surface dyslexia has been explained as a disruption of the semantic route. Deep dyslexia is characterized by frequent semantic paralexias, inability to read non-words, and profound effects of frequency and word category on the reading ability (substantive words such as nouns are read better than grammatical functors such as particles, and concrete words are read better than abstract words). Originally, deep dyslexia was interpreted as the disruption of the phonological route.

There have been a number of controversies regarding the symptomatology and theoretical explanations of surface and deep dyslexia (Shallice, 1988). An interesting question is how these conditions would appear in the unique dual writing system of Japanese.

The Japanese equivalence of surface dyslexia can be seen in a unique subtype of aphasia called Gogi (word-meaning) aphasia described by Imura and colleagues (Imura, 1943, Imura et al., 1971). Typical features of Gogi aphasia are 1) selective impairment of single word comprehension, 2) disproportionately severe impairment in reading kanji compared with kana, 3) peculiar paralexia in words that consist of several kanji characters (neglecting the meaning of words and reading each kanji character one by one).

The following is one example of kanji paralexia of Gogi aphasia. The word '土産' (gift) consists of two kanji characters and is pronounced *mi-ya-ge* in Japanese. This is a typical irregular word in terms of its pronunciation, because the usual pronunciation of the first Kanji '土' is *tsuchi* or *do* and that for the second '産' is *san*. A typical Gogi aphasia patient misreads this word as *do-san*. Such patterns of dyslexia are strikingly similar to the pattern of dyslexia shown by patients with surface dyslexia in some European languages, in which reading of irregular words is selectively disturbed and regularization errors occur frequently.

---

1. They also reported a third type, i.e. visual dyslexia, which won't be discussed in this section.

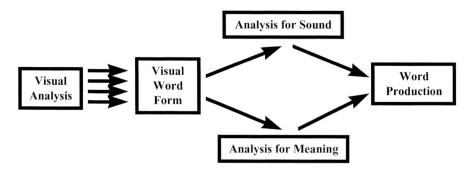

Figure 4. Dual route model of reading.

Another interesting parallel can be found between Gogi aphasia and semantic dementia (Table 4). Semantic dementia, described by Snowden et al. (1989) and Hodges et al. (1992) in patients with cortical atrophy, show a selective decline in semantic memory function while other cognitive functions such as episodic memory are relatively preserved. One of the striking features of semantic dementia is surface dyslexia. Since most of the reported Gogi aphasia patients suffered from progressive brain atrophy, we can see the similarity between semantic dementia and Gogi aphasia at the etiologic level, too. Hodges et al. regarded semantic dementia as a special form of memory impairment, whereas Imura and colleagues characterized Gogi aphasia as a subcategory of aphasia. However, both patient groups exhibited similar cognitive dysfunction and, possibly, the same underlying etiology (i.e. Pick's disease).

Table 4. Semantic dementia and Gogi aphasia

	English speaker	Japanese speaker
Neuropsychological syndrome	Semantic dementia	Gogi aphasia
Characteristics of reading impairment	Surface dyslexia	Surface-dyslexia-like kanji misreading
Frequently misread words	Irregularly spelled words	Irregularly spelled kanji words
Frequent etiology	Progressive brain atrophy (Pick's disease)	Progressive brain atrophy (Pick's disease)

An oversimplified view, which assumed kanji as ideograms showing clear contrast to kana, would predict that the Japanese parallel of surface dyslexia be kanji selective dyslexia. This assumption is partially true because patients with Gogi aphasia show disproportionately severe impairment in reading kanji characters compared with kana characters. However, it should also be noted that patients with Gogi aphasia read kanji with regular pronunciation relatively well. It is not the kanji/kana difference of a given word but the regularity of writing that determines the chance of correctly reading that word. Kanji/kana is a unique parameter to investigate and the partially relate to information-processing models of human reading in the European/American literature. However, caution again has to be taken when comparing the dual processing models of major European languages and the dual writing system of Japanese, because these two dichotomies are not exactly the same.

The occurrence of deep dyslexia has also been reported in Japanese aphasia (Asano et al., 1987, Hayashi et al., 1985). For example, a global aphasic patient reported by Asano et al. (1987) showed the typical syndrome of deep dyslexia with substantial semantic paralexia; relatively preserved reading of nouns, better reading of concrete nouns than abstract nouns, severely impaired in non-word readings, which corresponded to the characteristics of deep dyslexia in the European/American literature. In addition, they reported that typical semantic errors were much more prominent in kanji words than kana words. Different from surface dyslexia, there are still limited studies which have compared kanji/kana-reading performance among Japanese deep dyslexic patients.

6. Semantic priming effects in a Japanese speaker with surface dyslexia

As mentioned above, disruption of the semantic route is assumed in surface dyslexia. An interesting question is whether the semantic route is totally disrupted or only partially disrupted in these patients. Nakamura et al. (1997) investigated this issue using a semantic priming paradigm in a Japanese speaker with surface dyslexia.

They reported an 82-year-old female patient (diagnosed with senile dementia of the Alzheimer type) with frequent surface-dyslexic errors when reading words composed of kanji characters. The patient made errors consistently on a two-kanji character word reading '定規' as tei-ki instead of jou-gi. Since the most frequent pronunciations of these two kanji characters are tei and ki, the patient was making a regularization error. In addition, she defined the word as another word that was pronounced tei-ki (corresponding to the kanji orthography of '定期'). To investigate whether the semantic processing of these words is also disturbed at the level of automatic processing, the investigaters asked this patient to perform lexical decision tasks using the words which she misread with the pattern of surface-dyslexic error.

Three prime kanji words (A, B, C) were used for the target word '定規'. A was semantically related to '定規'. B was semantically related to

'定期'. C was semantically unrelated to both '定規' and '定期'. These three pairs of primes and targets (A-'定規', B-'定規', C-'定規'), along with one word–non-word pair, one non-word–word pair and three non-word–non-word pairs constituted the stimuli set. All stimuli were presented on a computer screen and the patient was requested to decide whether each presented kanji string was a word or a non-word. Each prime and target pair was presented pairwise sequentially, and the reaction time was recorded for each target stimulus. The experiment was repeated with the same stimuli set 12 times, and the mean reaction time for each prime-target pair was calculated.

Table 5 shows the findings. When the prime was semantically related to the target (A-'定規'), the mean lexical decision time was significantly shorter than the control condition (C-'定規'), whereas when the prime was semantically related to '定期' (B-'定規'), the mean lexical decision time was not significantly different from the control condition. Further experiments with other words also confirmed that when target words were primed semantically to related words, her reaction time was shorter than when the prime was semantically related to the wrong meaning derived from her misreading.

These findings suggest that despite reading errors, the patient could implicitly recognize the correct meaning of these kanji characters. The authors speculated that partial disruption of the semantic route would explain the dissociation between conscious and automatic reading.

7. Kanji-Kana problems in constructional agraphia

In the preceding section, we mainly described kanji/kana problems regarding reading impairments. Constructional agraphia is one of the writing impairments that involves kanji/kana differences in writing.

Constructional agraphia is one of the non-aphasic writing impairments after brain injury (Kleist, 1934). Constructional agraphia has been suggested to be an epiphenomenon of constructional apraxia, although not all patients with constructional apraxia show this condition. Constructional apraxia is the impairment of composing figures or objects from their elements. Similarly, constructional agraphia is the impairment of composing each letter from its elements despite intact motor ability in writing each part of the letter. The patients don't confuse a letter with another, thus a written letter

Table 5. Results of semantic priming task (Nakamura, H. et al., 1997)

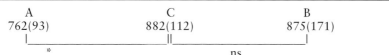

A	C	B
762(93)	882(112)	875(171)

Semantic priming task: the target word included '定規', and primes were semantically related to '定規' (A), semantically related to '定期' (B), or semantically unrelated to both words (C). Means (and SDs) of reaction times for the target '定規' for each prime are given in msec. *$p < 0.05$. ns: no significant difference.

has some similarity with the letter to be written. Characteristic findings are spatial mislocation of elements of a letter and distorted ratio among elements of a letter. Writing impairment in constructional agraphia is apparent both in dictation and copying.

It is important to distinguish constructional agraphia from other types of agraphias; aphasic, apraxic, visuospatial and pure agraphia. To identify the differential underlying mechanisms of agraphia, Asano et al. (1985) developed a simple test battery. In this battery of tests, patients are requested not to write but to combine the cards with parts of kanji characters to create correct kanji characters. In one agraphic patient, they found a pattern of errors (error of card arrangement) that was different from visuospatial error, supporting the existence of constructional agraphia (Fig. 5).

One of the characteristics of constructional agraphia is that writing impairments are severe in kanji and mild in kana (especially in hiragana). Kanji characters are generally composed of many elements (strokes) whereas each element is relatively simple. On the contrary, kana (hiragana) characters are composed of few elements whereas each stroke is often very complex, with frequent irregular curves and crossings (Fig. 6). Thus, the kanji/kana

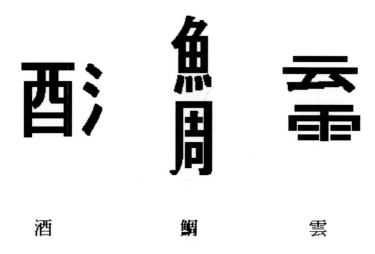

Fig. 5. Typical error pattern of constructional agraphia (Asano et al., 1985)
Many kanji–characters consist of two or more distinct parts. In this Kanji Character Constructive Test, patients are requested to compose given kanji characters correctly from the sets of cards on which parts of kanji characters are written. Errors patterns are variable from omission of parts of characters, wrong selection of components, etc. The type of errors shown in this figure was observed only in one patient among the reported seven patients. The characteristics of these errors are that the patient arranged components of each characters incorrectly, while selecting the correct components of each characters.
The upper part of the figure shows the patient's reactions and the lower the correct kanji characters.

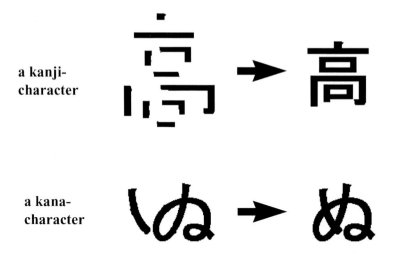

Fig. 6. Example of the structure of kanji characters and kana-characters
Kanji characters are generally composed of many strokes. Each component is relatively simple. Most of them are simple straight lines. On the contrary, kana (hiragana) characters are composed of few strokes. Some components are extremely complex, including irregular curves and crossings.

dissociation in patients with constructional agraphia could be explained by assuming impaired constructional ability (which is the ability to consciously arrange elements in a given space) and intact kinesthetic memory (which is required for realizing complex elements automatically) by these patients (Ohta & Koyabu, 1970).

8. Clinico-anatomical correlation and Kanji-Kana problems
In this section, a clinico-anatomical model of reading/writing will be discussed. Some Japanese brain-damaged patients with reading/writing disturbances have been reported to show disproportionate difficulty in either kanji or kana. Representative case reports are summarized in Table 6.

Yamadori (1975) reported a patient with alexia with agraphia due to angular gyrus lesion. This patient showed more prominent reading impairment in kana than kanji. Tanaka et al. (1987) reported a patient with selective agraphia for kana. There was a confirmed brain lesion in the left inferior parietal region. Several reports (Kawamura et al., 1987, Soma et al., 1989, Sakurai et al., 1994) confirm that the left posterior inferior temporal region is critical in kanji writing and possibly kanji reading.

In an attempt to integrate the findings of these case studies, Iwata (1986) proposed the following anatomical hypothesis (Fig. 7). Ventral pathways via the posterior part of the middle and inferior temporal gyrus are critical for ideogram reading, whereas the dorsal route passing through the angular

Table 6. Neuropsychological case studies showing disproportional reading/writing impairments either for kana or kanji.

Author(s)	Year	Etiology	Lesion	Reading/writing disturbance
Yamadori	1975	cerebral infarction	occlusion of the angular branch of the left middle cerebral (angiography)	agraphia with alexia, kanji-reading was better preserved
Tanaka et al.	1987	cerebral infarction	left inferior parietal lobule, and left corona radiata	selective agraphia for kana
Mochizuki & Ohtomo	1988	cerebral infarction	left occipital lobe and inferior temporal gyrus	pure alexia in kanji and kana, and agraphia in kanji
Yokota et al.	1990	haemorrhagic infarction (cortical vein thrombosis of Labbe)	left temporal lobe	pure agraphia of kanji
Kawamura et al.	1987	intracerebral haemorrhage	left posterior inferior temporal region	alexia with agraphia in kanji
Soma et al. (Case 1)	1989	intracerebral haemorrhage	left posterior inferior temporal region	pure agraphia for kanji
Soma et al. (Case 2)	1989	cerebral infarction	left posterior inferior temporal region	pure agraphia for kanji
Soma et al. (Case 3)	1989	cerebal contusion and intracerebral haemorrhage	left posterior inferior temporal region	pure agraphia for kanji
Sakurai et al.	1994	intracerebral haemorrhage	left posterior inferior temporal region	alexia with agraphia in kanji

gyrus is important for phonogram reading. The advantage of this anatomical hypothesis is that it explains not only the dissociation between kanji reading/kana reading but also several clinical combinations of kanji/kana reading/writing impairments in one scheme. Since patients with pure kanji or kana impairments are rare, the validity of this model should be further examined.

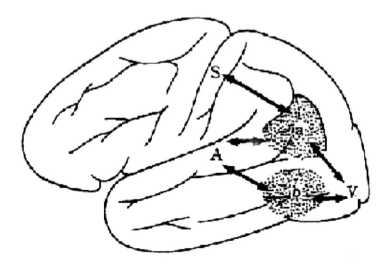

Figure 7. A neuroanatomical model of reading/writing disturbances in the Japanese language (Iwata, 1986).

A: Wernicke area, V: visual area, S: somatosensory area, a: left augular gyrus, b: left posterior inferior part of temporal lobe.

The reading process consists of a phonological process ("V→a→A") and a semantic process ("V→b→A"). Kana is decoded by the former, while kanji is decoded by both. The writing process consists of "A→a→S" and "A→b→V→a→S". Kana writing is realized by the former route, while kanji by the latter. The advantage of this hypothesis is that it explains not only the dissociation between kanji reading/kana reading but also several clinical combinations of kanji/kana reading/writing impairments in one scheme. For example, after lesion of the left posterior inferior temporal region (b), complete disruption of kanji writing and partial disruption of kanji reading is predicted from the model. This is in good accordance with frequent reports of "pure agraphia after left posterior inferior temporal lesion". After lesion of the left angular gyrus (a), total disruption of kana reading, partial disruption of kanji reading, and total disruption of kanji and kana writing are predicted from this model. This is in good accordance with reports of "alexia with agraphia, with relatively preserved kanji-reading, due to angular gyrus lesion" by Yamadori (1975).

9. Functional neuroimaging and Kanji-Kana problems

From the recent development of functional neuroimaging, such as positron emission tomography (PET), magnetoencephalography (MEG), or functional magnetic resonance imaging (fMRI), neurocognitive hypotheses, which were proposed based on brain damaged patients, can be tested using healthy subjects. Consequently, anatomical hypotheses regarding kanji/kana problems, such as Iwata's dual pathway model, can be tested using these new methods.

Sakurai et al. (1992,1993) investigated regional brain activation from either kanji or kana reading in a [15O]-PET study. In the first study (1992), subjects were instructed to read aloud words composed of two kanji characters. The comparison between the activations during kanji reading and gazing at a point on the screen (control task) showed that kanji reading produces a main cortical activation in the bilateral (left-side dominant) posterior inferior temporal area. Also, there was no significant activation in the parietal area. These findings support Iwata's dual route hypothesis. The authors argued that the left posterior inferior temporal area processes highly complex morphological features of kanji.

In a subsequent study (Sakurai et al., 1993), they conducted a similar [^{15}O]-PET study with kana-words and kana-non-words. In this study, main cortical activation was found bilaterally in the lateral and medial occipital gyri, and the left posterior inferior temporal area for both kana words and kana non-words. In addition, the kana word activated the right posterior inferior temporal area. Contrary to the prediction of Iwata's hypothesis (1986), no activation was found in angular/supramarginal gyri.

In a study of MEG, Koyama et al. (1998) showed no significant difference in magnetic responses between kanji and kana. In all the subjects, equivalent current dipoles were found in the posterior inferior temporal areas.

Kamada et al. (1998) conducted a MEG study using Japanese speakers and non-Japanese speakers. Kanji characters and meaningless figures were presented on the screen. When a kanji character was presented, the Japanese subjects were requested to read it in mind and imagine the object for the character. When a meaningless figure was presented, they were requested to specify it as "no kanji" in mind. The German subjects (non-Japanese speakers), having been trained to distinguish kanji and meaningless figures in advance, were requested to specify what was presented either as kanji or as "no kanji" in mind. Neuromagnetic fields obtained with meaningless figure stimuli were subtracted from those with kanji stimuli to demonstrate the semantic response. They found early responses in the right fusiform gyrus for both groups, whereas late responses were found in the left superior temporal gyrus and supramarginal gyrus only for Japanese speakers. Regarding the discrepancy with the PET studies of Sakurai et al. (1992), in which left posterior inferior temporal activation was demonstrated by kanji-word reading, Kamada et al. (1998) suspected that activations of the left posterior inferior temporal region observed in their own study might be concealed by simultaneous activities, which was one of the technical limitations of their methods.

Taken together, the findings of functional neuroimaging studies are mixed. Further studies, including fMRI, are needed to test the validity of the kanji/kana dual route model derived from neuropsychological studies.

Minority and Cross-Cultural Aspects of Bilingual Aphasia in the Japanese and Korean Languages

The preceding sections exclusively described issues of the Japanese language. However, it should be noted that Japanese is not the only language that is spoken in Japan. One of the other interesting topics of neuropsychological studies in Japan is the study of Japanese/Korean bilingual aphasics. Japanese and Korean share some basic similarities. Many characteristics of the Japanese language are shared with the Korean language: Both share SOV structure, postpositional characteristics and dual writing system (Sasanuma & Park, 1995).

Bilingual (or polyglot) aphasics attracted the attention of neuropsychologists, psychologists and linguists, because it is not always the case that two languages recover in parallel. Paradis (1989) identified six patterns of recovery from polyglot aphasia: parallel, differential, successive, antagonistic, selective and mixed. Several factors are involved in different patterns of recovery. They are 1) conditions of each language before onset (which language is dominant, when, how each language was learned, how often each language was used), 2) structural differences between the two languages, 3) initial symptomatology (locus and size of brain lesions, severity of aphasia), 4) environmental factors after brain injury, such as speech therapy (Takizawa, 1997).

Regarding the effect of structural differences of the two languages, many authors suggested that the patterns of recovery of two structurally similar languages tend to be similar, whereas the patterns of recovery of two structurally different languages tend to be dissimilar (Paradis, 1989). Investigations of Korean-Japanese bilingual aphasic patients provides a unique opportunity to test these hypotheses in non-European structurally-similar languages.

The case studies of Japanese-Korean bilingual aphasics are listed in Table 7 (Takizawa, 1997). Most patients showed the parallel pattern of recovery. In the four patients reported by Takizawa et al. (1995), speech therapy was conducted only in the Japanese language. The parallel recovery of Japanese and Korean in three of Takizawa et al.'s patients, as well as the parallel recovery in the second patient of Sasanuma and Park (1995) in which speech therapy was conducted only in the Korean language, supports the possibility of transfer of therapeutic effects to the non-trained language.

Concluding Remarks

In this chapter, the uniqueness of the Japanese language in neuropsychological problems was discussed. Although the Japanese language is unique, investigation of problems specific to the Japanese language may lead to understanding neuropsychological problems in general. Since language is often culture specific, this chapter focused on language based neuropsychological problems, excluding other possible cultural differences, such as memory, executive functions, or visual recognition.

Table 7. Case studies of Japanese-Korean bilingual aphasics (from Takizawa, 1998, modified)

Author(s)	Age of onset	sex	Handed-ness	Etiology	Side of lesion	Mother tongue	Other Languages	Age of acquisition	Type of symptoms	Pattern of recovery
Sugimoto et al. (1982)	58	M	R	stroke	L	Korean	Japanese	7	PA	D: Japanese> Korean
Takizawa et al. (1995)	64	M	R	stroke	L	Korean	Japanese	8	B	D: Japanese> Korean
	70	M	R	stroke	L	Korean	Japanese	7(?)	B	P
	66	F	R	stroke	L	Korean	Japanese	childhood	J	P
	66	M	R	stroke	L	Korean	Japanese	7(?)	W	P
Sasanuma & Park (1995)	62	M	R	stroke	L	Korean	Japanese	6	A	P
	29	M	R	stroke	L	Korean	Japanese	18	B?	P
Kijima et al. (1997)	65	M	R	stroke	L	Korean	Japanese	6	B(RU)	P
Fukunaga et al. (1997)	75	M	R	stroke	R	Korean	Japanese	6	G	Se

PA: pure alexia. B: Broca aphasia. J: jargon aphasia. A: amnestic aphasia. W: Wernicke aphasia. G: global aphasia. D: differential recovery. P: parallel recovery. Se: selective recovery.

References

Akimoto, H. (1976). *On apraxias*. Tokyo: Tokyo University Press (in Japanese, originally published in 1935).

Asano, K., Takizawa, T., Hadano, K., Morimune, S., & Hamanaka, T. (1985). Kanji character constructive test. *Shitsugosho Kenkyu (Higher Brain Function Research)*, 5, 810-816.

Asano, K., Takizawa, T., Hadano, K., & Hamanaka, T. (1987). Deep dyslexia: a case study. *Shinkeishinrigaku (Japanese Journal of Neuropsychology)*, 3, 209-215.

Blanken, G., Dittmann, J., Haas, J.C., & Wallesch, C.W. (1987). Spontaneous speech in senile dementia and aphasia: Implications for a neurolinguistic model of language production. *Cognition*, 27, 247-274.

Blanken, G., Dittmann, J., Haas, J.C., & Wallesch, C.W. (1988). Producing speech automatism (recurring utterances): Looking for what is left ? *Aphasiology*, 2, 545-556.

Broca, P. (1861). Rémarques sur le siège de la faculté de langage articulé, survies d'une observation d'aphémie (perte de la parole). *Bulletin de la Société Anatomique de Paris*, 36, 330-357.

Coney, J. (1998). The effect of complexity upon hemispheric specialization for reading Chinese characters. *Neuropsychologia*, 36, 149-153.

Fujita, I., & Miyake, T. (1984). *Test of Syntactic Processing in Aphasia (Trial 2A)*. Tokorozawa: Japanese Speech – Language – Hearing Association (in Japanese).

Fujita, I., & Miyake T. (1985). Syntactic processing in Broca's and Wernicke's aphasia. *Shinkeishinrigaku (Japanese Journal of Neuropsychology)*, 1, 129-137.

Fukunaga, S., Abe, H., Hatton, F., Setsu, K., & Kamei, H. (1997). A case of crossed aphasia in a right-handed Japanese – Korean bilingual, *Shitsugosho Kenkyu (Higher Brain Function Research)*, 17, 170-177 (in Japanese).

Grodzinsky, Y. (1995). A restrictive theory of agrammatic comprehension. *Brain and Language*, 50, 27-51.

Hadano, K. & Hamanaka, T. (1997). Semistereotypic speech. *Aphasiology*, 11, 1117-1125.

Hadano, K., Hayashi, M., Takizawa, T., Hamanaka, T., & Hirakawa, A. (1985). So-called "Kanji-Kana problem" in pure alexia. *Shinkeishinrigaku (Japanese Journal of Neuropsychology)*, 2, 91-96 (in Japanese).

Hadano, K., Morimune, S., Matsuda, Y., Hamanaka, T., & Hirakawa, A. (1986). A study of pure alexia by multivariate analyses. *Shinkeishinrigaku (Japanese Journal of Neuropsychology)*, 2, 135-143.

Hagiwara, H.. & Caplan, D. (1990). Syntactic comprehension in Japanese aphasics: effects of category and thematic role order. *Brain and Language*, 38, 159-170.

Hamanaka, T., Kato, N., Ohashi, H., Ohigashi, Y., Tomita, A., Hadano, K., & Asano, K. (1980). Kanji versus Kana problems in aphasiology. *Neurological Medicine*, 13, 213-221 (in Japanese).

Hamanaka, T. (1994). One hundred years of neuropsychology in Japan: retrospect and prospect. *Neuropsychological Review*, 4, 289-298.

Hartje, W., Hannen, P., & Willmes, K. (1986). Effect of visual complexity in tachistoscopic recognition of Kanji and Kana symbols by German subjects. *Neuropsychologia*, 24, 297-300.

Hatta, T. (1977). Recognition of Japanese kanji in the left and right visual fields. *Neuropsychologia*, 15, 685-688.

Hatta, T. (1983). Visual field differences in semantic comparative judgments with digits and Kanji stimulus materials. *Neuropsychologia*, 21, 669-678.

Hatta, T. (1992). The effects of Kanji attributes on visual field differences: examination with lexical decision, naming and semantic classification tasks. *Neuropsychologia*, 30, 361-371.

Hayashi, M.M., Ulatowska, H.K., & Sasanuma, S. (1985). Subcortical aphasia with deep dyslexia: a case study of Japanese patient. *Brain and Language, 25,* 293-313.

Hodges, J.R., Patterson, K., Oxbury, S., & Funnell, E. (1992). Semantic dementia: Progressive fluent aphasia with temporal lobe atrophy. *Brain, 115,* 1783-1806.

Imamura S. (1903). Ueber die corticalen Störungen des Sehactes und die Bedeutung des Balkens. *Pflügers Archiv, 100,* 495-531.

Imura, T. (1943). Aphasia: Characteristic symptoms in Japanese. *Psychiatria et Neurologia Japonica, 47,* 196-218 (in Japanese).

Imura, T., Nogami, Y., & Asagawa, K. (1971). Aphasia in Japanese language. *Nihon University Journal of Medicine, 13,* 69-90.

Iwata, M. (1986). Neural mechanism of reading and writing in the Japanese language. *Functional Neurology, 1,* 43-52.

Japanese Society of Aphasiology (1977). *Standard language test for aphasia.* Tokyo: Hohmeido (in Japanese).

Kamada, K., Kober, H., Saguer, M., Möller, M., Kaltenhäuser, M., & Vieth, J. (1998). Responses to silent Kanji reading of the native Japanese and German in task subtraction magnetoencephalography. *Cognitive Brain Research, 7,* 89-98.

Kawamura, M., Hirayama, K., Hasegawa, K., Takahashi, N., & Yamaura, A. (1987). Alexia with agraphia of kanji (Japanese morphograms). *Journal of Neurology, Neurosurgery and Psychiatry, 50,* 1125-1129.

Kijima, R., Yoshino, M., Kawamura, M., Kawachi, J., & Hakuno, A. (1997). Patterns of Kanji vs. Kana deficits in a Japanese–Korean bilingual aphasic patient: A case report. *Shitsugosho Kenkyu (Higher Brain Function Research), 17,* 1-9 (in Japanese).

Kleist, K. (1934). *Gehirnpathologie.* Leipzig: Johann Ambrosius Barth.

Koyama, S., Kakigi, R., Hoshiyama, M., & Kitamura, Y. (1998). Reading of Japanese Kanji (morphograms) and Kana (syllabograms): a magnetoencephalographic study. *Neuropsychologia, 36,* 83-98.

Marshall, J.C. & Newcombe, F. (1973). Patterns of paralexia: a psycholinguistic approach. *Journal of Psycholinguistic Research 2,* 175-199.

Mochizuki, H. & Ohtomo, R. (1988). Pure alexia in Japanese and agraphia without alexia in kanji. The ability dissociation between reading and writing in kanji vs kana. *Archives of Neurology, 45,* 1157-1159.

Nakamura, H., Nakanishi, M., Hamanaka, T., Nakaaki, S., Furukawa, T., & Masui, T. (1997). Dissociations between reading responses and semantic priming effects in a dyslexic patient. *Cortex, 33,* 753-761.

Ohashi, H. (1960). *Clinical neuropsychology.* Kyoto: Igaku-Shoin (in Japanese).

Ohta, Y., & Koyabu, S. (1970). A clinical study on constructional agraphia in Japanese language. *Seishin-Igaku (Clinical Psychiatry), 12,* 959-964 (in Japanese).

Paradis, M. (1989). Bilingual and polyglot aphasia. In F. Boller & J Grafman (Eds.), *Handbook of Neuropsychology,* Vol. 2, (pp. 117-140). Amsterdam: Elsevier.

Sakurai, Y., Momose, T., Iwata, M., Watanabe, T., Ishikawa, T., & Kanazawa, I. (1993). Semantic process in kana word reading: activation studies with positron emission tomography. *Neuroreport, 4,* 327-330.

Sakurai, Y., Momose, T., Iwata, M., Watanabe, T., Ishikawa, T., Takeda, K., & Kanazawa, I. (1992). Kanji word reading process analysed by positron emission tomography. *Neuroreport, 3,* 445-448.

Sakurai, Y., Sakai, K., Sakuta, M., & Iwata, M. (1994). Naming difficulties in alexia with agraphia for kanji after a left posterior inferior temporal lesion. *Journal of Neurology, Neurosurgery and Psychiatry, 57,* 609-13.

Sasanuma, S., Kamio, A., & Kubota, M. (1990). Agrammatism in Japanese: Two case studies. In L. Menn & L.K. Obler (Eds.), *Agrammatic aphasia: A cross-language narrative sourcebook* (pp. 1125-1307). Amsterdam: John Benjamins.

Sasanuma, S. & Park, H.S. (1995). Patterns of language deficits in two Korean-Japanese bilingual aphasic patients: A clinical report. In M. Paradis (Ed.), *Aspects of bilingual aphasia* (pp. 111-122), Oxford: Pergamon.

Shallice, T. (1988). *From neuropsychology to mental structure*. Cambridge: Cambridge University Press.

Shibatani, M. (1990). *The languages of Japan*. Cambridge: Cambridge University Press.

Snowden, J.S., Goulding, P.J., & Neary, D. (1989). Semantic dementia: a form of circumscribed cerebral atrophy. *Behavioural Neurology, 2*, 167-182.

Soma, Y., Sugishita, M., Kitamura, K., Maruyama, S., & Imanaga, H. (1989). Lexical agraphia in the Japanese language. Pure agraphia for Kanji due to left posteroinferior temporal lesions. *Brain, 112*, 1549-1561.

Sugishita, M., Otomo, K., Kabe, S., & Yunoki, K. (1992). A critical appraisal of neuropsychological correlates of Japanese ideogram (kanji) and phonogram (kana) reading. *Brain, 115*, 1563-1585.

Takewaka, Y., Kashiwagi, T., Hashitani, R., Matsubara, J., Kashiwagi, A. & Tanabe, H. (1995). A case report of aphasia with recurring utterance. *Shitsugosho Kenkyu (Higher Brain Function Research), 15*, 69-69 (in Japanese).

Takizawa, T. (1997). Bilingualism and aphasia. In K. Takakura & T. Miyamoto (Eds.). *Aphasia and neuroscience of language* (pp. 158-164). Tokyo: Medical View (in Japanese).

Takizawa, T., Asano, K., Hadano, K., Hamanaka, T., & Morimune, S. (1995). Korean-Japanese bilingual aphasics. *Shitsugosho Kenkyu (Higher Brain Function Research), 15*, 314-322 (in Japanese).

Tanaka, Y., Yamadori, A., & Murata, S. (1987). Selective kana agraphia: a case report. *Cortex, 23*, 679-684.

Tzeng, O.J.L., Hung, D.L., Cotton, B., & Wang, S.Y. (1979). Visual lateralization in reading Chinese characters. *Nature, 382*, 499-501.

Varney, N.R. (1984). Alexia for ideograms: implication for kanji alexia. *Cortex, 20*, 535-542.

Yamadori, A. (1975). Ideogram reading in alexia. *Brain, 98*, 231-238.

Yokota, T., Ishiai, S., Furukawa, T., & Tsukagoshi, H. (1990). Pure agraphia of kanji due to thrombosis of the Labbe vein. *Journal of Neurology, Neurosurgery and Psychiatry, 53*, 335-338.

Chapter 7

NEUROPSYCHOLOGICAL ASSESSMENT OF DEMENTIA ON GUAM

David P. Salmon
Department of Neurosciences, University of California, San Diego, California

Douglas Galasko
Department of Neurosciences, University of California, San Diego, California and Neurology Service, San Diego Veterans Affairs Medical Center, San Diego, California

Wigbert C. Wiederholt
Department of Neurosciences, University of California, San Diego

Abstract

Several common neurodegenerative diseases that lead to dementia occur with an unusually high prevalence in natives of the Marianas islands (particularly the Chamorros of Guam). The pathological manifestations of Parkinson-Dementia Complex (PDC) and Marianas dementia are similar to Alzheimer's disease (AD) in that both are characterized by neurofibrillary tangle formation in the entorhinal cortex, hippocampus, and the neocortex. Marianas dementia and PDC also involve degeneration in several sub-cortical nuclei (e.e., the substantia nigra and locus coeruleus) but, unlike AD, are not associated with neuritic plaque formation or abnormal amyloid deposition. Although both Marianas dementia and PDC lead to global cognitive deterioration, the specific features of the cognitive decline in the former have not been elucidated. In an ongoing, longitudinal study, we have compared the performances of patients with Marianas dementia, PDC, and non-affected individuals on neuropsychological tests of memory, attention, language, executive functions, and constructional abilities that have been translated and culturally adapted for this purpose. The utility of these tests for assessing dementia in the people of the Marianas islands is demonstrated and the pattern of cognitive deficits associated with Marianas dementia are described.

Introduction

In the early 1950s an unusually high prevalence and incidence of amyotrophic lateral sclerosis (ALS) was documented in the indigenous Chamorro population on the Marianas island of Guam (Arnold, Edgren, & Palladino, 1953). Prevalence estimates for the disease at that time (400 per 100,000 individuals) were 50 to 100 times the prevalence observed anywhere else in the world (4 to 6 per 100,000 individuals). The clinical presentation of the disease was essentially identical to that of sporadic ALS seen other places, but the pathology of the disease differed in several ways (Oyanagi et al., 1994). First, the corticospinal pathological changes in the ALS of Guam were more widespread than in sporadic ALS. Pathology occurred not only in the lateral columns and anterior horn cells as in sporadic ALS, but also in the spinocerebellar tracts and the posterior columns. Second, neurofibrillary tangles (NFT) that are morphologically and biochemically identical to those found in Alzheimer's disease (AD) were observed in the neocortex and hippocampal formation in the ALS of Guam, but are not seen in sporadic ALS.

   In the decade following the observation of the high prevalence of ALS on Guam, another neurodegenerative disease was identified on the island that was characterized by Parkinsonism and dementia (Hirano, Kurland, Krooth, & Lessel, 1961). This disorder, now known as the Parkinson-Dementia Complex (PDC), was characterized by the insidious and gradual progression of primary Parkinsonism and dementia. The Parkinsonism usually preceded the onset of dementia by several years and was essentially identical to that seen in idiopathic Parkinson's disease. Patients with PDC were likely to exhibit bradykinesia, increased muscle tone, dysarthria, hypophonic speech, loss of facial expression (i.e., masked facies), action or postural tremor, and impairment of gait. The dementia of PDC was not carefully characterized, but clinical reports suggested that it usually began with forgetfulness, disorientation, and difficulty with problem solving and calculations (Hirano et al., 1961). Language abilities appeared to remain intact until later stages of the disease. Apathy and lack of initiative were often observed in patients with PDC, but depression and other behavioral or psychiatric symptoms were rare.

The neuropathological changes that are associated with PDC include NFT, neuron loss, and depigmentation in the substantia nigra, locus ceruleus, and substantia innominata, and the widespread distribution of NFT in medial temporal lobe structures (e.g., entorhinal cortex, hippocampus) and the association cortices of the frontal and temporal lobes (Hirano, Malamud, & Kurland, 1961; Oyanagi et al., 1994; Hof et al., 1994). Although the NFT pathology of PDC resembles that of AD, there is little or no deposition of amyloid in PDC, either diffusely or as neuritic plaques. In addition, the Lewy body pathology that characterizes idiopathic Parkinson's disease is virtually absent in PDC.

A third highly prevalent neurodegenerative disease that was identified on Guam more recently is a disorder that produces a pure dementia syndrome without significant motor abnormality (Lavine et al., 1991). This dementia syndrome, sometimes known as Marianas Dementia, is similar in presentation to the dementia syndrome of AD (Galasko, Salmon, Craig, & Wiederholt, 2000). Marianas Dementia begins insidiously, usually with memory impairment as the earliest symptom. As the disorder gradually progresses, abstract reasoning, language, attention, and visuospatial abilities become impaired. Some patients have questionable or minimal Parkinsonism in the early stages of the disease, but most are free of motor dysfunction until the advanced stages, at a point when cognition is very severely impaired. About one-third of patients with Marianas Dementia report hallucinations and delusions, and physical or verbal agitation may occur as the dementia progresses. The neuropathological changes associated with Marianas Dementia are largely unknown, but may be similar to those of PDC or AD.

Over the past 45 years, the prevalence of ALS on Guam declined markedly for unknown reasons (Kurland, Radhakrishnan, Williams, & Waring, 1994; Reed & Brody, 1975), although the prevalence remains higher than for sporadic ALS in other parts of the world. The prevalence of PDC, in contrast, appears to have declined only slightly or to have remained steady over the years, possibly due to increases in life expectancy in the Chamorro population (Kurland et al., 1994). The prevalence of Marianas Dementia appears to be at least as high as for PDC (Galasko et al., 2000). Despite a considerable amount of neuroepidemiological research on Guam, the etiology and high prevalence of these disorders, and the changes in the patterns of prevalence among the three, has not been explained. A number of possible causative factors have been considered over the past 45 years, such as the ingestion of toxins released during the preparation of flour from local cycads (Spencer, Nunn, Hugon, Ludolph, & Roy, 1986; Spencer et al., 1987) and the absence of certain minerals (e.g., calcium and magnesium; for review, see Garruto, 1987) or excess of heavy metals (e.g., aluminum; Garruto, Yanagihara, Gajdusek, & Arion, 1984; Perl, Gajdusek, Garruto, Yanagihara, & Gibbs, 1982) in the water and soil on Guam. Genetic factors have also been considered since there is familial clustering of the disease (Plato, Garruto, Fox, & Gajdusek, 1986), although the disease does not follow an obvious pattern of inheritance (Reed, Torres, & Brody, 1975). Unfortunately, none of these possibilities have been conclusively proven.

Because of the occasional co-occurrence of the ALS and PDC forms of the disease in the same family (or even in the same individual), and the similarity in certain aspects of neuropathology (e.g., NFT), some investigators have proposed that the two disorders may be different manifestations of the same disease process (Hirano et al., 1961). Similarly, the clinical presentations of the dementia of PDC and Marianas Dementia are similar and it may be the case that Marianas Dementia represents a third form of the same disease. Alternatively, the disorders may have independent etiological and neuropathological determinants, but the key differences in the three diseases have yet to be identified. Ongoing studies of the genetic, environmental, neuropathological, and clinical aspects of the disorders may clarify the relationship among them, and may provide important information about the cause and potential cure for these devastating diseases.

One aspect of these neurodegenerative diseases on Guam that has received relatively little attention in the past is the nature of the cognitive deficits that characterize the dementia syndromes associated with PDC and Marianas Dementia. There has been very little clinical research that has attempted to identify or develop effective methods for detecting early cognitive changes in individuals who are in the beginning stages of PDC or Marianas Dementia, and there have been very few studies that have sought to delineate the pattern of cognitive deficits that occur in the two disorders. One of the few studies that examined cognitive deficits in patients with PDC or Marianas Dementia demonstrated that a short battery of tests known as the Cross-Cultural Cognitive Examination (CCCE) was very effective at differentiating between demented and non-demented Chamorro individuals on Guam (Glosser et al., 1993). Using failure on two or more of the brief tests of memory, attention, language, abstract thinking, visuospatial abilities, and psychomotor speed that constitute the CCSE as the criterion for dementia, the CCSE was found to have 94% sensitivity and 99% specificity for detecting dementia as identified by a full clinical evaluation. Because the performance of patients and non-demented control subjects on the individual tests of the CCSE were not reported, the specific patterns of cognitive deficits that might characterize PDC and Marianas Dementia could not be discerned.

Given the general paucity of neuropsychological research regarding the Guam neurodegenerative disorders, it is not known whether the dementia of PDC is identical to that of Marianas Dementia, or whether the two disorders produce different patterns of relatively impaired and spared cognitive abilities. There may indeed be differences in this aspect of the two disorders, as the virtual lack of motor dysfunction in Marianas Dementia suggests that the cognitive deficits may be typical of a so-called "cortical" dementia syndrome, whereas the combination of cortical and subcortical pathologic changes in

PDC may produce a dementia syndrome with subcortical as well as cortical features.

As part of our ongoing research into the neurodegenerative diseases that occur on Guam, we recently carried out studies of the effectiveness of cognitive screening procedures for detecting dementia on Guam, and we examined in some detail the cognitive deficits that occur in PDC and Marianas Dementia. The results of these efforts are described below. Before embarking upon this discussion, however, it is important to address some of the potential confounding factors that must be considered in performing cross-cultural neuropsychological research of this kind.

Cross-Cultural Considerations in Neuropsychological Research on Guam

It is well known that performance on most tests of cognitive ability can be markedly affected by the subject's level of education and cultural background. Significant relationships between level of education and neuropsychological test performance have been reported by a number of investigators in both healthy (Ardila, Rosselli, & Rosas, 1989; Heaton, Grant, & Matthews, 1986; Rosselli & Ardila, 1990) and brain damaged subjects (Benton, Levin, & Van Allen, 1974; Finlayson, Johnson, & Reitan, 1977; Lecours et al., 1987). Similarly, cultural variables which affect the performance of subjects on tests of intellectual abilities have been described by numerous investigators, and include such factors as familiarity with test taking, previous exposure to the test materials, and familiarity with writing implements (for review, see Ardila et al., 1989; Pick, 1980; Segall, 1986). In addition, cultural differences in the emphasis placed on particular cognitive abilities during development, and the stage of development in which certain cognitive abilities are learned, may affect later performance on neuropsychological tests (Berry, 1979; Cole, Gay, Click, & Sharp, 1971).

Because of the potential influence of cultural and educational factors on neuropsychological test performance, tests sensitive to dementia in one culture may not be effective in differentiating between demented and nondemented individuals in another cultural setting, particularly if the two cultures differ greatly in median level of education. Therefore, a test adapted for the assessment of dementia in a new cultural setting must be evaluated in terms of both sensitivity to dementia and susceptibility to the effects of education.

In light of these potentially confounding factors, we were cautious in our application of cognitive tests for the assessment of dementia in the Chamorro population of Guam. Tests were translated into Chamorro and back translated into English to check their linguistic accuracy. Testing was carried out in either English or Chamorro as requested by the subject. Because English is widely spoken on Guam and is the language used in the school system, most subjects chose to be tested in English. Tests were screened for cultural appropriateness by a group of knowledgeable health-care workers at the University of Guam and were modified as needed. To control for the affects of age and education on cognitive test perform-ance, normative data were collected for each test from a group of healthy, functionally-intact, elderly Chamorro individuals with the same general age and education level as the patients with suspected dementia. With these normative data, we were able to detect the presence of cognitive dysfunction in elderly Chamorro individuals and to delineate the pattern of deficits associated with PDC and Marianas Dementia.

Cognitive Screening on Guam

The ability to detect and stage cognitive impairment is greatly facilitated by the use of objective and structured mental status examinations. The most effective mental status examinations are those that: (1) can differentiate between the beginning of a dementing disorder and normal aging; (2) can assess a wide range of cognitive functions that are likely to be affected in a dementing disorder; (3) are sensitive to change in mental status over time and quantify this change in an interval or ordinal manner so that remission or progression of a cognitive disorder can be measured; and (4) are not so difficult as to preclude any meaningful measurement of cognitive abilities in severely impaired patients.

As mentioned above, performance on most structured mental status exam-inations can be influenced by level of education and literacy and these fac-tors must be taken into consideration when interpreting test results (Ritchie, 1988; Schmitt, Ranseen, & DeKosky, 1989). On the one hand, poor edu-cation or illiteracy can lead to poor test performance by non-cognitively impaired individuals with the consequence of a false positive classification of cognitive dysfunction. On the other hand, highly educated individuals may have a true decline in cognitive functioning but still perform within the normal range on these tests, leading to a false negative classification of no cognitive dysfunction. This problem in interpretation can be ameliorated to some extent by the use of education-adjusted normative data or cut-off scores for impairment. While race and socioeconomic status do not seem to have a notable effect on mental status examination performance once the effect of education is accounted for, most of the tests do have cultural idiosyncrasies that must be considered when the test is adopted for use with a non-English speaking population.

With these factors in mind, we chose to screen for cognitive dysfunction indicative of PDC or Marianas Dementia with the Cognitive Abilities Screen-ing Instrument (CASI; Teng et al., 1994). The CASI is a relatively brief screen-ing instrument that consists of subscales for attention, concentration, orienta-tion, short-term and long-term memory, language, visual construction, and abstraction and judgment. The total score on the test ranges from 0 to 100 points and scores for the Mini-Mental State Examination (MMSE) and the Hasegawa Dementia Screening Scale can be generated from subsets of the CASI items. The test's cross-cultural applicability in screening for dementia has been demonstrated in studies in the United States and Japan.

Before implementing the CASI for the assessment of dementia on Guam, pilot testing of a version of the test that was translated and culturally adapted for use with the Chamorro population was completed in San Diego, California. Twenty-seven Chamorro individuals were tested with the CASI and then received detailed neurological and neuropsychological evaluations. Of the 27 subjects, 21 were judged to be neurologically and cognitively normal, and six were found to be demented according to DSM-IV criteria (American Psychiatric Association, 1994). The non-demented individuals achieved an average CASI score of 86.6 (SD=6.9) with scores ranging from 80 to 96. The demented individuals scored significantly lower than the non-demented subjects with an average CASI score of 47.7 (SD=11.3) and a range of scores from 37 to 66. When a CASI cut-off score for impairment of 75 was applied (approximately 2 standard deviations below the mean score), the test achieved 95% accuracy in distinguishing between the demented and non-demented individuals.

Given the success of the CASI in distinguishing between demented and non-demented Chamorro individuals in pilot testing, the test was adopted as the main cognitive screening instrument in our study of dementia on Guam. A cutoff score of 75 was selected as the threshold for triggering a more detailed dementia evaluation. Individuals scoring above 75 on the CASI and having no reported functional impairment or evidence of motor dysfunction were considered normal and not further evaluated. Those scoring below 75 on the CASI or reporting functional impairment or exhibiting motor dysfunction received a standardized neurological evaluation and detailed neuropsychological testing (described below). Depending upon the results of this detailed evaluation, a neurologic diagnosis was made or the subject was classified as normal.

To determine the affects of age and education on CASI performance on Guam, we recently completed a study that included 217 normal control subjects who ranged in age from 20 to 84 (mean age = 55), and had completed from 2 to more than 20 years of education (Wiederholt, Galasko, Salmon, & Craig, 1998). The total CASI score is presented as a function of age in Fig. 1 and as a function of level of education in Fig. 2. Simple linear regression analyses showed that CASI scores were significantly negatively correlated with increasing age (r = -0.4462) and positively correlated with increasing levels of education (r = 0.5062). While not unexpected, these results suggest that age- and education-adjusted cut-off scores might be more effective than a generic cut-off score for the detection of mild cognitive impairment in the Chamorro population on Guam.

It should be noted, however, that the CASI cut-off score of 75 that was adopted for our dementia studies on Guam provides reasonable sensitivity

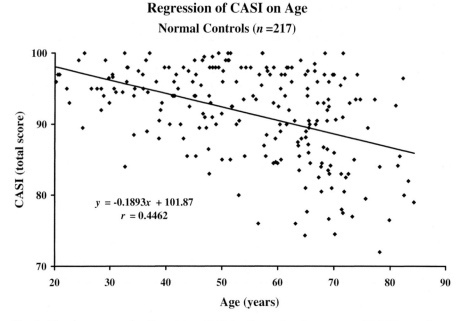

Fig. 1. Total score on the Cognitive Abilities Screening Instrument (CASI) as a function of age in non-demented Chamorro individuals on Guam.

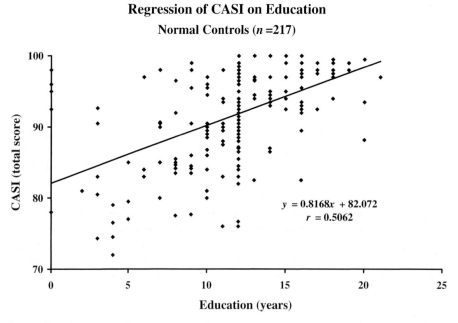

Fig. 2. Total score on the Cognitive Abilities Screening Instrument (CASI) as a function of years of education in non-demented Chamorro individuals on Guam.

and specificity for the detection of cognitive impairment. We recently compared the CASI performances of 58 demented and 34 non-demented elderly subjects on Guam who all had less than 12 years of education. The classification of subjects as demented or non-demented was made independently of the CASI score on the basis of the neurological evaluation and assessment of functional status. A cut-off score on the CASI of less than 75 provided 93% specificity and 82% sensitivity for the detection of dementia in these groups.

Neuropsychological Testing on Guam

Although brief mental status examinations such as the CASI are useful in screening for cognitive impairment and for staging the severity of cognitive dysfunction in demented patients, a much more detailed neuropsychological evaluation is necessary to confirm cognitive impairment in very mildly affected patients and to discern patterns of deficits that may be indicative of a particular dementia syndrome. Unfortunately, very little detailed neuropsychological testing has been carried out with demented patients with PDC or Marianas Dementia on Guam, and the nature of the dementia in the two disorders remains unknown. It is not known, for example, whether these dementing disorders produce different patterns of cognitive deficits, or if one or the other of these disorders conforms to a pattern of deficits indicative of a so-called "cortical" or "subcortical" dementia syndrome (Salmon & Heindel, 1998).

The distinction between cortical and subcortical dementia syndromes is exemplified by a comparison of the cognitive deficits associated with AD which produces a prototypical cortical dementia syndrome, and those associated with Huntington's disease (HD) or Parkinson's disease (PD) which produce a prototypical subcortical dementia syndrome. The dementia of AD is characterized by prominent amnesia with additional deficits in language and semantic knowledge (i.e., aphasia), abstract reasoning, other "executive" functions, attention, and constructional and visuospatial abilities (Corkin, 1982; Moss & Albert, 1988). The severe amnesia that is a cardinal feature of AD has been attributed to the early and pronounced damage that occurs in the hippocampus and related structures (e.g., the entorhinal cortex; Hyman et al., 1984). Deficits in language and semantic knowledge are thought to be associated with deterioration of the neocortical association areas of the temporal and parietal lobes (Hodges et al., 1994), while impaired abstract reasoning and "executive" functions (e.g., the ability to monitor two cognitive tasks simultaneously) are believed to occur as a consequence of frontal lobe neocortical degeneration (Morris, 1996). Impaired attention is also attributed to frontal lobe deterioration in AD (Parasuraman & Haxby, 1993) and may be heightened by neocortical depletion of norepinephrine following damage to the locus ceruleus. The visuospatial and visuoconstructional deficits that typically occur in AD are thought to be mediated by neocortical deterioration in the parietal lobe (Martin, 1987), but may be influenced by damage in the frontal cortex (Nielson et al., 1996). All of the cortical features of the dementia of AD might be exacerbated by the severe reduction in neocortical acetylcholine that occurs as a result of significant pathology in basal forebrain structures.

Huntington's disease and PD, in contrast, produce a dementia syndrome that is characterized by slowness of thought, impaired attention, a mild or moderate memory disturbance, a deficiency in planning and problem solving, and visuoperceptual and constructional deficits (Bondi & Kaszniak, 1991; Brandt & Butters, 1986; Butters, Sax, Montgomery, & Tarlow, 1978). Personality changes such as depression and apathy also often occur as part of the sub-cortical dementia syndrome (Cummings, 1990). Because neocortical regions are minimally damaged, subcortical degenerative diseases usually result in little or no aphasia or semantic memory impairment; however, dysarthria may be present due to motor dysfunction. The cognitive and neuropsychiatric deficits that form the subcortical dementia syndrome are similar to the changes that occur with frontal lobe damage and are thought to be a consequence of the disruption of the fronto-striatal circuits that link the frontal lobes with subcortical structures (Alexander, DeLong, & Strick, 1986; Cummings, 1990). In HD, for example, the fronto-striatal circuits are interrupted by direct atrophy of the neostriatum. In PD, on the other hand, fronto-striatal circuits are disrupted by the loss of dopaminergic innervation of the neostriatum and cortex. These differences in the specific site of disruption within the circuits, and variations in the additional neuropathological and neurochemical changes associated with each disease (e.g., neocortical dopamine loss in PD), account for the subtle differences in the cognitive and neuropsychiatric presentation of each subcortical neurodegenerative disorder.

To characterize the neuropsychological deficits associated with Guam PDC and Marianas Dementia, we recently completed a study in which Chamorro patients with clinically-diagnosed PDC, Marianas Dementia, or idiopathic PD were administered a battery of neuropsychological tests that assessed all major cognitive domains (Salmon et al., submitted). The performances of these patient groups were compared to that of a group of Chamorro normal control (NC) subjects. The PDC and Marianas Dementia groups were matched for age, level of education, and global level of dementia as measured by the CASI. The NC and PD patients were matched for age with the other two groups, but were slightly more educated, and as expected, scored higher on the CASI. The CASI scores of the NC subjects and PD patients were not significantly different.

The battery of neuropsychological tests used in this study is shown in Table 1. The battery consisted of several tests of each major cognitive ability affected in various dementing disorders, including memory, "executive" functions, attention, language, visuospatial abilities and constructional praxis, and psychomotor speed. The test battery was designed to be sensitive to

Table 1. Neuropsychological tests used in the Guam dementia study.

Attention	Memory
– Digit Span Test	– CERAD Memory Test
– Letter and Symbol Cancellation Test	
Executive Functions	**Language**
– Odd-Man Out Test	– Boston Naming Test (15-item)
– Trails A and B	– Letter and Category Fluency
– Symbol-Digit Substitution Test	
Visuospatial Functions	**Psychomotor Speed**
– Block Design Test	– Grooved Pegboard Test
– Clock Drawing Test	

the predominant cognitive deficits that occur in AD and in PD and other subcortical dementias. Test measures sensitive to early AD include immediate and delayed recall and recognition memory tasks, confrontation naming and category fluency tasks, tests of abstract reasoning, and tests of visuoconstructive ability. Tests sensitive to the cognitive changes associated with PD and other fronto-subcortical dementias included free recall memory tasks, tests of attention, rule learning and set shifting tasks, tests of psychomotor speed and manual dexterity, and visuospatial processing tasks. The proposed tests have been shown in previous studies to be quite sensitive for detecting dementia in its early stages and to effectively differentiate between patients with "cortical" and "subcortical" dementia.

The neuropsychological tests were translated (and back translated) into Chamorro and culturally adapted, when necessary, for use with the Chamorro population. The validity and effectiveness of the tests was then verified through pilot testing of the sample of Guam-born Chamorro individuals who currently reside in San Diego. This pilot investigation also provided preliminary normative data for the various tests with relatively low educated Chamorro individuals.

The results of our study showed that the PDC and Marianas Dementia patients exhibited overall poorer memory and a slower rate of learning across trials than the NC subjects and PD patients on the CERAD Memory Test. In addition, both of the demented patient groups exhibited abnormally rapid forgetting of information over the ten-minute delay interval. Patients with PD, in contrast, had a rate of forgetting on this task that was similar to that of the NC subjects. The abnormally rapid forgetting exhibited by the PDC and Marianas Dementia patients is similar to the rapid forgetting that characterizes the memory deficit of AD and suggests that both disorders produce a frank amnesia due to ineffective encoding or consolidation of information into memory.

In addition to a pronounced amnesia, patients with PDC and Marianas Dementia were found to have a significant language deficit that was evident on tests of confrontation naming and verbal fluency. The PDC and Marianas

Dementia patients performed significantly worse than the NC subjects and PD patients on the Boston Naming Test and the Letter and Category Fluency Tests. The dementia groups did not differ from each other on any of these tests of language ability. The PD patients were impaired relative to the NC subjects only on the Letter Fluency task. The pattern of language deficits exhibited by the PDC and Marianas Dementia patients were identical and were indicative of semantic memory dysfunction. In addition to the anomia that was evident in their confrontation naming test performances, these patients tended to be more impaired, relative to NC subjects, on the semantically-demanding Category Fluency Test than on the phonemically-driven Letter Fluency Test. This pattern of naming and fluency test performance is common in patients with AD and has been attributed to the deterioration of cortical association cortices in that disease. The patients with PD, in contrast, produced a pattern of performance on the language tasks that is commonly observed in patients with subcortical dysfunction. These patients retained relatively intact naming ability and performed well on the semantically-demanding, but structured Category Fluency Test. However, when the fluency test was less structured and required greater self-initiated effortful retrieval, the patients with PD were impaired.

The PDC and Marianas Dementia patients exhibited a significant degree of constructional apraxia. Both patients groups performed worse than the NC subjects and PD patients on the Block Design Test and the Clock Drawing Tests. Furthermore, the deficits they exhibited on these tests were equivalent in the two dementia groups. Although deficits in constructional abilities occur in both cortical and subcortical dementia syndromes, studies have shown that qualitative aspects of the deficit may differ in the two syndromes. In performing the Clock Drawing Test, for example, patients with a cortical dementia syndrome such as AD often produce conceptual errors that appear to be indicative of a loss of semantic knowledge (e.g., leaving out significant aspects of the clock such as hands or numbers). Patients with a subcortical dementia such as HD, in contrast, often make visuospatial or planning errors when drawing or copying clocks. A qualitative analysis of the types of errors produced by Chamorro patients with PDC or Marianas Dementia has not yet been carried out, but may reveal differences in the two groups and provide important information about the underlying pathological basis of their deficits on the Clock Drawing Test.

Executive dysfunction was prominent in both PDC and Marianas Dementia patients. Both groups were equally impaired compared to NC subjects on two tests that required the ability to shift between cognitive sets: the Odd-Man Out Test and Part B of the Trail-Making Test. This type of executive dysfunction often occurs relatively early in the course of AD (Lafleche & Albert, 1996), most likely due to direct pathology in the association cortex of the frontal lobes. A similar executive dysfunction can also occur in subcortical dementia syndromes, however, and has been attributed to an interruption of the fronto-striatal circuits that form a closed-loop connection that flows from specific sections of the frontal cortex to the basal ganglia, the basal ganglia to the thalamus, and the thalamus back to the frontal cortex (Alexander et al., 1986).

Finally, both demented patient groups were impaired on tests of attention, scoring significantly worse than control subjects on the Digit Span Test and the Letter and Symbol Cancellation Tests. The PDC and Marianas Dementia patients performed similarly on these tests of attention. Patients with PD performed worse than the NC subjects on the Letter and Symbol Cancellation Tests, but not on the Digit Span Test. Similarly, both PDC patients and patients with Marianas Dementia exhibited a significant reduction in psychomotor speed relative to NC subjects on the Grooved Pegboard Test and Part A of the Trail-Making Test. Interestingly, the two demented groups did not differ from each other and were as impaired as the patients with PD on these tests.

Summary

When considered as a whole, the results of our neuropsychological studies on Guam demonstrate that patients with PDC and Marianas Dementia have remarkably similar patterns of cognitive deficits when they are at a comparable stage of disease. Despite marked differences in the severity of motor dysfunction, the groups did not differ significantly on tests of memory, language, attention, executive functions, visuospatial abilities, or psychomotor speed. Furthermore, the qualitative aspects of their deficits on tests of memory and verbal fluency were virtually identical. These findings suggest that the cognitive deficits that occur in PDC and Marianas Dementia may arise from similar distributions of pathology in the brain. However, verification of this possibility awaits detailed clinico-pathologic studies of patients with Marianas Dementia.

It is also important to note that the pattern of deficits produced by the PDC patients and by patients with Marianas Dementia was consistent with the cortical dementia syndrome of AD. Like patients with AD, PDC and Marianas Dementia patients exhibited severe amnesia characterized by rapid forgetting of information over time, a language deficit that appears to be due to semantic memory dysfunction, executive dysfunction on tests that require shifting cognitive set, deficits in attention, and constructional apraxia. These deficits are consistent with the extensive pathology that is known to occur in the medial temporal lobe structures (e.g., hippocampus, entorhinal cortex) and the frontal and temporal lobe association cortices in patients with PDC. Whether the cognitive deficits exhibited by patients with Marianas Dementia arise from a comparable distribution of PDC-type pathology (i.e., neurofibrillary tangles) or AD pathology (i.e., neuritic plaques and neurofibrillary tangles) remains a question for further study.

Acknowledgements

We are saddened to report that Dr. Bert Wiederholt died on March 9, 2000. This chapter is dedicated to his memory. The preparation of this chapter was supported by National Institute on Aging grant AG-14382 to the University of California, San Diego.

References

Alexander, G.E., DeLong, M.R., & Strick, P.L. (1986). Parallel organization of functionally segregated circuits linking basal ganglia and cortex. *Annual Review of Neuroscience, 9,* 357-381.

American Psychiatric Association (1994). *Diagnostic and Statistical Manual of Mental Disorders (4th ed.).* Washington D.C.: American Psychiatric Association.

Ardila, A., Rosselli, M., & Rosas, P. (1989). Neuropsychological assessment of illiterates: Visuospatial and memory abilities. *Brain and Cognition, 11,* 147-166.

Arnold, A., Edgren, D.C., & Palladino, V.S. (1953). Amyotrophic lateral sclerosis: Fifty cases observed on Guam. *Journal of Nervous and Mental Diseases, 117,* 135-139.

Benton, A.L., Levin, H.H., & Van Allen, W.V. (1974). Geographic orientation in patients with unilateral brain disease. *Neuropsychologia, 12,* 183-191.

Berry, J.W. (1979). Culture and cognitive style. In A. Marsella, R. Tharp, & T. Ciborowsli (Eds.), *Perspectives on cross-cultural psychology* (pp. 117-135). New York: Academic Press.

Bondi, M.W., & Kaszniak, A.W. (1991). Implicit and explicit memory in Alzheimer's disease and Parkinson's disease. *Journal of Clinical and Experimental Neuropsychology, 13,* 339-358.

Brandt, J., & Butters, N. (1986). The neuropsychology of Huntington's disease. *Trends in Neuroscience, 9,* 118-120.

Butters, N., Sax, D.S., Montgomery, K., & Tarlow, S. (1978). Comparison of the neuropsychological deficits associated with early and advanced Huntington's disease. *Archives of Neurology, 35,* 585-589.

Cole, M., Gay, J., Glick, J., & Sharp, D. (1971). *The Cultural Context of Learning and Thinking.* New York: Basic Books.

Corkin, S. (1982). Some relationships between global amnesias and the memory impairments in Alzheimer's disease. In S. Corkin, K.L. Davis, J.H. Growdon, & E. Usdin (Eds.), *Alzheimer's disease: A report of progress in research* (pp. 149-164). New York: Raven Press.

Cummings, J.L. (1990). *Subcortical Dementia.* New York: Oxford University Press.

Finlayson, N.A., Johnson, K.A., & Reitan, R.M. (1977). Relation of level of education to neuropsychological measures in brain damaged and non-brain damaged adults. *Journal of Consulting and Clinical Psychology, 45,* 536-542.

Galasko, D., Salmon, D.P., Craig, U.-K., & Wiederholt, W.C. (2000). The clinical spectrum of Guam ALS and Parkinson-dementia complex; 1997-199. *Annals of the New York Academy of Sciences, 920,* 120-125.

Garruto, R.M. (1987). Neurotoxicity of trace and essential elements: Factors provoking the high incidence of motor neuron disease, Parkinsonism and dementia in the Western Pacific. In M. Gourie-Devi (Ed.), *Motor neuron disease: Global clinical patterns and international research* (pp. 73-82). New Delhi: Oxford and IBH Publishing.

Garruto, R.M., Yanagihara, R., Gajdusek, D.C., & Arion, D.M. (1984). Concentration of heavy metals and essential minerals in garden soil and drinking water in the Western Pacific. In K.M. Chen & Y. Yase (Eds.), *Amyotrophic Lateral Sclerosis in Asia and Oceania* (pp. 265-329). Taipei: National Taiwan University.

Glosser, G., Wolfe, N., Albert, M.L., Lavine, L., Steele, J.C., Calne, D.B., & Schoenberg, B.S. (1993). Cross-cultural cognitive examination: Validation of a dementia-screening instrument for neuroepidemiological research. *Journal of the American Geriatric Society, 41,* 931-939.

Heaton, R.K., Grant, I., & Matthews, C.G. (1986). Differences in neuropsychological test performance associated with age, education, and sex. In I. Grant & K. Adams (Eds.), *Neuropsychological assessment of neuropsychiatric disorders* (pp. 100-120). New York: Oxford University Press.

Hirano, A., Kurland, L.T., Krooth, R.S., & Lessell, S. (1961). Parkinsonism-dementia complex, an endemic disease on the island of Guam. I. Clinical features. *Brain, 84,* 642-661.

Hirano, A., Malamud, N., & Kurland, L.T. (1961). Parkinsonism-dementia complex, an endemic disease on the island of Guam. II. Pathological features. *Brain, 84,* 662-679.

Hodges, J.R., Patterson, K., & Tyler, L.K. (1994). Loss of semantic memory: Implications for the modularity of mind. *Cognitive Neuropsychology, 11,* 505-542.

Hof, P.R., Nimchinsky, E.A., Buee-Scherrer, V., Buee, L., Nasrallah, J., Hottinger, A.F., Purohit, D.P., Loerzel, A.J., Steele, J.C., Delacourte, A., Bouras, C., Morrison, J.H., & Perl, D.P. (1994). Amyotrophic lateral sclerosis/parkinsonism-dementia complex of Guam; quantitative neuropathology, immunohistochemical analysis of neuronal vulnerability, and comparison with related neurodegenerative disorders. *Acta Neuropathologica, 88,* 397-404.

Hyman, B.T., Van Hoesen, G.W., Damasio, A., & Barnes, C. (1984). Alzheimer's disease: Cell-specific pathology isolates the hippocampal formation. *Science, 225,* 1168-1170.

Kurland, L.T., Radhakrishnan, K., Williams, D.B., & Waring, S. (1994). Amyotrophic lateral sclerosis-parkinsonism-dementia complex on Guam: epidemiologic and etiological perspectives. In A.C. Williams (Ed.), *Motor neuron disease* (pp. 109-130). London: Chapman and Hall Medical.

Lafleche, G. & Albert, M.S. (1995). Executive function deficits in mild Alzheimer's disease. *Neuropsychology, 9,* 313-320.

Lavine, L., Steele, J.C., Wolfe, N., Calne, D.B., O'Brien, P.C., Williams, D.B., Kurland, L.T., & Schoenberg, B.S. (1991). Amyotrophic lateral sclerosis/parkinsonism-dementia complex in southern Guam: Is it disappearing? In L.P. Roland (Ed.), *Amyotrophic lateral sclerosis and other motor neuron diseases. Advances in Neurology, 56,* 271-285. New York: Raven Press.

Lecours, A., Mehler, J., Parente, M., Caldeira, A., Cary, L., Castro, M., Dehaout, F., Delgado, R., Gurd, J., Karmann, D., Jakubovitz, R., Osorio, Z., Cabral, L., & Junqueira, M. (1987). Illiteracy and brain damage: 1. Aphasia testing in culturally contrasted populations (control subjects). *Neuropsychologia, 25,* 231-245.

Martin, A. (1987). Representation of semantic and spatial knowledge in Alzheimer's patients: Implications for models of preserved learning in amnesia. *Journal of Clinical and Experimental Neuropsychology, 9,* 191-224.

Morris, R.G. (1996). Attentional and executive dysfunction. In R.G. Morris (Ed.), *The cognitive neuropsychology of Alzheimer-type dementia* (pp. 49-70). Oxford: Oxford University Press.

Moss, M.B. & Albert, M.S. (1988). Alzheimer's disease and other dementing disorders. In M.S. Albert & M.B. Moss (Eds.), *Geriatric neuropsychology* (pp. 145-178). New York: Guilford Press.

Nielson, K.A., Cummings, B.J., & Cotman, C.W. (1996). Constructional apraxia in Alzheimer's disease correlates with neuritic neuropathology in occipital cortex. *Brain Research, 741*, 284-293.

Oyanagi, K., Makifuchi, T., Ohtoh, T., Ikuta, F., Chen, K.-M., Chase, T.N., & Gajdusek, D.C. (1994). Topographic investigation of brain atrophy in Parkinson-dementia complex of Guam: A comparison with Alzheimer's disease and progressive supranuclear palsy. *Neurodegeneration, 3*, 301-304.

Parasuraman, R. & Haxby, J.V. (1993). Attention and brain function in Alzheimer's disease: A review. *Neuropsychology, 7*, 242-272.

Perl, D.P., Gajdusek, D.C., Garruto, R.M., Yanagihara, R., & Gibbs, C.J. (1982). Intraneuronal aluminum accumulation in amyotrophic lateral sclerosis and parkinsonism-dementia complex of Guam. *Science, 217*, 1053-1055.

Pick, A.D. (1980). Cognition: Psychological perspective. In H. Triandis & W. Lonner (Eds.), *Handbook of cross-cultural psychology: Basic processes, Vol. 3* (pp. 177-153). Boston: Allyn & Bacon.

Plato, C.C., Garruto, R.M., Fox, K.M., & Gajdusek, D.C. (1986). Amyotrophic lateral sclerosis and Parkinsonism-dementia on Guam: A 25-year prospective case-control study. *American Journal of Epidemiology, 124*, 643-656.

Reed, D.M. & Brody, J.A. (1975). Amyotrophic lateral sclerosis and Parkinsonism-dementia complex on Guam, 1945-1972. I. Descriptive epidemiology. *American Journal of Epidemiology, 101*, 287-301.

Reed, D.M., Torres, J.M., & Brody, J.A. (1975). Amyotrophic lateral sclerosis and Parkinsonism-dementia complex on Guam, 1945-1972. II. Familial and genetic studies. *American Journal of Epidemiology, 101*, 302-310.

Ritchie, K. (1988). The Screening of Cognitive Impairment in the Elderly: A Critical Review of Current Methods. *Journal of Clinical Epidemiology, 41*, 635-643.

Rosselli, M & Ardila, A. (1990). Neuropsychological assessment of illiterates: II. Language and praxic abilities. *Brain and Cognition, 12*, 281-296.

Salmon, D.P., Galasko, D., Craig, U.-K., San Nicolas, P., Gamst, A., & Wiederholt, W.C. (2000). *Patterns of neuropsychological deficits associated with Parkinson-dementia complex and Marianas dementia in the Chamorro population of Guam.* Submitted for publication.

Salmon, D.P. & Heindel, W.C. (1998). The effects of cortical and subcortical brain dysfunction on the cognitive presentation of dementing disorders. *Neuroscience News, 1*, 36-42.

Schmitt, F.A., Ranseen, J.D., & DeKosky, S.T. (1989). Cognitive Mental Status Examinations. *Clinics in Geriatric Medicine, 5*, 545-564.

Segall, M.H. (1986). Culture and behavior: Psychology in global perspective. *Annual Review of Psychology, 37*, 523-564.

Spencer, P.S., Nunn, P.B., Hugon, J., Ludolph, A., Ross, S.M., Roy, D.N., & Robertson, R.C. (1987). Guam amyotrophic lateral sclerosis-parkinsonism-dementia linked to a plant excitant neurotoxin. *Science, 237*, 517-522.

Spencer, P.S., Nunn, P.B., Hugon, J., Ludolph, A., & Roy, D.N. (1986). Motor neuron disease on Guam: Possible role of a food neurotoxin. *Lancet, ii*, 965.

Teng, E.L., Hasegawa, K., Homma, A., Imai, Y., Larson, E., Graves, A., Sugimoto, K., Yamaguchi, T., Sasaki, H., Chiu, D., & White, L.R. (1994). The Cognitive Abilities Screening Instrument (CASI): A practical test for cross-cultural epidemiological studies of dementia. *International Psychogeriatrics, 6*, 45-58.

Wiederholt, W.C., Galasko, D., Salmon, D.P., & Craig, U.-K. (1998). The utility of the Cognitive Abilities Screening Instrument (CASI) in the Chamorro population. *Neurobiology of Aging, 19* (Supplement), S9.

Chapter 8

CHALLENGES IN PROVIDING NEUROPSYCHOLOGICAL AND PSYCHOLOGICAL SERVICES IN GUAM AND THE COMMONWEALTH OF THE NORTHERN MARIANA ISLANDS (CNMI)

Frederick W. Bylsma, Ph.D.
Department of Psychiatry, University of Chicago, Chicago, Illinois

Catherine A. Ostendorf, M.A.
Private Practice, Chicago, Illinois

Pamina J. Hofer, Ph.D.
Private Practice, Guam and University of Guam, Guam

Abstract

The degree of westernization of the population on Guam is varied. The indigenous Chamorros (43.3% of the population) are now a minority due to the immigration of US military personnel and support staff, Filipinos, Micronesians, Chinese, Korean and Caucasians. While English has become the predominant common language, each ethnic group maintains its language within their own community. Cultural tensions are also prevalent. The population is predominantly literate and is of young average age. There is a wide variation in the degree of acceptance of western medicine and many, particularly indigenous, individuals may turn to the local traditional healer for treatment of illnesses of all kinds, particularly mental disorders. Neuropsychological service providers in Guam and the CNMI must be sensitive to all of these issues when providing service. Adding these factors to the more typical concerns of facility with the English language, degree of acculturation of the patient, and applicability of established test norms (typically of white, middle class, Caucasian, American origin) to the inhabitants of Guam makes the provision of adequate neuropsychological and psychological services a substantial challenge. Still, a small cadre of psychologists manages to provide academic assessments, forensic assessments, general clinical assessments, and appropriate treatments to both the indigenous and immigrant residents of the islands. This chapter will address how this is currently accomplished

Introduction

Almost exactly half way around the world from the mainland United States is a little-known bit of the U.S. – the Unincorporated Territory of Guam and the Commonwealth of the Northern Mariana Islands (comprised of Saipan, Rota, and Tinian). Residents of these islands are citizens of the U.S., although they don't vote in national elections. Representation in congress is limited to non-voting observer status, although both Guam and the CNMI lobby and make presentations. The CNMI has only held its Commonwealth status since 1975, however Guam has been a territory of the United States for in excess of 50 years. Across these islands, the degree of westernization of the population is extremely varied – from Rota, which was nearly untouched by WWII, is almost exclusively inhabited by indigenous Chamorros, and is relatively unspoiled, quiet and friendly, to Saipan and Guam, which are bustling mini-metropoli with everything from first-run movies to friendly arches. The percentage of the population which is indigenous varies from island to island, as well, with Guam housing only around 30% indigenous Chamorro while Saipan boasts 43%.

One commonality across these islands is that the indigenous Chamorro people are now a minority. An influx of U.S. military personnel and support staff, Filipinos, Japanese, Korean, Chinese, East Indian, Vietnamese, and Micronesians (from the 607 islands of Federated States of Micronesia, and the more than 1,000 coral islands of the Marshall Islands) has resulted in this state of affairs. While English has become the predominant common language, each ethnic group maintains its own language and customs. There are many individuals whose proficiency with English is below the level of the conversationally functional – or who do not speak English at all. Cross-cultural tensions are also prevalent. Still, the population is predominantly literate and is of young average age, although the older indigenous residents may have only 2 – 3 years of formal education.

Mental health services are quite well developed in some areas but less so in others. For instance, there are more numerous services available on Saipan than on Guam. Mental and physical health care is typically provided free of charge, primarily through government programs although private clinics are also available. Fee for service providers and thirdparty payers – including PPOs and HMOs – are becoming more prevalent as well. Inpatient and outpatient services as well as community outreach programs are provided, although the ease with which individuals can avail themselves of these services varies greatly, due to geographical distance, and to community customs and pressures. There is a wide variation in the degree of acceptance of western medicine, and many individuals – particularly the older indigenous persons – may turn to the local traditional healer or "suruhano" for treatment of illnesses of all kinds, particularly mental disorders (Wilson, 1980).

Psychological and neuropsychological service providers on Guam and the CNMI must be sensitive to all of these issues when providing service. There are also many aspects of the clinical encounter that must be attended to (Hinkle, 1994; Prediger, 1994), and cultural differences in the degree of personal disclosure to the clinician by the patient, and reciprocal disclosure by the clinician, must also be taken into account. Confidentiality of patient and encounter information is not always easy to maintain, for it is not unusual in the relatively closed communities for everyone to know everyone else, and to openly inquire about and discuss a patient's problems. In the same vein, care must be taken not to induce feelings of "shame" on the part of the patient in the eyes of the community. Therapeutic assessment techniques are a must, as most clients are the first in their family to ever receive mental health services. The length of the assessment is also important, as anything over two hours may be considered excessive. Adding these factors to the more typical concerns of facility with the English language, degree of acculturation of the patient, and applicability of established test norms (typically of white, middleclass, Caucasian-American origin) to the inhabitants of Guam and the CNMI makes the provision of adequate neuropsychological and psychological services a substantial challenge. Still, a small cadre of clinical psychologists and other mental health care providers manage to provide academic assessments, forensic assessments, general clinical assessments, and appropriate treatments to both the indigenous and immigrant residents of the islands.

The following service descriptions encompass, but are not exhaustive of, the available mental health and social service resources available to individuals in the CNMI and Guam since 1997. Many psychologists and psychiatrists perform several functions, and may work simultaneously for two or more of the listed mental health organizations. Staffing issues, including few appropriately trained professionals, a small and restricted number of available referral resources, and the lack of competent specialists to whom more complex cases can be referred, are prominent difficulties directly affecting daily clinical care of patients requiring mental health treatment. In addition, access to modern technological medicine which is taken for granted on the mainland USA – functional brain imaging with PET or SPECT techniques, modern EEG machines and methods, post traumatic-injury rehabilitation services – is quite restricted to residents of Guam and the CNMI, and may require expensive travel to Hawaii or the mainland. Specialty services, such as neuropsychological testing, neurological consultations and neuroimaging including CT and MRI structural brain or other internal imaging, are not immediately available in the CNMI unless specialists are brought to the islands and/or patients are sent to Guam.

Mental Health Activities on Guam

Information on mental health activities on Guam was limited, and in general, services are less well developed than in the CNMI. In 1997, the Guam Department of Mental Health and Substance Abuse had four part-time psychiatrists, 12 social workers and 26 other staff providing direct clinical care (Wilton, 1998). Currently, because of staff turnover and departures, there are fewer providers than there were in 1997. The Department currently employs one licensed clinical psychologist and three master-level service providers. The number of social workers and psychiatrists was not reported.

The Superior Court of Guam is a consumer of mental health services in conjunction with the adjudication of civil and criminal cases. The court has available a staff of three licensed clinical psychologists, two licensed master-level social workers, one master-level counselor, two master-level social workers, four part-time master-level social workers, two student interns, and one retired, master-level volunteer.

Information on other mental health resources and the qualifications of those providing services was limited. According to the Guam Board of Allied Health, there are six psychiatrists, three clinical psychologists, two counseling psychologists, and one counseling service offering masters-level social work mental health services in private practices. The Department of Education employs one masters-level school psychologist, but also offers Head Start programs, Children's Development Assistance Center (CDAC), and educational counseling through school counselors. The University of Guam offers masters-level training in educational testing, counseling, and mental health career training, and job placement assistance through three counseling staff. With regard to the mental health training programs, it should be noted though, that this a free-access University with no academic entrance requirements, not even facility with English (the language of instruction). As such many of the students graduating with degrees from the University of Guam would not likely be considered for acceptance in mainland colleges or universities. The University has recently been placed on provisional accreditation status by the Western Association of Schools and Colleges (WASC).

Mental Health Activities in the Commonwealth of the Northern Mariana Islands

The CNMI Department of Public Health, Division of Mental Health and Social Services has provided mental health services in five major areas since 1999: community mental health, behavioral health, addiction treatment, illness prevention and research, and mental health provider training. Typically, either a licensed psychiatrist or a licensed psychologist manages each of the three major clinical service teams and is assisted by nurses, other licensed mental health counselors, licensed therapists, social workers and/or substance abuse specialists. The majority of the *licensed* professionals are from mainland United States and Canada, whereas more of the social workers and substance abuse specialists are indigenous residents who have been trained locally. All members -- licensed or not -- provide direct services to individuals in the community.

Mental health resources and services in the CNMI have become more numerous and prominent over the last two decades. Resources have expanded from one main federal grant funded institution -- whose clinical encounters were described as "teaching" ones (Wilson, 1980) -- to several local and federally supported services, non-profit entities, and privately-funded operations that provide a wide variety of mental health care services. Prior to 1980, there was one psychiatrist, one psychologist, and six registered nurse mental health coordinators providing services to the entire Trust Territory of the Pacific Islands through the Department of Health Services, Division of Mental Health (Wilson, 1980). As of 1999, the CNMI Department of Pubic Health, Division of Mental Health and Social Services continues to provide the bulk of mental health services, but these are now buttressed by other psychiatrists, psychologists, social workers and mental health counselors who work for other CNMI government agencies, Federal agencies, non-profit entities, or privately funded organizations.

These operations service the general community on the islands of Saipan, Tinian, and Rota. The Division also provides clinical services for other local and federal government agencies. Each agency's operation has one manager and several team members that provide specific services to specific identified populations within the community. For example, the community mental health team, behavioral health team, and addiction services teams each provide specific clinical services to individuals in the community that require them. Educational services are provided by both the prevention services and addiction services teams, although most health care professionals also incorporate some form of education within their clinical encounters or through public speaking engagements or invited addresses.

The community mental health team provides services for the chronically mentally ill population, through an inpatient treatment facility for acutely ill individuals, and an outpatient medication management program for all Division of Mental Health patients. The team organization includes a psychiatrist as the manager, a community mental health nurse, a recreational therapist, and a social worker/case manager.

The behavioral health team provides outpatient psychological assessment and counseling. The organization is divided into three areas of practice: intake assessment of individuals new to the behavioral health system, continuing outpatient care for adult patients, and continuing outpatient child and family care. The intake team is lead by a coordinator and involves three social workers. The adult care team, lead by a licensed clinical psychologist, involves two mental health counselors and one child-and-family therapist. The child and family team is led by a licensed clinical psychologist and includes one mental health counselor and two child and family therapists.

The addiction services team consists of a manager, an addictions specialist, a community prevention specialist, three "professionals" who specialize in the treatment of substance abuse patients, and two assistants (information above provided by the CNMI Government, 1997, 1999).

A limited number of private practice mental health professionals are available at present. Currently, there are two licensed clinical psychologists and one psychiatrist that provide psychological and psychiatric assessments, counseling, and consultative services. Typically, their clients are local and federal government agencies through contractual work, and to a lesser extent to private individuals. Recently, self-help support groups have begun in the CNMI. There are several independent groups including Alcoholics Anonymous, AL-ANON, S.A.F.E (support group for adult survivors of sexual abuse), Rally for Life Association (for families of suicide victims), and Young Christian Life (Ayuda Network, 1997).

Other human resource operations in the CNMI provide primarily assessment, social services and/or religious, supportive or educational counseling services to the public. The Commonwealth Health Center Social Services Department provides psychosocial assessments, social services and counseling. The Children's Developmental Assistance Center (CDAC) provides infant screening, counseling and education for high-risk cases and children with developmental disabilities. The Public School system offers Head Start programs on each island, early childhood special education programs, educational assessments by an educational psychologist and supportive and school counseling through counselors located at each school. The Department of

Community and Cultural Affairs, Division of Youth services offers social services, counseling, and education to victims of child abuse, neglect, and domestic violence, and also intervene in cases of delinquency and school truancy. Northern Mariana College offers educational testing and educational counseling services. Karidat, formerly CNMI Catholic Social Services, offers social services to victims of crime and the indigent, as well as offering youth programs and a crisis hotline. Several churches offer theological and supportive counseling. Critical incident (disaster) crisis counseling is offered through the Northern Mariana Islands American Red Cross. The Commonwealth Health Center also supports a HIV/AIDS and sexually transmitted disease section that offers testing and disease-specific counseling. Other organizations provide social services to the public are the Carolinian Affairs office, Department of Public Safety, Northern Mariana Protection and Advocacy System, the CNMI and Federal court systems, and the CNMI Public Defender's office (Ayuda Network, 1997).

Staffing Problems Common to Guam and the CNMI

Much has been accomplished over the last 20 years and the expansion of human resource services has broadened the once primarily teaching-oriented encounters to more clinical patient-service oriented practices. There is much yet to be done (Untalan & Comacho, 1997) to ensure adequate and consistent access to mental health services here, though. Often, the economy, and influx and outflow of professionals influence mental health resources both in the CNMI and on Guam. Though resources have become more numerous and prominent since the 1980s, the availability of daily clinical care continues to be influenced by staffing issues, few available referral resources and the lack of specialists. Often, a single psychologist or psychiatrist may serve on several government committees related to health care, service many populations on different islands, and hold several positions across several provider organizations. It is not uncommon for one psychologist to work for one agency and provide services through that agency to other agencies, privately funded operations and non-profit organizations while serving on several community boards. For example, only two psychiatrists, one at the Department of Public Health, Division of Mental Health and Social Services and the other in private practice, service the entire CNMI population.

As such, when a single psychologist, psychiatrist or licensed therapist/counselor retires or leaves the islands, several provider services suffer, referral choices become markedly limited, and case loads for the remaining providers become larger. Often, services are placed on hold, patients are placed on waiting lists and/or the service is not offered until the vacancy has been filled. These repercussions from a vacancy may persist for months until a qualified candidate is found. For instance, the success of a recent government early-retirement program resulted in the loss of most of the Mental Health

Counselors at a free mental health clinic in Guam. This resulted in a communication by the Department of Mental Health and Substance Abuse to school counselors that individuals in crisis should no longer be referred to the clinic because there were very few counselors left to treat the patients.

Neuropsychological Services on Guam and the CNMI

The providing of neuropsychological assessment services to residents of Guam and the CNMI requires attention to all of the details as noted above, in addition to many that are more specific to neuropsychology. First, there are very few psychologists who have had training specifically in neuropsychology, but many who claim to provide neuropsychological services. This is, in part, due to the small number of available trained providers for a large number of patients spread over a large geographical area, but also in part to individuals practicing beyond the scope of their training. (This is not unique to provision of neuropsychological services).

The current training programs for mental health providers at the University of Guam – currently only Bachelor of Arts and Master of Arts degrees – do not allow graduates sufficient exposure to the theory and practice of clinical assessment. The psychologists on Guam and the CNMI do have available a large number of currently used standardized assessment instruments for both cognitive and psychological status (Table 1). In their undergraduate training, students may learn *about* current testing instruments, but are given

Table 1. Standardized tests of neuropsychological and psychological functioning that are in use by psychologists in Guam and the CNMI.

Neuropsychological and Cognitive Assessment Instruments

Adult	*Child*
Booklet Category Test	Conner's Continuous Performance Test
Finger Tapping Test	Developmental Test of Visual Motor Integration (VMI)
Test of Nonverbal Intelligence-3 (TONI-3)	Kaufman Assessment Battery for Children
Wechsler Memory Scale-III (WMS-III)	Test of Nonverbal Intellegence-3 (TONI-3)
Hand Dynamometer	Wechsler Individual Achievement Test (WIAT)
Tactile Perception Test (TPT)	Wechsler Intelligence Scale for Children-R (WISC-R)
Rey Complex Figure Test (CFT)	Wide Range Achievement Test-3 (WRAT-III)
Wechsler Adult Intelligence Scales-III (WAIS-III)	Bender Gestalt
Wide Range Achievement Test-3 (WRAT-III)	Bergance
Wisconsin Card Sorting Test	California Verbal Learning Test-Child version

Table 1, continued.

Grooved Pegboard	Children's Auditory Verbal Learning Test (CAVLT)
Developmental Test of Visual Motor Integration (VMI)	Children's Trail Making Test
Benton Visual Retention Test	Children's Booklet Category Test
Cognistat	Comprehensive Test of Nonverbal Intelligence
Comprehensive Test of Nonverbal Intelligence	Speech sounds/Seashore rhythm
Controlled Oral Word Association Test	Aphasia Screen/Sensory Perception
Dementia Rating Scale (DRS)	KTEA Achievement
Aphasia Screen/Sensory Perception	Leiter Battery
Trail Making Test	Mullen Scales of Early learning
Peabody Individual Achievement Test-R	NEPSY
Raven's Progressive Matrices	Peabody Individual Achievement Test-R
Repeatable Episodic Memory Test	Peabody Individual Picture Vocabulary Test
Stroop Color/Word	Raven's Colored Progressive Matrices
Wechsler Adult Intelligence Scale-R	Stanford Binet
Woodcock Johnson Basic and Battery	Test of Oral Language Development-3 Extended (TOLD-3)
	Wechsler Intelligence Scale for Children-III
	Woodcock Johnson Basic and Supplemental

Psychological Assessment Tests

Adult	*Child*
Minnesota Multiphasic Personality Inventory (MMPI-II)	Minnesota Multiphasic Personality Inventory – Adolescent (MMPI-A)
Rorschach Test	Conner's Rating Scales-Revised
Thematic Apperception Test	Adolescent Drinking INDE scale
Substance Abuse Subtle Screening Inventory	Attention Deficit Disorders Evaluation Scale
16 PF	Behavioral Assessment for Children
Beck Depression Inventory	CAT (animal) and (human)
Brief Symptom Inventory	Child Behavior Checklist
Forer Structured Sentence Completion	Childhood Autism Rating Scale
Marital Evaluation Checklist	Children's Depression Inventory
MCMI-III	Developmental History Checklist
Personal History and Problems Inventory	Developmental Profile II
Psychosocial Pain Inventory	Forer Structured Sentence Completion
Roger's Criminal Responsibility Assessment Scale	HTP/DAP
Sentence Completion	MACI
State-Trait Anxiety Inventory	Parenting Stress Index
	Personality Inventory for Children
	Preschool Behavioral Checklist
	Revised Behavioral Problem Checklist
	Rotter Sentence Completion
	State-Trait Anxiety Inventory for Children
	Stress Index Parents of Adolescents

limited hands-on experience in their administration or interpretation in clinical settings. Some exposure is given to Mental Health Interns on the island of Saipan, though. This process, however, does not afford students sufficient opportunity to become sufficiently skillful at clinical-test administration and interpretation at the time of graduation.

Persons performing neuropsychological assessments in the Northern Mariana Islands must consider many cultural factors when conducting evaluations (Hinkle, 1994; Loewenstein *et al.*, 1994; Mayer & Bauman, 1986; Prediger, 1994). For example, most measures developed on the mainland U.S. include questions regarding seasons, which are inappropriate (or, at least foreign) to tropical-dwelling residents. If the client *can* accurately answer the query, this is a likely indication of either higher intellect or greater geographical experience than typical for this level question for persons in the indigenous Guamanian population. Care must be taken when attempting to use technology-based test equipment with the indigenous patients. The use of computers and other typical mechanical devices such as tape recorders or timers, may make the patient quite afraid and they may "freeze," and no longer co-operate with the examiner. The provision of snacks or drinks as reinforcement for continued co-operation is often necessary. Other aspects of the clinical setting are important, and complicating for the examiner who attempts to follow mainland test administration techniques when assessing the indigenous patient. First, it is imperative that you sit beside them, not across from them. Having a table between you and the patient will not be tolerated. Ways must be devised to provide the patient and the examiner each a work area without placing any "barriers" between them. Also, patients are likely to bring their children to the clinic visit, so having the resources to provide childcare while the assessment is going on is often necessary (although the children can be helpful sources of collateral information at times!).

The range of clinical conditions that the neuropsychologist on Guam and the CNMI is typically asked to evaluate is no less diverse than on the mainland. In fact, due to the lack of qualified specialists and specialty clinics (*e.g.*, memory clinic, schizophrenia clinic, head-injury clinic, *etc.*), a wider range of patients might be encountered. Despite the tourist brochures that suggest an idyllic life style, the people of the islands are quite hard-working and high-pressured, and stroke- and MI-prone individuals abound. In addition, there are few "mild" injuries that result in an individual visiting a mental health clinic. Moderate to severe head injuries in adults and children are common, and many result from falling from the back of moving pick-up trucks (a favorite local means of transportation). Dementia due to vascular disease and to primary progressive conditions, such as Alzheimer's disease, is also often seen. Other neurological conditions such as Parkinson's disease and amytrophic lateral sclerosis (ALS) are also encountered. The sequelae of chronic alcohol abuse and dependence may also bring a patient to the clinic for assessment. Psychiatric disorders such as depression, bipolar disorder or schizophrenia are also encountered. Suicide is also prevalent. School truancy, delinquency, and teen pregnancy are also prevalent.

Evaluating the client's claims and statements about personal medical history is also an area in which cultural awareness is imperative. For example, most interviews include some question of alcohol usage. Most evaluators on the U.S. mainland are aware of their clients' propensity to diminish their actual level of drinking. However, an Asian male is far more likely to exaggerate his alcohol usage. Additionally, most mainland evaluators would accept a response of "I only drink socially" to mean the individual seldom drinks. "Social occasions" where alcohol is prolific are at least a weekend, and sometimes a daily, occurrence in the islands. One local custom dictates a more than two-week wake-like period of mourning after a death (referred to simply as "the Rosary"), and another typical social occasion is the huge adult get-togethers to celebrate an infant's birthday, and significant alcohol consumption is prevalent at each. Anecdotally, one of my (PH) favorite responses to, *What does this saying mean: "One swallow doesn't mean a summer?"* was *"One drink doesn't mean a party."*

Even so-called "culture-free," non-verbal measures of intellectual potential (IQ) typically demand top-down, left-to right visual processing in order to accurately complete the sequences. Many Asian-educated residents of Guam and the CNMI scan top-down, right to left. Additionally, persons who have little formal education are frequently found to be bottom-up processors. Also, many individuals are bilingual or multilingual, with English being a second or third acquired language. The majority of neuropsychological assessment instruments available to psychologists on Guam and the CNMI were developed on the mainland with middle-class Caucasian individuals with an average education as the target population, and with normative data typically derived from a group of such people. Thus, while facility with the English language of the average indigenous Guamanian resident may be adequate for casual conversation, it is not likely to be at the level typically expected for good performance on current neurocognitive tasks. Often, despite completing formal education, a person's functional level in English is well below the grade level attained. As such, the normative data in manuals for those tests is relatively useless for helping the clinician interpret test data generated by typical patients in Guam or the CNMI. The clinician must rely more on clinical impressions, and an acquired, experience-based knowledge about how the indigenous peoples perform these tasks in order to interpret a given person's performance. There have been some attempts to gather normative data for the indigenous populations of Guam and the CNMI, but even those data are largely lacking in scientific rigor. Often the data are based upon convenience samples of patients, and not population-stratified normal non-patient samples from the community. Currently, more rigorous studies are under way to establish normative data for two standardized tests – the *Comprehensive Test of Nonverbal Intelligence* (computerized format), and the *Woodcock-Johnson Revised Tests of Achievement*. However, clinically applicable data will not be available for some time, and will leave many more tests that require culturally appropriate normative data.

Guam has one of the first laws allowing psychologists to prescribe, administer, and dispense *any* licensed medications, and some psychologists are doing so. There are as yet no established criteria for required minimal training by psychologists in psychopharmacology. The Guam Department of Education is currently employing two individuals who have yet to complete their *undergraduate* education to administer, score and interpret – without supervision – tests administered to individuals requiring special education and accommodations in the school system. As such, some of the violations of minimal training guidelines, that are more strictly adhered to on the mainland, are due to systemic issues related to providing much-needed services without adequate numbers of qualified providers, and may not reflect the conscious actions and desires of the junior practitioners themselves.

Lastly, neuropsychologists on Guam and the CNMI are no less likely to encounter difficulty in receiving payment for or authorization for assessment services they provide. This may be one of the few things that neuropsychologists on the mainland USA and their counterparts on Guam and the CNMI have in common in attempting to provide services to their patients.

Conclusion

In providing clinical service to the culturally and ethnically varied population of Guam and the CNMI, neuropsychologists, clinical psychologists and other mental health providers are likely to encounter numerous challenges. That environment presents challenges due to language, cultural and societal expectations, challenges to confidentiality of findings, modified testing situations, use of tests with culturally and even geographically inappropriate items, and inapplicable or unavailable normative data. In this microcosm are all of the things that might go wrong with a given patient on the mainland. However, these challenges are a daily struggle for providers on Guam and the CNMI, and they are to be applauded for their efforts and treatment successes in spite of them. Clearly, the neuropsychological community – providers and those who develop and market testing materials – must attend more to cultural variations, and strive to provide better and more easily applicable instruments to those practitioners who ply their trade in any place other than the mainland United States.

References

Ayuda Network (1997). *An alliance of human/social service providers, Common-wealth of the Northern Mariana Islands, 1997 Directory.* Commonwealth of the Northern Mariana Islands: Ayuda.

Commonwealth of the Northern Mariana Islands Government (1997, 1999). Structural and functional chart for the CNMI Department of Public Health, Division of Mental Health and Social Services.

Hinkle J.S. (1994). Practitioners and cross-cultural assessment: A practical guide to information and training. *Measurement and Evaluation in Counseling and Development, 27,* 103-115.

Loewenstein, D.A., Arguelles, T., Arguelles, S., & Linn-Fuentes, P. (1994). Potential cultural bias in the neuropsychological assessment of the older adult. *Journal of Clinical and Experimental Neuropsychology, 16,* 623-629.

Mayer, P.A., & Bauman, K.A. (1986). Health practices, problems, and needs in a population of Micronesian adolescents. *Journal of Adolescent Health Care, 7,* 338-341, 1986.

Prediger, D.L. (1994). Multicultural assessment standards: A compilation for counselors. *Measurement and Evaluation in Counseling and Development, 27,* 68-73.

Untalan, F.F., & Comacho, J.M. (1997). Children of Micronesia. In G. Johnson-Powell, J. Yamammoto (Eds.). *Transcultural child development: Psychological assessment and treatment.* New York: John Wiley & Sons, Inc. (pp 305-327).

Wilson, L.G. (1980). Community psychiatry in Oceana: Fifteen months' experience in Micronesia. *Social Psychology, 15,* 175-179.

Wilton, N.M. (1998). Survey conducted on the *Legal Aspects of Mental Health Care in Guam.* Unpublished manuscript.

PART IV

HISPANIC / LATINO

Chapter 9

CURRENT ISSUES IN NEUROPSYCHOLOGICAL ASSESSMENT WITH HISPANICS/LATINOS

Alfredo Ardila
Memorial Regional Hospital, Hollywood, Florida

Gerardo Rodríguez-Menéndez
Carlos Albizu University, Miami, Florida

Mónica Rosselli
Florida Atlantic University, Davie, Florida

Abstract

In this chapter, initially an analysis of cultural and linguistic issues on Hispanics will be presented. Major difficulties with translations and using interpreters, and cultural attitudes toward testing will be analyzed. This will be followed by a presentation of the neuropsychological instruments available in Spanish for children, adults, and the elderly. Final conclusions and general recommendations will then be presented.

What is a Hispanic/Latino?

Neuropsychological assessment with Hispanic populations entails a complex process due in part to variability among subjects in terms of linguistic

(Spanish/English) competence, heterogeneity of Latino culture, and differences in cultural assimilation in the U.S. To gain an understanding of the
intricacies underlying the neuropsychological assessment of Latinos, one must
first begin by defining the parameters of the term "Hispanic".

Webster's New Collegiate Dictionary defines the term Hispanic as relating to the people, speech or culture of Spain, Spain and Portugal, or Latin
America. The *Diccionario de la Lengua Española* (The Dictionary of the
Spanish Language, 1984) edited by the Royal Spanish Academy, defines the
word Hispanic as pertaining to (or relative to) Spain or the nations of Latin
America. There is a basic agreement in terminology even though according
to the New Collegiate Dictionary Portugal and Brazil would be included
as Hispanic nations. The Current Population Survey (U.S. Census Bureau,
1997) defines the concept of Hispanic Origin noting, "Persons of Hispanic
origin, in particular, are those who indicated that their origin was Mexican-
American, Chicano, Mexican, Puerto Rican, Cuban, Central or South American, or other Hispanic." It behooves the practitioner to note that persons
from some Caribbean countries generally prefer to be called "Hispanics",
whereas those of Mexico, Central or South American origin generally preferred to be called "Latinos", because they identify themselves as "Latin
Americans". Throughout this chapter, the terms Hispanic and Latino will be
used interchangeably.

Once having defined the term Hispanic, it also becomes important to discuss what a Hispanic is not. The word Hispanic should not be confused as
constituting a particular race. In the U.S. it has become increasingly common to refer to Hispanics as a separate racial entity (e.g., Whites or Caucasians, Blacks and Hispanics). This trend is partially attributable to the growing constituency of Hispanics on the U.S. mainland. The word Hispanic is
more correctly used to denote a general ethnicity. Hispanics can be of any
race: Caucasian, Black, Mongolian, or mixtures thereof (U.S. Census Bureau,
1999). It makes no more sense to regard Hispanics/Latinos as constituting a
separate race than it would to regard all persons in North America as having
one racial identity.

Demographic Variables

Similarly to the U.S., the peoples of the Spanish Caribbean, Mexico, Central
and South America represent an international melting pot of cultural, racial,
and ethnic identities. Interestingly, the U.S. is the fifth largest Spanish-speaking country in the world (following Mexico, Spain, Colombia and Argentina).
According to the U.S. Census Bureau (1998) the total Latino/Hispanic population of the U.S. currently accounts for over 29 million people (11% of
the total U.S. population). Of these Hispanics, 63% are of Mexican origin,
14.4% are of other Central and South American origin, 10.6% are mainland
Puerto Ricans (persons residing in the Commonwealth of Puerto Rico are

not included in these statistics), 4.2% are of Cuban ancestry, and 7.4% are classified as being of "Other origin". By 2050, the U.S. Hispanic population is projected to comprise one quarter of the nation's total population (U.S. Bureau of the Census, 1997). Taking into account not only the significant number of Spanish-speakers, but also the fact that there is one Spanish-speaking US Associate State (Puerto Rico), the US can be regarded to a certain extent as a Latin American country and as partially Spanish-speaking country. Spanish, however, is not socially, academically, economically, and politically at the same level as English and frequently is maintained as a marginal language. Native Spanish speakers are usually required to speak English at work and in general everyday activities. Children attend English-speaking schools. Spanish books are very limited, and in general cultural activities in Spanish are scarce. Psychological and neuropsychological services provided in Spanish are limited.

History and Current Status of Neuropsychology with Hispanics/Latinos

Neuropsychology in Latin America has a marked European influence. Its roots date back to the 1950s when Carlos Mendilaharsu created a division devoted to the analysis of the higher cortical functions at the Montevideo Neurological Institute (Uruguay). During the 1960s and 1970s, a growing interest in neuropsychology was observed in Latin America, particularly in Peru and Mexico (for a review on the history of neuropsychology in Latin America, see Ardila, 1990). The International Congress of Neuropsychology held in Bogota (August, 1981), and attended by over 700 people from 14 countries, represented a decisive milestone in the development of neuropsychology in Latin America. This was a historical meeting because it allowed its participants to become aware of each other's work, it facilitated the interchange of ideas at several levels, and it provided the groundwork for the development of a formal organization of Latin American neuropsychologists. During the following years, a *Boletín* of the emerging Latin American Society of Neuropsychology was published. The *Sociedad Latinoamericana de Neuropsicología* (SLAN) was formally founded in 1989.

During the 1983 Meeting of the International Neuropsychological Society (INS) held in Mexico City, a group of Latin American representatives proposed the creation of a Latin American Branch of the INS. It was further proposed during that meeting that a joint new journal in neuropsychology be developed, however, it never materialized

During the 1980s and 1990s in Latin America, over half a dozen graduate programs were developed (e.g., Mexico, Colombia, Argentina) in neuropsychology. In 1995 the first issue of *Neuropsychologia Latina* was published jointly by the *Sociedad Latinoamericana de Neuropsicología, Sociedad Catalana de Neuropsicología, Sociedade Brasilera de Neuropsicología*, and *Asociaçao Portuguesa de Neuropsicología*.

In 1999 a second Latin American society, the *Asociación Latinoamericana de Neuropsicología* (ALAN) was created. The *Asociacíon* ALAN, jointly with the *Asociacíon Colombiana de Neuropsicología, Sociedad Neuropsicologica Antioqueña* and the Antioquia Neuroscience Center (Colombia) proceeded in April 1999 to publish the journal *Neuropsicología, Neuropsiquiatria y Neurociencias*.

During the last 20 years, a tremendous effort has been devoted, especially in Colombia and Mexico to the development and normalization of neuropsychological instruments (e.g., Ardila, Rosselli, & Puente, 1994; Ostrosky, Ardila, & Rosselli, 1999). Today in Latin American, most of basic neuropsychological tests have local norms (see below).

Since the advent of neuropsychology and behavioral neurology as professional activities in the U.S., Hispanics have been actively participating in the field. Joaquín Fuster, Ismael Mena, Alberto Galaburda, Antonio Puente, and Mario Mendez are examples of this involvement of Hispanics in the behavioral neurosciences.

Limitations of Current Neuropsychological Tests with Latinos

Problems Encountered With Bilingualism

As previously mentioned, the issue of bilingualism must be addressed by the neuropsychologist, in order to understand the nuances inherent in the assessment of Hispanics/Latinos. As noted by Pontón and Ardila (1999) whereas Spanish or English monolingualism facilitates the assessment of cognitive faculties, bilingualism does not. A question of immense research potential is: how does bilingualism affect neuropsychological performance? The possible interaction effects are highly diverse, given that bilingualism comprises many shades within a wide linguistic spectrum.

The concept of bilingualism has been approached along a variety of dimensions. For example, Earle (1967) introduced the concept of compound bilingualism (an individual who learns more than one language in a sequential fashion) vs. coordinate bilingualism (the learning of two languages simultaneously). For our purposes (relative to the English and Spanish languages) it helps to understand the concept of balanced bilingualism (Albert & Obler, 1978). According to this paradigm, at one extreme of the bilingual spectrum is the individual who is Spanish-dominant, and has limited proficiency in English. At the other extreme is the English-dominant bilingual who has a limited mastery of Spanish. Individuals at both extremes, while bilingual, would be regarded as unbalanced, in that their education is lacking in a given area of oral or (more commonly) written language competency. An individual at the middle of the continuum would be considered a balanced bilingual, having mastery over all language modalities in both languages.

It should be noted that the positions on the continuum occupied by the clinician and patient may be either congruent or incongruent. In the former case both the practitioner and the client occupy adjacent positions along the continuum (e.g., both are balanced, or are unbalanced toward the same extreme). In the latter case, the clinician and patient are on opposite sides of the spectrum (e.g., the clinician may be Spanish-dominant and have limited English mastery, whereas the patient may be English-dominant with some Spanish mastery or vice-versa). There will be a greater chance of increased error variance.

Linguistic Aspects

As noted by Cuellar (1998) neuropsychological assessment has failed to discern the powerful role of culture in the assessment of psychological functioning. The field as a whole has largely ignored the importance of ethnicity, culture, language, and education, erroneously assuming that such variables have little effect on cognitive processes.

To further complicate the issue of neuropsychological assessment with Hispanics, regionalisms or vernacular idiosyncrasies with respect to vocabulary exist in the use of Spanish. This is valid with any large language, such as English, Chinese and Russian. Realize that Spanish is the primary language spoken in at least nineteen countries within the Western Hemisphere. Given the expansive geographic distribution and the huge number of speakers (some 400 million), regionalisms in vocabulary usage are common. For example, in virtually every Spanish speaking country, the word for orange is "naranja". However, in Puerto Rico, the word for orange is "china" (pronounced "cheé-nah"). The word "china" in Spanish-speaking countries refers to the nation of China or to the Chinese; whereas in Puerto Rico the word can have either meaning (orange or China). A Puerto-Rican colleague was testing a Cuban child and used the word "china", meaning to ask, "In what way are an orange and a banana alike?" Instead the child understood "In what way is a Chinese woman and a banana alike?" To which the child quickly responded, "Chinese women eat bananas!" leaving the examiner a bit bewildered.

Each country will also have its own slang terms which are commonly used in conversational speech. The meanings of words such as "chévere" (nice, good), and "chin-chin" (expression used when toasting) will not be found in a standard Spanish dictionary. The meanings will only be gained through inquiry and cultural exposure. Moreover, at times even apparently innocuous words in most Hispanic cultures can be associated with vulgar profanity in others. Such regionalisms will no doubt cause perplexing, albeit humorous moments in assessment and/or psychotherapy. Due to limited space, however, this aspect will not be explored further in the current chapter.

Acculturation

Culture includes behaviors, beliefs, values, and cultural elements. Patterns of behavior of Hispanics living in the US tend to become progressively more similar to traditional middle-American standards. Beliefs and values (i.e., the values system and the interpretation of the world) also tend to progressively be more similar to the English speakers. Most Hispanics living in the US present mixed patterns of behaviors and make attempts to integrate the Latin values with the traditional middle American values. Sometimes, integration is not easy, and conflict can result.

Differences between English and Latin cultures affect not only the way to approach the purpose of life, the general interpretation of the world, and the style to relate with other people, but also the way of behaving during a medical or psychological exam. Further, English-speakers have usually grown up with a very intensive training in testing. For them usually it is evident that testing is a challenge, he or she must perform at best, and speed may be crucial. For Hispanics, it may be more important establishing a good rapport than performing well. It may be significant to have the opportunity to talk and exchange ideas. The personal relationship with the examiner may be more important than the results. Speed may be not so important: Good products are usually the result of a careful process, and quality and rush may be contradictory. Because of these differences, Hispanics frequently do not feel totally comfortable with English-speaking examiners. Flexible approaches in testing can be more successful with Hispanic clients.

Hispanic culture in the U.S. is strongly linked to the Spanish language. The use of the Spanish language is frequently perceived as a kind of Hispanic cultural identification. Spanish and English usually represent everyday languages, and mixtures can be anticipated. A phenomenon can occur that Cobos (1983) has referred to as the "Hispanicizing" of English terms. Examples include "washetera" (laundry mat); "carpeta" (carpet), "norsa" (nurse), "troca" (truck) and "el parking" (parking lot). The most blatant examples of Hispanicized English occurs among second-generation Hispanics who are members of the lower socioeconomic status. According to the American Council on Education, 1996 high school completion rates among 18 to 24 year old Hispanics (57.5%) lagged far behind those of African Americans (75.3%), and Non-Hispanic Whites (82.3%). Concurrently, Hispanics had the highest dropout rate (30%) of the three major ethnic groups (Wilds & Wilson, 1998). For many individuals who fail to receive a rudimentary education in either English or Spanish, an inevitable outcome is that many Hispanics live in a linguistic twilight in which neither language is completely mastered across basic language modalities (i.e., articulation, vocabulary, reading, spelling, literature, and composition). Hispanicized English also occurs among second-generation Hispanics in higher socioeconomic levels who feel pressured to assimilate the dominant culture. Moreover, in both the former and latter cases, such persons will often resort to using what has been dubbed as "Spanglish", a form of Spanish-English using blends and code switchings. When a word (or an expression) is more retrievable in one language as compared to another, code-switching is triggered. For example, "Más tarde te encontraré en el amusement park" (I'll meet you later at the amusement park). Interestingly, this phenomenon occurs among the educated and uneducated alike. It is not uncommon for the media to exploit such linguistic blends in the promotion of commercial products for public usage (e.g., "Las mejores cheeseburgers!"; "Mudanzas and deliveries").

Normative Variables

As noted by Cervantes and Acosta (1992), the lack of published studies on the use of existing neuropsychological tests for Hispanics is a neglected area which will assume critical importance in the coming years, given the increasing numbers of Latinos in the U.S. It is not uncommon to find clinicians engaging in the practice of using poorly translated instruments with Hispanic subjects and scoring protocols with norms designed for the U.S. mainstream. Neuropsychological evaluations performed without adequate psychometric instruments and standardized norms are likely to be fraught with error. It is all the more disturbing that such practices are being used to determine the nature and extent of brain injury in rehabilitative and forensic settings (e.g., workman's compensation, Social Security disability evaluations, criminal and civil court litigation).

López and Romero (1988) note that the practice of translating tests during simultaneous administration constitutes an ethical violation and should therefore not be undertaken. According to the Standards for Educational and Psychological Testing (American Educational Research Association, American Psychological Association, National Council on Measurement in Education, 1996), "When a test is translated from one language or dialect to another, its reliability and validity for the uses intended in the linguistic groups to be tested should be established" (Standard 13.4, p. 75).

Given the complexities of bilingualism and culture among Hispanics, the problem of obtaining representative normative samples arises. As noted by Ardila, Rosselli, and Puente (1994) while over 3,000 articles on neuropsychological assessment were published during the 1980s, fewer than 20 dealt with subject variables (apart from age and education). This problem is compounded by a dearth of adequate translations of neuropsychological instruments and the development of normative scales for Spanish speakers. Whereas the Halstead-Reitan and the Luria-Nebraska Neuropsychological Batteries have been translated into Spanish, these works represent pioneering efforts and by no means contain representative normative data for the various Hispanic/Latino cultures found in the U.S. Furthermore, Ponton and Ardila (1999) cite that the current trend is to translate English tests into Spanish as a means of assessing cognitive functioning. The authors note that a number of potentially faulty assumptions are inherently made using this approach. Specifically, (a) existing tests are the best predictors of the domain to be measured, regardless of cultural context, (b) exact translations provide an equivalent measure of a given domain as assessed in the original language, and (c) psychometric properties of the original test will transfer along with the items into the new language. Ardila (1995) advances the position that culture determines what is and is not contextually relevant. Hence, emphasis must be placed on the development of culturally

appropriate measures as opposed to the mere exercise of obtaining translations of widely used tests.

Professional Qualifications

Whenever possible, the neuropsychological evaluation of a Hispanic/Latino
client should be performed by a qualified bilingual (Spanish/English) clinician. Whereas the federal courts require that an interpreter pass a proficiency
examination as a necessary condition for employment, no such qualification
process is legally required to administer psychological tests. As previously
noted, bilingualism is a complex phenomenon which may be conceived as
a continuum of language mastery. Presently, it is therefore left to the clinicians' ethical and professional judgement as to whether they are linguistically
competent to perform bilingual neuropsychological assessments in Spanish
and English. We foresee the need to create a proficiency examination at the
national level to ensure that Spanish/English psychological examiners have at
least a minimal linguistic competency to conduct such evaluations.

Given the shortage of competent bilingual (English/Spanish) neuropsychologists, the need to use translators will probably arise in either urban or
rural areas with a large Hispanic constituency. The practice of using translators in neuropsychological evaluations can result in serious errors affecting
both scoring and interpretation. As noted by Cervantes and Acosta (1992),
"It is often difficult for an evaluator to distinguish between what is a direct
translation of the patient's reports and what is a personal and edited interpretation on the part of the translator" (p. 215). Similarly, the authors assert
that qualitative linguistic aspects in reference to patients with language disturbances (i.e., aphasia) would be lost. In order to minimize such problems,
Woodcock and Muñoz-Sandoval (1996) discuss a team approach between
a *primary examiner* (a qualified English-speaking practitioner) and an *ancillary examiner* (a Spanish speaker who is trained to administer a particular
test). The authors provide a six-step protocol which addresses the Batería
Woodcock-Muñoz-Revisada, but can also be adapted for use with any psychological assessment instrument.

Cognitive Changes During Aging

General intelligence-test batteries and mini-mental status examinations are
commonly used by neuropsychologists to assess general cognitive performance. The term "general intelligence", however, is a construct that is difficult to define. Perez-Arce and Puente (1996) defined general intelligence by
a set of test scores that are heavily correlated with America's definition of
scholastic success. Individual differences in intelligence as assessed by standardized tests relate to what individuals learn in school (Brody, 1992). The
determinants of "normal" or "abnormal" may be established by the cultural
group that develops the intelligence test (Ardila, 1995).

The most common test of intelligence in adults, independent of their ethnic origin, is the Wechsler Adult Intelligence Scale (WAIS). The original version has been adapted to Spanish *(Escala de Inteligencia de Wechsler para Adultos*, EIWA; Wechsler, 1968). Currently the WAIS-III Spanish is in the developmental process. Lopez and Taussig (1991) found that the cognitive-intellectual functioning of Hispanic adults is prone to be underestimated when using the WAIS-R and overestimated when using the EIWA. In their study, the WAIS-R subtests indicated cognitive impairment in normal Spanish speakers and the EIWA subtests indicated less cognitive impairment in Spanish speakers suffering from Alzheimer's disease. Jacobs et al. (1997) compared the performance of English- and Spanish-speaking elders, matched by age and level of education, on a brief neuropsychological test battery. Spanish and English speakers scored comparably in many of the language tests including the Similarities subtest from the WAIS-R; Spanish speakers scored significantly lower, however, on non-verbal reasoning and visuoperceptual skills subtests (e.g., Benton Visual Retention Test-Matching and Identities and Oddities from the Mattis Dementia Rating Scale). The authors hypothesized that the geometric nature of the stimuli on these non-verbal measures may have conferred an advantage to the English speakers, perhaps by virtue of differences on educational emphasis or exposure. In general, however, it can be expected that bilinguals will show a higher Performance than Verbal IQ (Puente & Salazar, 1998).

Although it is well-known that visuospatial and constructional abilities, including drawing figures, are affected by the subject's culture (Deregowski, 1989; Pontius, 1989), and level of education (Ardila, Rosselli & Rosas, 1989; Ponton et al., 1996), neuropsychologists do not always take this into account when performing neuropsychological evaluation. This is reflected in the limited norms available with visuospatial and constructional tests for different cultural and educational groups. In American urban society, training in drawing skills is basically provided through formal education. Then, level of schooling is a critical variable with important impact on cognitive test performance.

Aging is characterized by a decline in visuospatial and visuomotor abilities (Albert, 1988; Ardila & Rosselli, 1989; La Rue, 1992). The test best measuring the visuospatial aging factor, in the Ardila and Rosselli (1989) study was the Rey-Osterrieth Complex Figure (ROCF). Some norms are available in current literature for Spanish speakers (e.g., Ardila, Rosselli, & Puente, 1994; Ardila & Rosselli, in press; Ponton et al., 1996) and English speakers (Spreen & Strauss, 1997). A similar effect of age and education on the ROCF has been observed for both Spanish and English speakers.

Performance in language ability tests is strongly associated with the subject's educational level (Ardila, Rosselli, & Ostrosky, 1992; Heaton, Grant, & Matthews, 1986; Lantz, 1979; Ostrosky et al., 1985; Ponton et al., 1996; Rey, 1990). And this educational-level effect on language tests can even be more significant than the aging effect (Rosselli et al., 1990;

Benton & Hamsher, 1978; Wertz, 1979). The effects of education may be so strong that, when education is controlled, there is no longer evidence of an age-related decline in verbal intelligence (Albert & Heaton, 1988). Level of education significantly correlates with IQ (Matarazzo, 1979). In Latin-American countries low educational levels are more often the result of economical limitations than academic failures, and therefore the correlation value between level of education and IQ is expected to be lower than what has been reported in more developed countries.

Few studies have compared the language test performance in bilingual Hispanics when performing in Spanish and English. No differences have been reported in repetition and naming. Differences between Spanish and English speakers in category fluency but not in letter fluency have been reported (Rosselli et al., 2000b). Jacobs et al. (1997) found significantly lower scores in Spanish elderly living in New York city, in semantic fluency (cloth, fruits and animals) when compared to matched English speakers. Rosselli et al. (2000a) found semantically but not phonologically decreased fluency in Spanish/English bilinguals as a result of the interfering effect between both languages. Exposure to a second language in Hispanics may account for the verbal fluency differences reported by Jacobs et al. (1997).

Neuropsychological Tests

Several neuropsychological tests have been developed or adapted to Spanish in the last decades and have been normalized in Hispanic populations. Some of the neuropsychological tests that are available in Spanish are listed in Table 1. The corresponding source is indicated.

Some studies have approached the normalization of neuropsychological instruments in children. The WISC-R (Escala de Inteligencia Wechsler para Niños–Revisada, EIWN-R) has been translated and adapted to the Spanish language (Wechsler, 1983). The Woodcock-Johnson Psychoeducational

Table 1. Some neuropsychological tests with norms for Spanish speakers.

Test	Age range	Source
CHILDREN		
EIWN-R	6-16	Wechsler, 1983
Batería-R	2>90	Woodcock & Muñoz-Sandoval, 1996
TVIP (Peabody Picture)	2-18	Dunn et al., 1986
Boston Naming Test	5-12	Ardila & Rosselli, 1994
Token Test	5-12	Ardila & Rosselli, 1994
Verbal fluency	5-12	Ardila & Rosselli, 1994
WMS	5-12	Ardila & Rosselli, 1994
Rey-Osterrieth Figure	5-12	Ardila & Rosselli, 1994
Wisconsin Card Sorting Test	5-12	Rosselli & Ardila, 1993

Table 1, continued.

Test	Age range	Source
ADULTS		
General Cognitive Performance		
Neuropsi	20-100	Ostrosky et al., 1997
MMSE	55-85	Ardila et al., 1994
		Bird et al., 1987
		Escobar et al., 1986
		Gurland et al., 1992
		Mungas et al., 1996
		Ostrosky-Solis et al., 2000
		Taussig et al., 1992
EIWA	18-64	Wechsler, 1968
Batería-R	2>90	Woodcock-Muñoz, 1996
NeSBHIS	16-75	Ponton et al., 1996
Raven	16-75	Ponton et al., 1996
MDRS	60-75	Taussig et al., 1992
Attention		
Cancelation test	55-85	Ardila et al., 1994
Digit-Span	55-85	Ardila et al., 1994
		Olazaran et al., 1996
		Ponton et al., 1996
		Loewenstein et al., 1995
Memory		
Fuld Object Memory	70-85	Loewenstein et al., 1995
	60-75	Taussig et al., 1992
WHO-UCLA-AVLT	16-75	Ponton et al., 1996
WMS	55-85	Ardila et al., 1994
	70-85	Loewenstein et al., 1995
	20-100	Ostrosky-Solis et al., 2000
Serial Verbal Learn	55-85	Ardila et al., 1994
ROCF: Memory	20-85	Ardila et al., in press
	16-75	Ponton et al., 1996
Languge		
Boston Naming	55-85	Ardila et al., 1994
	70-85	Loewenstein et al., 1995
	16-75	Ponton et al., 1996
Multilingual Aphasia Exam-Spanish	6-69	Rey & Benton, 1991
Verbal Fluency	55-85	Ardila et al., 1994
	70-85	Loeweintein et al., 1995
	16-75	Ponton et al., 1996
Token Test	55-85	Ardila et al., 1994
Visospatial and Constructional		
ROCF: Copy	20-80	Ardila & Rosselli, in press
	55-85	Ardila et al., 1994
	16-75	Ponton et al., 1996
	20-100	Ostrosky et al., in press
Block design	60-75	Taussig et al., 1992
	16-75	Ponton et al., 1996
Functional Scales		
DAFS	65-85	Loewenstein et al., 1992

Battery (1977) is also available in Spanish (Woodcock & Muñoz-Sandoval, 1996). The McCarthy Scales for Children's Abilities (McCarthy, 1972) was also published in Spanish. Nonetheless, in recent catalogs of the Psychological Corporation it is not announced any more. Currently a child neuropsychological assessment test battery is under development in Mexico (Matute, Rosselli, Ardila & Ostrosky, unpublished).

Ardila and Rosselli (1994) administered some common neuropsychological instruments to five- to 12-year old normal Colombian children. They included the Boston Naming Test, the Token Test, Verbal fluency (semantic and phonologic), Wechsler Memory Scale and Rey-Osterrieth Complex Figure. The Wisconsin Card Sorting Test (Heaton, 1981) has also been normalized in children (Rosselli & Ardila, 1993).

The mini-mental status exam by Folstein et al. (1975) is frequently used in the assessment of Spanish speakers. Several Spanish versions are available (e.g., Ostrosky-Solis, Lopez-Arango, & Ardila, 2000; Rosselli et al., 2000a). Ostrosky, Ardila and Rosselli (1997) developed a Spanish extended mini-mental evaluation named Neuropsi. The normalization of this test among 800 normal Mexican subjects between the ages of 16-85 and AD patients is presented elsewhere (Ostrosky, Ardila, & Rosselli, 1999).

Several studies have approached the question of assessing intellectual functioning in bilingual Spanish-English populations in the U.S. It has been emphasized that cultural and language bias against Spanish-speaking demented as well as non-demented patients may impact upon performance on neuropsychological and functional variables (Loewenstein et al., 1992, 1995; Lopez & Taussig, 1991; Olmedo, 1981). Difficulties with the use of standard intellectual function assessment instruments developed for American English speakers have been pointed out in a previous section of this chapter. Lopez and Romero (1988), and Melendez (1994) have raised serious concerns about the use of the WAIS Spanish version (EIWA) when testing Spanish populations. Lopez and Taussig (1991) have emphasized the necessity to use functional measures (activities of daily living) in addition to the standard psychometric measures. According to the authors, the WAIS-R or the EIWA should be used depending upon the specific conditions of the testee: age, level of education, proficiency in English, general cognitive functioning, etc. Ponton et al. (1996) used the Raven Progressive Matrices as a test of reasoning or non verbal intelligence. Ardila, Rosselli and Puente (1994) adapted most of the common neuropsychological tests to Spanish and administered them to a large Colombian population. Ponton et al. (1996) provide norms stratified by age, education and gender for memory, visuospatial skills, concentration, psychomotor skills, and reasoning. Taussig, Henderson and Mack (1992) administered, to a sample of normal Spanish-speaking elderly and to AD patients, an extensive neuropsychological battery, plus a behavior checklist and depression inventory. Although the sample was small, the authors report means and standard deviations. Artiola i Fortuny, Hermosillo, Heaton and Pardee (1999) administered a battery comprised of eight tests designed to measure attention, learning and memory, and executive function skills. Normative data is presented for a combined group of 185 individuals living in either Mexico or the U.S. Additional normative data is presented for 205 Spaniards living in Madrid.

It is important to include in the neuropsychological evaluation of the elderly a scale of functional assessment. Neurological conditions (i.e. dementia) may influence daily living skills and the degree of impairment may correlate with the severity of the neurological condition. Functional assessment includes activities of daily living (ADLs) and instrumental activities of daily living (IADLs). ADLs include self-care skills (i.e. toileting, bathing, etc). IADLs require planning and experience (i.e cooking) (Lawton & Brody, 1969).

Functional assessment is obtained through direct observation or by patient's or significant other's report. The detection of ADLs is easy and may not be influenced by cultural factors. The assessment of IADLs may be influenced by gender, education and culture. For example, in the old Hispanics managing money may be considered mainly a male task while cooking and cleaning are considered mainly female responsibilities. Loeweinstein et al., (1992, 1995) recommend the use of functional measures (activities of daily living) in addition to the psychometric measures. They propose a functional battery, the Direct Assessment of Functional Status (DAFS) to be used with demented and nondemented patients with different cultural and linguistic backgrounds (Loeweinstein et al., 1989a, 1989b). Loewenstein et al. (1995) determined the extent to which various neuropsychological tests were predictive of performance on functional measures administered within the clinical setting (Loewenstein et al., 1989a, 1989b). Among English-speaking AD patients, Block Design and Digit Span, as well as tests of language were among the stronger predictors of functional performance. For Spanish-speakers Block Design, Digit Span and the Mini-Mental had the highest predictive power.

In summary, there have been efforts to develop norms for elderly Spanish speakers and better neuropsychological instruments that are more appropriate for Spanish-speaking populations. Currently, there are some norms available for Hispanic populations living in the US and in Latin America. More research is needed, however, to increase the ecological validity of the neuropsychological evaluation.

Future Directions

The population of Hispanics is increasing and the need for culturally appropriate instruments to measure cognition in this population is increasing too. Some studies have demonstrated the significant influence of cultural factors on neuropsychological test performance. Variables that should be studied as possible factors affecting test performance are acculturation, learning opportunities, relevance of different cognitive abilities and non-specific factors of the testing situation. Another very important variable is the subject knowledge of more than one language. Some studies have shown that bilingual subjects may perform below monolingual subjects in some cognitive tests (Grosjean, 1989).

The issue of testing language with Hispanics deserves special consideration: Spanish-English bilinguals may be at a disadvantage when using either language. Both languages can be active languages, if the functional language is not either Spanish or English, but a mixture of both. Interference is expected to be high. To use either Spanish or English testing materials and norms can penalize US Spanish-English bilinguals. No clear solution to this difficulty is available.

Three procedures, however, could at least reduce the *bilingualism effect* in psychological and neuropsychological testing (1) to have special norms for Spanish-English bilinguals. This solution does not seem easy, taking into consideration the tremendous heterogeneity of U.S. bilingualism; (2) the examiner could be a bilingual mastering a similar type of bilingualism. Testing could be performed in Spanish, English, and any combination of both languages. Instructions and answers in either language or any mixture of both languages could be acceptable; both English and Spanish norms could be used, preferring the one favoring the subject; and (3) to "adjust" the scores in order to neutralize the penalizing effect of bilingualism. The problem is that we do not know how much the test scores should be adjusted in order to be "fair at best". Of course, it depends on the test, the idiosyncrasies of the client's bilingualism, and the testing situation, including the examiner's language. None of these three solutions alone or combined seem easy to put in action.

Therefore it is advisable that upon commencing an evaluation of a bilingual individual, a test of receptive language ability be conducted in each language. This is particularly important with children and with the aged, where erroneous assumptions of language dominance are most likely to occur. Based on the results of the receptive language testing, the evaluation should continue using as the primary language that in which the patient exhibits greatest strength. Tests commonly used for this purpose include the Peabody Picture Vocabulary Test and its Spanish Counterpart: Test de Vocabulario en Imagenes Peabody. Alternatively, the receptive vocabulary tests of the Batería-R could be used (Woodcock & Muñoz-Sandoval, 1996). The Batería-R has the added advantage of incorporating a Language Use Survey and comparative language (Spanish/English) indices.

Moreover, when testing U.S. Hispanic bilinguals, it be should emphasized that "current results may not necessarily reflect the subject's real abilities, and his/her real performance may be higher than observed". Obviously, any neuropsychological report of a bilingual individual should mention the subject's degree of bilingualism (at least: age of acquisition of the second language, schooling language, and use of both languages in everyday life), language used in testing, norms used, and caution regarding the potentially penalizing effect of bilingualism.

We opine that neuropsychological tests used with Hispanics in the U.S. should (a) contain an adequate sample of subjects representative of Hispanic subgroups living in the U.S. as reported by national census figures, (b) contain items and instructions that are applicable to all Spanish-speaking subgroups, (c) undergo a content and item analysis to control for potential cultural bias, (d) have published data concerning the instruments' reliability, validity, and measures of central tendency, (e) provide age- and education-corrected scale scores, and (f) provide specific Hispanic subgroup (e.g., Mexican-Americans) and overall group norms. To date there is a paucity of tests available on the market which meet these criteria. It is doubtful that any one research center could finance the cost and satisfy the scientific criteria in standardizing neuropsychological instruments for the growing Hispanic populace in the U.S. Therefore, we advocate the creation of a national task force to establish clear priorities, foster regional collaboration, and develop protocols for the ethical guidelines, subject selection, and standardization of neuropsychological instruments in Spanish.

References

Albert, M.S. (1988). Cognitive function. In M.S. Albert & M.B. Moss (Eds.), *Geriatric neuropsychology*. New York: The Guilford Press.

Albert, M.S., & Heaton, R.K. (1988). Intelligence testing. In M.S. Albert & M.B. Moss (Eds.), *Geriatric neuropsychology* (pp. 10-32). New York: The Guilford Press.

Albert, M., & Obler, L. (1978). *The bilingual brain*. New York: Academic Press.

American Educational Research Association, American Psychological Association, National Council on Measurement in Education (1996). *Standards for educational and psychological testing*. Washington, D.C.: America Psychological Association.

Ardila, A. (1990). Neuropsychology in Latin America. *The Clinical Neuropsychologist, 4,* 121-132.

Ardila, A. (1995.). Directions of research in cross-cultural neuropsychology. *Journal of Clinical and Experimental Neuropsychology, 17,* 143-150.

Ardila, A., & Rosselli, M. (1989) Neuropsychological characteristics of normal aging. *Developmental Neuropsychology, 5,* 307-320.

Ardila, A., & Rosselli, M. (1994). Development of language, memory and visuospatial abilities in 5-to 12-year-old children using a neuropsychological battery. *Developmental Neuropsychology, 10,* 97-120.

Ardila, A., & Rosselli, M. (In press). Educational effects on the Rey-Osterrieth Complex Figure. In J. Knight & E. Kaplan (Eds.). *Handbook of Rey-Osterrieth Complex Figure usage: Clinical and research applications.*

Ardila, A., Rosselli, M., & Ostrosky, F. (1992). Socioeducational. In A.E. Puente & R.J. McCaffrey (Eds.), *Handbook of neuropsychological assessment: A biopsychosocial perspective* (pp. 181-192). New York: Plenum Press.

Ardila, A., Rosselli, M., & Puente, A. (1994). *Neuropsychological evaluation of the Spanish speaker*. New York: Plenum Press.

Ardila, A., Rosselli, M., & Rosas, P. (1989). Neuropsychological assessment in illiterates: Visuospatial and memory abilities. *Brain and Cognition, 11,* 147-166.

Artiola i Fortuny, L., Hermosillo, H., Heaton, R. K., & Pardee, D. (1999). *Batería Neuropsicológica en Español.* Odessa, FL: Psychological Assessment Resources.

Benton, A.L., & Hamsher, K. (1978). *Multilingual Aphasia Examination.* Iowa City: University of Iowa Press.

Bird, H. R., Canino, G., Stippec, M. R., & Shrout, P. (1987). Use of the Mini-Mental State Examination in a probabilistic sample of a Hispanic population. *Journal of Nervous and Mental Diseases, 175,* 731–737.

Brody, N. (1992). *Intelligence.* New York: Academic Press.

Cervantes, R.C., & Acosta, F.X. (1992). Psychological testing for Hispanics. *Applied and Preventive Psychology, 1,* 209-219.

Cobos, R. (1983). *A dictionary of New Mexico and Southern Colorado Spanish.* Santa Fe: Museum of New Mexico Press.

Cuellar, I. (1998). Cross-cultural clinical psychological assessment of Hispanic americans. *Journal of Personality Assessment, 70,* 71-86.

Deregowski, J.B. (1989). Real space and represented space: Cross-cultural perspectives. *Behavioral and Brain Sciences, 12,* 51-119.

Dunn, L.M., Padilla, E.R., Lugo, D.E., & Dunn, L.M. (1986). *Test de vocabulario en imagenes Peabody* (Peabody picture vocabulary test), Adaptacion Hispanoamericana. Circle Pines: American Guidance Service.

Earle, M. J. (1967). Bilingual semantic merging and an aspect of acculturation. *Journal of Personality and Social Psychology , 6,* 304-312.

Escobar, J. I., Burman, R., & Marno M. (1986). Use of the Mini-Mental State Examination (MMSE) in a community population of mixed ethnicity: Cultural and linguistic artifacts. *Journal of Nervous and Mental Diseases, 174,* 607-614.

Folstein, M.F., Folstein S.E., & McHugh, P.R. (1975). Mini-Mental State. *Journal of Psychiatric Research, 12,* 189-198

Grosjean, F. (1989). Neurolinguistics beware! The bilingual is not two monolinguals in one person. *Brain and Language, 36,* 3-15.

Gulard, B. L., Wilder, D. E., Cross, P., Teresi, J., & Barret, V. W. (1992). Screening scales for dementia: toward a reconciliation of conflicting cross-cultural findings. *International Journal of Geriatric Psychiatry, 7,* 105-113.

Heaton, R. (1981). *Wisconsin Card Sorting Test: Manual.* Odessa: Psychological Assessment Resources, Inc.

Heaton, R.K., Grant, I., & Matthews, C. (1986). Differences in neuropsychological test performance associated with age, education and sex. In I. Grant & K.M. Adams (Eds.), *Neuropsychological assessment in neuropsychiatric disorders* (pp. 108-120). New York: Oxford University Press.

Jacobs, D.M., Sano, M., Albert, S., Schofield, P., Dooneief, G. & Stern, Y. (1997). Cross-cultural neuropsychological assessment: A comparison of randomly selected, demographically matched cohorts of English- and Spanish- Speaking older adults. *Journal of Clinical and Experimental Neuropsychology, 19, 3,* 331-339.

Lantz, D. (1979). A cross-cultural comparison of communication abilities: Some effects of age, schooling, and culture. *International Journal of Psychology, 14,* 171-183.

La Rue, A. (1992) Adult Development. In A.E. Puente & R.J. McCaffrey (Eds.), *Handbook of neuropsychological assessment: A biopsychosocial perspective.* New York: The Plenum Press.

Lawton, M. P., & Brocky, E. M. (1969). Assessment of older people: Self maintained and instrumental activities of daily living. *Gerontologist, 9,* 179-186.

Loewenstein , D.A., Amigo, E., Duara, R., Guterman, A., Hurwitz, D., Berkowitz, N., Wilkie, F., Weinberg, G., Black, B., & Gittelman, B. (1989a). A new scale for the assessment of functional status in Alzheimer's disease and related disorders. *The Journal of Gerontology, 4,* 114-121.

Loewenstein, D.A., Ardila, A., Rosselli, M., Hayden, S., Duara, R., Berkowitz, N., Linn-Fuentes, P., Mintzer, J., Norville, M., & Eisdorfer, C. (1992). A comparative analysis of functional status among Spanish and English-speaking patients with dementia. *Journal of Gerontology, 47,* 389-394.

Loewenstein, D.A., Ardila, A., Rosselli, M., Hayden, S., & Eisdorfer, C. (1989b). A comparative analysis of Spanish and English-speaking patients with dementia and normal controls. *Gerontological Society of America Meeting.* Minneapolis, Minnesota.

Loewenstein, D.A., Rubert, M.P., Arguelles, T., & Duara, R. (1995). Neuropsychological test performance and prediction of functional capacities among Spanish-speaking and English speaking patients with dementia. *Archives of Clinical Neuropsychology, 16,* 75-88.

Lopez, S., & Romero, A. (1988). Assessing the intellectual functioning of Spanish speaking adults: Comparisons of the EIWA and the WAIS. *Professional Psychology: Research and Practice, 19,* 263-270.

Lopez, S., & Taussig I.M. (1991). Cognitive-Intellectual functioning of Spanish-speaking impaired and non-impaired elderly: implications for culturally sensitive assessment. *Psychological Assessment, 3,* 448-454.

Lopez-Aquires, J.N., Kemp, B., Plopper, M., Staples, F.R., & Brummel-Smith, K. (1984). Health needs of the Hispanic elderly. *Journal of the American Geriatrics Society, 32,* 191-197.

Matarazzo, J.D. (1979). *Wechsler's measurement and appraisal of adult intelligence.* New York: Oxford University Press.

Matute, E., Rosselli, M., Ardila, A., & Ostrosky, F. **Examen Neuropsicologico Infantil (ENI).** Unpublished manuscript.

McCarthy, D. (1972). *McCarthy scales for children's abilities.* New York: The Psychological Corporation.

Melendez, F. (1994). The Spanish version of the WAIS: Some ethical considerations. *The Clinical Neuropsychologist, 8,* 388-393.

Mungas, D., Marshall, S.C., Weldon, M., Haan, M., & Reed, B.R. (1996). Age and education correction of Mini-Mental State Examination for English and Spanish-speaking elderly. *Neurology, 46,* 700-706.

Olazaran J., Jacobs, D., & Stern Y. (1996). Comparative study of visual and verbal short term memory in English and Spanish spekers: testing a linguistic hypothesis. *Journal of the International Neuropsychological Society, 2,* 105-110.

Olmedo, E.L. (1991). Testing linguistic minorities. *American Psychologist, 36,* 1078-1085.

Ostrosky, F., Ardila, A., & Rosselli M. (1997). *Neuropsi: Un examen neuropsicologico breve en Espanol.* Mexico: Bayer.

Ostrosky, F., Ardila, A., & Rosselli, M. (1999) Neuropsi: A brief neuropsychological test battery in Spanish with norms by age and educational level. *Journal of the International Neuropsychological Society, 5,* 413-433.

Ostrosky, F., Canseco, E., Quintanar, L., Navarro, E., Meneses, S., & Ardila, A. (1985). Sociocultural effects in neuropsychological assessment. *International Journal of Neuroscience, 27,* 53-66.

Ostrosky-Solis, F., Lopez-Arango, G., & Ardila, A. (2000). Sensitivity and specificity of the Mini-Mental State Examination in a Spanish-speaking population. *Applied Neuropsychology, 7,* 47-60.

Padilla, A.M. (1979). Critical factors in the testing of Hispanic-Americans: A review and some suggestions for the future. In R.W. Tyler & S.H. White (Eds.), *Test-*

ing, teaching and learning: Report of a conference on testing. Washington, D.C.: National Institute of Education.

Perez-Arce, P., & Puente, A.E. (1996). Neuropsychological assessment of ethnic minorities: The case of assessing Hispanics living in North America. In R.J. Sbordone & C.J. Long (Eds.), *Ecological validity of neuropsychological testing.* Delray Beach: GR Press/St. Lucie Press.

Pontius, A.A. (1989). Color and spatial error in block design in stone age Auca: ecological underuse of occipital-parietal system in men and of frontal lobe in women. *Brain and Cognition, 10,* 54-75.

Pontón, M.O., & Ardila, A. (1999). The future of neuropsychology with Hispanic populations in the U.S. *Archives of Clinical Neuropsychology, 14,* 565-580

Ponton, M., Satz, P., Herrera, L., Ortiz, F., Urrutia, C.P., Young R., D'Ellia, L.F., Furst, C.J. & Nameron, N. (1996). Normative data stratified by age and education for the Neuropsychological Screening Battery for Hispanics (NeSB-HIS): Initial report. *Journal of the International Neuropsychological Society, 2,* 96-104.

Puente, A.E., & Salazar, G. (1998). Assessment of minority and culturally diverse children. In A. Prifetera & D. Saklokske (Eds.). *WISC-III: clinical use and interpretation.* New York: Academic Press.

Real Academia Española (1984). *Diccionario de la lengua Española* (vigésima ed., Tomo II). Madrid: Espasa-Calpe.

Rey, G. (1990). Multilingual Aphasia Examination-Spanish development and normative data. *Dissertation Abstracts International, 50,* 5892.

Rey, G., & Benton, A. (1991). *Examen de afasia multilingue (Multilingual Aphasia Examination-Spanish).* Iowa City: AFA Associates, Inc.

Rosselli, D., Ardila, A., Pradilla, G., Morilla, L., Bautista, L., Rey, O., Camacho, M., & Geneco (2000a). El examen mental abreviado como prueba de tamizaje para el diagnóstico de la demencia: Estudio poblacional colombiano. *Revista de Neurologia, 30,* 428-432.

Rosselli, M., & Ardila, A. (1993). Developmental norms for the Wisconsin Card Sorting Test in 5-to 12-year-old children. *The Clinical Neuropsychologist, 7,* 145-154.

Rosselli, M., Ardila, A., Florez, A. & Castro, C. (1990a). Normative data on the Boston Diagnostic Aphasia Examination. *Journal of Clinical and Experimental Neuropsychology, 12,* 313-322.

Rosselli, M., Ardila, A., Araujo, K., Weekes, V.A., Caracciolo, V., Pradilla, M., & Ostrosky, F. (2000b). Verbal fluency and repetition skills in healthy older Spanish-English bilinguals. *Applied Neuropsychology, 7,* 17-24.

Rosselli, M., Ardila, A. & Rosas, P. (1990b). Neuropsychological assessment in illiterates II: Language and praxic abilities. *Brain and Cognition, 12,* 281-296.

Spreen, O., & Strauss, E. (1997). *A compendium of neuropsychological tests.* New York: Oxford University Press.

Taussig, I.M., Henderson, V.,W., & Mack, W. (1992). Spanish translation and validation of a neuropsychological battery: performance of Spanish- and English-speaking Alzheimer's disease patients and normal comparison subjects. *Clinical Gerontologist, 11,* 95-108.

U.S. Bureau of the Census (1996). *Current Population Reports, Special Studies,* pp. 23-190, 65+ in the United States, US Government Printing Office, Washington, D.C.

U.S. Bureau of the Census (1997). *Census Facts for Hispanic Heritage Month* (Press release CB97-fs. 10, issued 9/11/97).

U.S. Census Bureau (1990). Statistical Abstract of the United States (110th ed.). Washington, D.C.: Bureau of Census.

U.S. Census Bureau (1997). *The current population survey: Hispanic origin, Appendix A: Definitions and explanations.* Retrieved from the World Wide Web February 20, 1999: http://www.census.gov/population/www/socdemo/hispanic/hispdef97.html

U.S. Census Bureau (1998). *Selected social characteristics of all persons and Hispanic persons, by type of origin.* Retrieved from the World Wide Web February 20, 1999: http://www.census.gov/population /socdemo/hispanic/cps97/sumtab01.txt

U.S. Census Bureau (1999). *United States census 2000, race, Hispanic origin, and ancestry: Why, what and how.* Washington, D.C.: U.S. Dept. of Commerce.

Wertz, R.T. (1979). Review of the word fluency measures (WF). In F.L. Darley (Ed.), *Evaluation and appraisal techniques in speech and language pathology.* Reading: Addison-Wesley.

Wechsler, D. (1968). *Escala de Inteligencia Wechsler para Adultos.* New York: The Plenum Press.

Wechsler, D. (1983). *Escala de Inteligencia Wechsler para Ninos-Revisada.* New York: Psychological Corporation.

Wilds, D.J., & Wilson, R. (1998). *Minorities in higher education 1997-98: Sixteenth annual status report.* Washington, D.C.: American Council on Education.

Woodcock, R.W. & Johnson, M.B. (1977). *Woodcock-Johnson Psychoeducational Battery.* Hingham, MA: Teaching Resources.

Woodcock R.W., & Muñoz-Sandoval, A.F. (1996). *Batería Woodcock-Muñoz: Pruebas de habilidad cognitiva-Revisada, Supplemental Manual.* Chicago: Riverside Publishing Company.

Chapter 10

NEUROPSYCHOLOGICAL ASSESSMENT OF LATINO CHILDREN

Rubén J. Echemendía and Laura Julian
Department of Psychology, The Pennsylvania State University, University Park, Pennsylvania

Abstract

In this paper, the authors will provide a review of the empirical literature regarding the assessment of Spanish-speaking children in the United States. This review will include the state of the field of neuropsychology in the development of methodologically sound and appropriate instruments to use with this group. Specific test instruments used for intellectual, achievement, and neurocognitive assessment will be reviewed in terms of the utility, development, standardization, and appropriateness for use with this population. In addition to a review of the literature to date and status of test instruments, this chapter will provide guidelines for assessing this population. Factors including the initial interview, use of technicians, familial considerations, and the implications of school involvement will also be discussed. It will become clear that the state of the field in the assessment of Spanish speaking children is in need of increased test development, and empirical validation. Suggestions for future directions are also included in this chapter.

Introduction

It has been widely reported that the Hispanic population will increase dramatically within the next fifty years to become the largest "minority" group within the United States. Indeed, the U.S. Census Bureau estimates (U.S. Census Bureau, 2000) that the Hispanic population will number 98,229,000 by the year 2050 which represents an increase of 213% from the year 2000 estimates. In contrast, it is estimated that during the same time period non-Hispanic Whites will increase by 9%, Blacks by 61%, American Indian/Eskimo/Aleut by 60%, and Asian or Pacific Islanders by 248%. In 2050, Hispanics will comprise 24% of the U.S. population, non-Hispanic Whites will constitute 53%, Blacks will account for 13%, American Indian/Eskimo/Aleut will comprise less than 1 percent, and Asians or Pacific Islanders will comprise 9% of the U.S. population.

Hispanics have a higher percentage of children under the age of 18 than any of the ethnic minority groups tracked by the U.S. Census Bureau. According to the year 2000 census estimates, there are 12,815,000 Hispanic children under the age of 18 in the U.S., accounting for 31% of the U.S. Hispanic population. Taken together, these data make clear that individuals who identify themselves as Hispanic or Latino will constitute a sizable group within the U.S. in the next 50 years.

Unfortunately, psychology in general, and neuropsychology in particular, has done little to prepare for these changing demographic patterns. The purpose of this chapter is to review many of the issues that are pertinent to the assessment of Hispanic individuals, with particular attention paid to the issue of assessing Latino children. As a matter of convention, we will use the terms Hispanic and Latino interchangeably. However, it is important to recognize that some groups prefer to be called Hispanic while others prefer the use of the term Latino. We will also use Latino and Latina interchangeably, recognizing that many Latina women prefer the use of the feminine form of the word.

The statements above regarding the use of ethnic descriptors are a simple reflection of the complexity and heterogeneity that comprise Latino culture and language. Hispanics in the U.S. come from a wide range of countries (e.g., Mexico, Cuba, Puerto Rico, Columbia, Costa Rica, etc.) and represent a broad range of sociocultural and sociopolitical differences. They are unified by their common use of the Spanish language but vary significantly in their use of that language. Slang expressions, idiosyncratic words, and differences in intonation and inflection, all combine to create subtle, but often significant changes in language (see Chapter 9, this volume).

Latinas vary in their level of education and the emphasis that is placed on education in their culture. For example, Hispanics originating in rural cultures may place significantly more emphasis on collective work than on education. Latinos differ in their immigration patterns and the economic and political factors that led them to emigrate. There are even differences within

Hispanic subgroups. For example, within the Cuban population there are significant educational, political, and economic differences between those Cubans who emigrated to the U.S. in the late fifties and early sixties when compared to the recent exodus of the "Marielitos."

In short, there is considerable heterogeneity within and between Spanish-speaking cultures. The scope of this chapter will not allow for a thorough discussion of these differences. Thus, the reader is cautioned that general statements about differences between Latino and Anglo-Saxon cultures may not be accurate for the specific child that is before them for an evaluation. Our goal is simply to point out the issues that exist and hope that they are taken into consideration in the neuropsychological evaluation of Latino children.

The Child in Context

The neuropsychological evaluation of bilingual and bicultural adults is a difficult task. One cannot assume that the adult being assessed has the same cultural values, beliefs, language, etc. as the examiner. Often there are questions as to whether the tests are valid for a given population or whether the norms are appropriate for the individual who is being assessed. The assessment of bilingual and bicultural children (with a bilingual or monolingual family) is even more difficult because of the added complexity of developmental variables. Puente and Salazar (1998) argue that differences in intelligence and cognitive functioning across individuals from various cultures are largely a function of cultural variables. They note that culture plays a more prominent role in intelligence that does race. Moore (1987) elaborates further by asserting that not only is family ethnicity related to IQ differences, but that the environment in which the child interacts on a daily basis is also significantly related to IQ differences. Thus, the neuropsychologist must come to understand the neurocognitive functioning of the child, but he or she must do so while also understanding the culture and background of the family as well as the child's overall environment. In order to reach this understanding, several factors need to be addressed, including language use, acculturation, education, socioeconomic variables, and developmental factors.

Language
Does the child speak English? This is often the first question asked of a Latino child who is being evaluated in the U.S. It is a critically important question, yet it assumes that if the child speaks English, it is "OK" to go ahead with the evaluation using a standard battery of tests. Although the child may speak English, it is important to know how well the child speaks English, the context in which the child speaks English (e.g., home, school, church), the proportion of time that the child spends speaking English, who the child speaks English with, and how well the child is able to write and read in English.

Also important, particularly in a neuropsychological evaluation, is how well the child speaks Spanish. An erroneous assumption can easily be made that the child has simply not been exposed to enough English, when, in fact, the child exhibits a significant developmental delay in language which is evident in both Spanish and English.

Even if the child does speak English, it cannot be assumed that the child speaks English and Spanish equally well. In actuality, the "balanced bilingual" may be relatively rare (if they exist at all), with most bilinguals demonstrating greater facility with one of the two languages (Manuel-Dupont, Ardila, Rosselli, & Puente, 1992). Hickey (1972) documented that Mexican-American bilingual children had trouble matching pictures with English nouns because of the differences between the languages. Harris, Cullum, and Puente (1995) created Spanish and English modifications of the California Verbal Learning Test to examine differences between bilingual Hispanic adults and White English speakers. They found that when Spanish dominant bilinguals were assessed in English they learned fewer words and had poorer retention than monolinguals. When assessed in their dominant language no differences were found between groups.

Acculturation

The impact of culture on the neuropsychological assessment process cannot be considered constant and equal among children and adolescents from widely different backgrounds. The child's level of acculturation can influence test performance in many ways. The likelihood of a child's ability to perform adequately on tests developed within the United States is highly dependent upon his or her familiarity with the testing practices used commonly in the U.S. (Pontón & Ardila, 1999). Marín (1992) suggests that acculturation is a process of attitudinal and behavioral change undergone by those who come in contact with a new culture. These processes consist of both psychological and social changes dependent upon the characteristics of the individual. For example, the level of identification with the values or the culture of origin as well as the intensity of contact between cultural groups may mediate level of acculturation for a child. The critical issue is the understanding that acculturation is multi-faceted, dynamic, and highly individualized.

Marín (1992) differentiates among distinct operational definitions of acculturation. A common perception is that acculturation consists of a learning process that is unidimensional, i.e. the movement away from the original culture towards the new culture. This process appears to be better identified as assimilation. Secondly, Marín posits that biculturality is a process by which one will learn qualities of the new culture while retaining some or all of the cultural components of the original group. He describes a bicultural Hispanic as one who feels comfortable within the Hispanic culture, and could switch easily to a non-Hispanic perspective when interacting with non-Hispanics.

Berry et al. (1988) posits six areas in which acculturation has a direct effect on psychological functioning: language, cognitive styles, personality, identity, attitudes, and acculturative stress. Given the complexity inherent in the acculturation process, it is unlikely that unidimensional measures of language use, dominance or preference will serve as a reliable proxy for acculturation. Yet, despite a sizable literature on the multidimensional nature of acculturation, most current research studies continue to operationalize acculturation as a unidimensional phenomenon (scales moving from the "Spanish only" end of the continuum to the "English only" end). Pontón & Ardila (1999) have suggested that the G. Marín et al. (1987) scale of acculturation may be the most useful tool for neuropsychologists conducting research. This scale is composed of 12 items that evaluate acculturation on the three factors of Language Use, Media, and Ethnic Social Relations (ethnicity of friends). Normative data were initially acquired on 363 Hispanics and 228 Anglos and the subscales were found to correlate highly with the following variables: generation, length of residence in the U.S., age at arrival, and ethnic self-identification.

For children, the measurement of acculturation may be more complex than it is for adults. First, it may be possible for both children and adults to exist in a host culture without the loss of their original cultural values, language, and customs. For example, children living in areas that are predominately Hispanic in the United States may be isolated from many of the influences of the majority culture. Although the parents may have significant contact with English-speakers at their jobs, they may only speak Spanish at home. Children may have only Spanish-speaking friends and their circle of social contacts may all be Spanish. The music they listen to is Spanish, the TV shows are in Spanish and the corner grocery store is run by Spanish-speakers. In this example, the children's level of acculturation is different from the parents' level of acculturation.

As noted earlier, it is important for neuropsychologists to become cognizant of many factors not only related to the child, but also related to the family and the socio-cultural factors of the home and neighborhood environment. For example, a child that lives in a primarily Hispanic neighborhood and attends a primarily Hispanic school has a distinctly different experience than a child who has recently been transplanted from a predominantly Latino environment to a non-Hispanic one. In addition, the employment status, socioeconomic status (SES), and the relative acculturation of the family with which the child lives are important variables to assess. Not only does the child's current SES level relate to test performance but Golding and Burnam (1990) suggested that the best predictor of immigrants' acculturation to the United States culture is the SES of the immigrant prior to entrance to the new culture.

The most pertinent issue here is that in the assessment of a child or adolescent, not only is the level of acculturation of the child important, but the family context must also be thoroughly explored. This will provide the neuropsychologist with important information regarding the child's (and family's) familiarity with various aspects of the assessment process such as formal testing procedures, service providers, and doctors.

Acculturation is also difficult to assess among adolescents. Not only are adolescents grappling with identity issues regarding adulthood vs. childhood, but they may also be struggling with their ethnic and/or racial identity. The struggle over their ethnic identity may give rise to many behaviors ranging from an uncritical acceptance of the host culture and adamant refusal to acknowledge their culture of origin, to a fervent retention of the culture of origin and refusal to engage in activities associated with the host culture. These factors should be examined within the clinical interview of both adolescent and family.

Measures of acculturation have not been widely used clinically by neuropsychologists. In part, the lack of use may be related to the fact that there are very few scales that can be used with Latino children. Barona and Miller (1994) designed an acculturation scale for use with Hispanic youth. This scale is a short, self –report scale that primarily evaluates aspects of extrafamilial language use, familial language use, and ethnic social relations. Although the scale has been normed on both Hispanic and Caucasian students, the norms are only for grades 5 through 8.

Cuellar, Harris, Lorwen, and Jasso (1980) developed a scale that has been used with Mexican-American seventh graders to assess behavioral correlates of acculturation (Deosaransingh, Moreno, Woodruff, et al., 1995). The scale contained seven items from Cuellar's original scale that were chosen based on an exploratory factor analysis which revealed a group of items that measured "general acculturation" (e.g., language use, media preferences) and another group of items that assessed the ethnicity of friends and elements of "Latino pride". All items consisted of a five-point Likert-type scale with the exception of the Latino pride item which used a four-point scale (very proud to little pride). Although this scale appeared to measure salient constructs of adolescent acculturation, the scale was originally developed for adult populations. The use of adult norms may limit conclusions that can be drawn when the scale is used with children or adolescents.

Epstein, Botvin, Dusenbury, and Diaz (1996) studied acculturation in Hispanic sixth and seventh graders living in New York City. These authors suggested that language use was the best predictor of acculturation among youth. Adolescents were asked to complete a single-item language use measure which was found to correlate significantly (.49) with a 10-item measure used with adults. Although these authors caution against utilizing language as the only measure of acculturation, they considered it a "reliable shorthand measure" that has construct validity, accounts for the greatest proportion of variance when related to acculturation scales, and has a low misclassification rate of 12% (Marín & Marín, 1991; Ramirez, Cousins, Santos, & Supik, 1986). Epstein et al. (1996) suggested that this single-item method is particularly useful when measuring acculturation along with other behaviors or clinical variables (e.g., alcohol use). They argue that acculturation measures which include items that are less salient to clinical variables (e.g., food preferences, music) may obscure the components of acculturation related to a behavioral process.

More recently, the Psychological Acculturation Scale (PAS) was developed to assess psychological acculturation in Puerto-Rican adolescents and adults (Tropp, Erkut, Coll, Alarcón, & Vázquez-García, 1999). This measure holds promise in the assessment of acculturation beyond specific behavioral markers of acculturation (i.e. language preference, language use, media preferences, etc.). Although language preferences and behavioral factors of acculturation are important to assess when conducting cognitive evaluations, measures that assess the psychological aspects of adjustment may provide the clinician with a multi-faceted picture of how well the child or adolescent has adjusted. The PAS assesses variables such as, "which group(s) of people do you feel you share most of your beliefs and values?" and "In which culture do you feel confident that you know how to act?" The PAS has been used only with Puerto-Rican individuals living in the Boston area. It appears to have fairly equivalent Spanish and English versions with internal consistencies of .83 and .85, respectively.

In addition to using empirically derived scales, a thorough clinical interview of the child and family is necessary for the neuropsychologist to develop an understanding of the role of acculturation in any evaluation. Variables that need to be assessed include age of immigration, means of arrival in the U.S., ethnic composition of the child's neighborhood, orientation of the school district towards Latinos, school resources for dealing with bilingual children, years in U.S. school, language proficiency in both languages, level of "switching" required between the home and school setting, familiarity and attitude towards "doctors" and formal testing procedures, and attitudes towards school. From the parents, it will be important to obtain information regarding: occupational history, languages used in the home, level of education, attitudes towards education, familiarity with U.S. school systems, financial stability, SES in host country, reasons for immigrating to U.S., existence of a support network, access to healthcare, familiarity with service providers, childcare situation, and attitudes towards formal testing and evaluations. It is essential that this information be used to inform the entire evaluation process and be integrated into the final report and feedback to both the family, school, and referral source.

Education

Formal education is easier to operationally define and measure than is acculturation. Yet, the apparent ease of measuring years of education is complicated by cultural differences in educational systems. Puente, Sol Mora, and Muno-Cespedes (1997) warn that for children who have completed some schooling outside of the U.S., the number of years of schooling are not always equivalent. Not only are the educational systems markedly different between Latino countries and the U.S., there are many differences in school systems within countries. Urban private schools offer many more resources than do poor rural schools. For example, affluent schools in Latin America often begin teaching children how to speak English at a very early age.

Students also are exposed to U.S. fashion, music, and pop culture to a much greater degree than are their counterparts in rural, often poor, areas of the country.

Using the Neuropsychological Screening Battery for Hispanics (NeSBHIS) with adults, Pontón et al. (1996) found that formal education, as measured by years, was the most important factor in test performance. Education level has also been strongly associated with language ability (Ardila, Rosselli & Otrosky, 1992) and fine visuomotor movements (Rosselli, Ardila, & Rosas, 1990). Ardila and Rosselli (1989) compared completely illiterate normal and highly educated subjects. They found that language test performance differed significantly between the two groups for measures including language comprehension, phonological discrimination, naming, repetition, and verbal fluency. Even visuo-spatial and motor skills, often considered independent of educational level, are influenced by education. For example, Ardila, Rosselli, and Rosas (1989) found that illiterate subjects demonstrated significant differences in performance on tasks such as three-dimensional drawings and recognition of super-imposed figures when compared to highly educated professionals. Ostrosky et al. (1985) found that individuals with low levels of education had difficulties on tasks requiring fine motor movements and coordinated movements. Similarly, Rosselli et al. (1990) found that education was a significant variable predicting performance on praxic ability tests consisting of finger alternating movements, meaningless movements, coordination of both hands, and cancellation tests.

Formal education does not only directly affect performance on the cognitive tests given by neuropsychologists, it also provides qualitative information regarding familiarity with U.S. testing procedures and test-taking skills. For example, a child who has not been exposed to formal education may not be accustomed to sitting in a chair while having a stranger require him to remain attentive and focused on a task that is unfamiliar. She may not know how to hold a pencil, use blocks or complete puzzles. This observational information not only sheds light on the interpretation of test data, it also adds greater dimension to the neuropsychologists' understanding of the child's level of acculturation.

Education also plays a pivotal role in the cognitive development of the child. Perez-Arce and Puente (1996) use concepts borrowed from educational psychology to discuss maturation of functional scholastic behaviors. These include a stage of "readiness to learn," or readiness to acquire literary skills. This readiness includes the processes of stimulating the thinking process of young children to prepare them for understanding information presented at

who have been raised in illiterate and often transient environments that leads them to be significantly delayed when enrolled in U.S. schools. Not only have these children not had the opportunity to learn to analyze and understand multiple levels of meaning, they are unfamiliar with tasks related to school, and even more unfamiliar with neuropsychological testing.

discussion is warranted. Bernal (1983) broadly defines bias as occurring when a "circumstance or condition – usually one which has no relevance to the intended purpose of the measurement – works systematically to distort the results enough to misrepresent the true condition of an individual or a definable group of individuals" (p. 4). Due to the infrequency of studies investigating the utility of neuropsychological tests with children and adolescents, neuropsychologists have not placed much emphasis on this issue. A demonstration of the occurrence of bias can be found in a study described earlier by Harris et al. (1995) who evaluated balanced Spanish-English bilinguals, non-balanced Spanish-English bilinguals, and monolingual English Speakers using the California Verbal Learning Test (CVLT) and an equivalent Spanish version of this test. The results of this study suggested that the degree of bilingualism was a significant factor that systematically altered the learning and retention of verbal information. No differences were found in performance when the test was administered in the participants' dominant language. The non-balanced bilinguals (although they were assessed to have adequate knowledge of the language for conversational purposes) learned fewer words and had lower retention scores when tested in English as compared to Spanish. When assessed in their dominant language, no significant differences were found among the groups. This study demonstrates that even when individuals have language skills in both languages, reduced proficiency in one language may easily be interpreted as neurological impairment. This investigation also highlights the advantage of using both languages in assessment as much as possible.

In what language to assess?

The ideal assessment conducted by a neuropsychologist would include the flexibility for both the examiner and the child to utilize both Spanish and English throughout the testing with the bilingual child. Bernal (1990) suggests the use of Spanish and English "judiciously" during individualized testing to enhance the understanding of the test procedures and maximize the effort and performance of the child. Correct answers in Spanish, English, or both should be accepted. Encourage the child to articulate his or her thoughts in either language so that the examiner may obtain as much information as possible regarding the abilities and cognitive styles of the child. However, it should be kept in mind that alterations in the standardized administration of a test may render the norms from that test inappropriate. Violations of standard administration practices should be noted in the neuropsychological evaluation report and cautions regarding the appropriateness of the norms should be issued.

The clinical interview

Given the paucity of reliable and valid instruments for the assessment of Spanish-speaking children and adolescents, the clinical interview may be the single most valuable source of information for the evaluation. The interview allows the neuropsychologist to question, explore, and observe without the necessary constraints that come with standardized testing. Information regarding the child's developmental history, family history, immigration history, academic achievement, peer relations, among others, can be obtained from the parents and child.

The interview also allows for a period of time during which the neuropsychologist seeks to establish rapport with the child and the family. Latino cultures place a great deal of emphasis on interpersonal relationships. Trust and security arise from knowing each other and this practice is extended to professional relationships. Latino parents will generally want to "know" and feel comfortable with the doctor that is treating their child, particularly when the testing process seems alien to them. Failure to secure this trust may lead to an incomplete and uninformative evaluation. Because of the additional time needed to build rapport, Puente (1990) suggested that interviews with minority group members may be 1.5 to 2 times longer than interviews with individuals from the majority culture, especially when the evaluation involves children.

Early in the evaluation process the neuropsychologist should carefully explain the purposes of the evaluation, the procedures of the evaluation, and the implications of the findings for the child in terms of academic and non-academic areas. It is helpful for the parents (and child) to understand that the evaluation is being undertaken in order to identify optimal ways for the child to negotiate successfully his or her environment (e.g. U.S. school system, learning-support system, rehabilitation setting, home, future occupational functioning, etc.).

Differences between Anglo children and Latino children also have implications for the interview process. Whereas the Anglo child is encouraged to be independent, self-assured, and curious, there is greater emphasis on cooperation and social interaction among Latino children (Kagan, 1984). The interview becomes an excellent forum for the establishment of a relationship with the child and the parents that in turn will help to lay the foundation for a productive evaluation experience.

In addition to the formal assessments of language proficiency mentioned earlier in this chapter, Bernal (1990) suggests that the examiner can also informally assess the child's language proficiency and fluency during the interview. The examiner may invite the child to discuss familiar topics such as school activities (Politzer et al., 1983), or implement role-playing or storytelling techniques. These procedures not only provide the opportunity for the child to discuss his or her experience with the examiner, but also allow the examiner to observe the child's imagination and cognitive abilities to conceptualize a theme and discuss it with others. Mendoza (1983) suggests that older children may be asked to fill in the blanks in a sentence test, engage in oral dictation, or write a composition. In addition, any work samples that can be obtained that the child or adolescent has completed at school may be helpful.

Assessment Instruments

Intelligence measures

Intelligence tests are the most widely used of all psychological tests (cf. Putnam & DeLuca, 1990) with Latino children generally performing better on performance tasks than verbal ones (Kaufman, 1990). The Wechsler Intelligence Scale for Children – Revised (WISC-R) has been translated into Spanish (Escala de Inteligencia Wechsler para Ninos-Revisada – EIWN-R). The test publishers (The Psychological Corporation) consider the EIWN-R to be a research edition and it is published without normative data (Psychological Corporation, 1983). Another version of the WISC-R was translated into Spanish in Puerto Rico. The Escala de Inteligencia Para Ninos – Revisada de Puerto Rico (EIWN-R PR) was normed on 2,200 Puerto-Rican children between the ages of 6 and 16.11 years (Psychological Corporation, 1993). Because of the narrow norming base, this test may not be appropriate for most Hispanic groups in the U.S.

Neuropsychological measures

There has been surprisingly little attention paid to the development of neuropsychological tests and norms for Latino children and adolescents. Ardila and Rosselli (1994) compiled normative data on five to twelve year-old Colombian children on a range of neuropsychological measures assessing several domains. Language was assessed with Spanish translations of the Boston Naming Test, Token Test-Shortened Version, and Verbal Fluency (both semantic and phonologic). Visual-spatial abilities were evaluated with the Rey-Osterrieth Complex Figure Copy, reproduction, and recognition tasks. Memory was assessed with the Wechsler Memory scale and a sequential verbal memory test. The preliminary normative study found SES significantly related to test performance and sex differences. Rosselli (1993) administered the Wisconsin Card Sorting Test to 233 normal children (aged 5-12 years). She demonstrated a relationship between academic achievement (as measured by a questionnaire) and indices of the WCST. There were no significant differences between SES and gender on the WCST, unlike the other language, memory and visual-spatial tests utilized in the later study.

Although these studies are limited in that they only assessed Colombian children, they are an excellent example of the types of investigations that will lead to a growing knowledge base of how language and culture affect neuropsychological test performance. Additional studies with different populations will help to build a normative database that will be clinically useful.

Test batteries

Psychoeducational

Emerging from the educational psychology realm, the Batería-R Woodcock-Muñoz Pruebas de Aprovechamiento-Revisada (Batería-R ACH) holds much promise as a measure of achievement. Similarly, the Batería-R Wood-cock-Muñoz Pruebas de Habilidad Cognitiva-Revisada (Batería-R COG) is designed to measure a broad range of cognitive abilities. These measures were designed and normed with children, adolescents and adults from the ages of two to 79. They are the parallel Spanish versions of the Woodcock-Johnson Tests of Achievement-Revised (WJ-R ACH), and the Woodcock-Johnson Tests of Cognitive Ability-Revised (WJR-COG; Woodcock & Johnson, 1989).

The Batería-R ACH is intended for use as a wide-range, comprehensive set of tests to measure achievement in reading, mathematics, written language, and knowledge in the content areas of science, social studies, and humani-ties. The Batería-R COG was developed to measure cognitive abilities, scho-lastic aptitudes, and Spanish oral Language. The Batería-R ACH and COG also include a rating of reading and writing proficiency levels based on pre-dicted performance in instructional situations requiring cognitive-academic language proficiency (CALP) (Cummins, 1984; Woodcock & Muñoz-San-doval, 1993a, 1993b, 1993c). In addition, there exists a Comparative Lan-guage Index/Índice de comparación de idiomas (CLI) that allows direct com-parison of Spanish and English reading or writing proficiencies in a single index (Woodcock & Muñoz-Sandoval, 1993b, 1993c).

The Batería begins with a *Language Use Survey*, which includes a number of questions about the individual's language use (i.e., first language, lan-guage primarily spoken by individual at home, primary languages spoken by others at home, primary language spoken by individual in social settings such as playground or cafeteria, primary language spoken by individual in classroom). The Comparative Language Index/ Índica de Comparación de Idiomas (CLI) is a combination of the Spanish Relative Proficiency Index (RPI) and an English Relative Mastery Index (RMI). This index produces a proportion (the CLI) signifying proficiency in Spanish over the relative proficiency in English. An example provided by the test developers dem-onstrates this procedure. A child obtaining an RMI for the English Oral Language cluster of 15/90 indicates that if the child is given oral language tasks performed with 90% proficiency by average beginning second-graders in the U.S., he is predicted to perform these tasks with 15% proficiency in English. His RPI for Spanish Oral Language/ Lenguaje oral cluster was 66/90 (suggesting that he is predicted to perform parallel oral language tasks with 66% proficiency when those tasks are presented in Spanish). The final CLI is 66/15, indicating a predicted 66% proficiency in Spanish and a 15% proficiency in English. This index allows the clinician to assess the child's relative mastery of the English language compared to English-speaking peers enrolled in U.S. schools. The closer the proportion is to one, the greater the relative English mastery.

This CLI provides the neuropsychologist with rich information base regarding the child's language. First, there exists comparative information demonstrating which of the two languages is stronger or dominant (i.e., Spanish in the demonstration case). Secondly, this index produces information regarding proficiency in *each* language compared to others at the same age or grade level.

In addition to the added language-related assessment subtests, the Batería measures similar abilities as the original WJ-R Tests of Achievement used to assess several domains of cognitive functioning including attention, visual perception/ processing, auditory perception/ processing, memory and learning, language, reasoning and problem solving, and academic achievement. These domains and the tests of the WJ-R and the Batería are presented in Table 1.

Test development of the Batería
In development of the test items, the authors of the Batería-R utilized a Spanish-speaking sample consisting of 1,325 individuals from Arizona, California, Florida, New York, and Texas. In addition, 2586 individuals were recruited from countries other than the U.S. including Costa Rica, Mexico, Peru, Puerto Rico, and Spain. The norms for the Batería-R were based on two general requirements: 1) To be based on a cross-section of the general U.S. population with respect to demographic variables (e.g., race, gender, geographic location, and size of community), and 2) participants included reflect the general normal course of development in Spanish (Woodcock & Muñoz-Sandoval, 1996). The test developers prepared norms based on a detailed test calibrating-equating and norming procedure by application of the Rasch model technology (Rasch, 1960). This procedure produced a Spanish version of the WJ-R ACH and COG psychometrically similar to the original English version.

Recommendations for future research
The field of clinical neuropsychology is still very early within its developmental trajectory and cross-cultural neuropsychology, particularly within the U.S., is even less developed. As with any new and developing field, there are many challenges as well as many intriguing possibilities; only a few of which can be discussed within the scope of this paper. The possibilities that exist include the basic science of neuropsychology as well as its clinical applications. For example, at a basic level, the work of Judy Kroll and her colleagues (c.f., Kroll, Michael, & Sankaranarayanan, 1998) underscores the importance of understanding how bilingualism is represented in cognitive and structural models.

Clinically, there is an urgent need for the development of normative data across a wide spectrum of Latino/Spanish-speaking cultures. Importantly, these norms must be adequately stratified developmentally with tightly bound age cohorts. As discussed earlier, tests and norms need to be developed that will allow for the flexibility to examine the child in both English and Spanish and allow the child to provide answers in whichever language is most comfortable. Lastly, most of the test development that has occurred to date

Table 1. Neuropsychological domains for WJ-R/ BAT-R cognitive and achievement subtests.

Domain	WJ-R Subtest/ BAT-R Subtest
Attention	
Sustained and Selective Attention	Visual Matching/ Pareo Visual** Cross Out/ Tachar**
Sustained Attention	Writing Fluency/ Fluidez in la redacción*
Attentional Capacity	Memory for Words/ Memoria para palabras** Memory for Sentences/ Memoria para frases** Numbers Reversed/ Inversión de números**
Visual Perception/ Processing	Visual Closure/ Integración visual** Spatial Relations/ Relaciones espaciales** Picture Recognition/Reconocimiento de dibujos**
Auditory Perception/ Processing	Incomplete Words/ Palabras incompletas** Sound Blending/ Interación de sonidos** Sound Patters/ Configuración de sonidos**
Memory and Learning	
Short-Term Memory	Memory for Words/ Memoria para palabras** Memory for Sentences/ Memoria para frases** Numbers Reversed/ Inversión de números** Picture Recognition/ Reconocimiento de dibujos**
Long-Term Retrieval	Memory for Names (and Delayed Recall)/ Memoria para nombres (y Memoria diferida)** Visual-Auditory Learning (and Delayed Recall)/ Aprendizaje visual-auditivo (y Memoria diferida)**
Remote Memory	Science/ Ciencia* Social Studies/ Estudios sociales* Humanities/ Humanidades*
Oral Language	Picture Vocabulary/ Vocabulario sobre dibujos** Oral Vocabulary/ Vocabulario oral** Memory for Sentences/ Memoria para frases** Listening Comprehension/ Comprensión de oraciones** Verbal Analogies/ Analogías verbales**
Reasoning and Problem Solving	Analysis-Synthesis/ Análisis-Sintesis** Concept Formation/ Formación de conceptos** Verbal Analogies/ Analogías verbales** Spatial Relations/ Relaciones espaciales** Numbers Reversed/ Inversión de números** Calculation/ Cálculo* Applied Problems/ Problemas aplicados*

Table 1, continued.

Domain	WJ-R Subtest/ BAT-R Subtest
Reading Achievement	Letter-Word Identification/ Identificación de letras y palabras* Word Attack/ Análisis de palabras* Reading Vocabulary/ Vocabulario de lectura* Passage Comprehension/ Comprensión de textos*
Writing Ability	Dictation/ Dictado* Proofing/ Corrección de textos* Writing Fluency/ Fluidez en redacción* Writing Samples/ Muestras de redacción*
Mathematics Achievement	Calculation/ Cálculo* Applied Problems/ Problemas aplicados* Quantitative Concepts/ Conceptos cuantitavos*
Curricular Knowledge	Science/ Ciencia* Social Studies/ Estudios sociales* Humanities/ Humanidades*

From *The WJ-R and Batería-R in Neuropsychological Assessment: Research Report Number 1*. (pp. 11-18), by R.W. Woodcock, Riverside Publishing Company.
* Included in Batería-R ACH. ** Included in Batería-R COG.

has involved the translation and adaptation of existing English-language neuropsychological instruments. Although this is an important and very useful endeavor, it also seems important that tests be developed within Latino cultures that assess the subtle (and perhaps not so subtle) differences between cultures.

The type of research discussed above is expensive and requires access to many different populations. In the absence of large multi-center grants, data collection will require the cooperation of many neuropsychologists who are working with Spanish-speaking populations. If a group of neuropsychologists joined forces, perhaps through an organization like the Hispanic Neuropsychological Society, very useful and informative data could be gathered. For example, a core group of five neuropsychological tests could be chosen. The neuropsychologists would agree to administer them in a standardized manner to the population that they work with. The data can then be aggregated and published for others to use. Although such an endeavor will require effort and a spirit of cooperation, the benefits to child neuropsychology are invaluable.

Lastly, test publishers need to be at the forefront of test development and lead efforts to collect data on clinical populations. Cooperation between test publishers and the Latino neuropsychology community could lead to the development of projects that are both clinically useful and fiscally rewarding.

Concluding Remarks

Demographic data clearly demonstrate that Latinos constitute a significant proportion of the U.S. population. Projected growth rates indicate that Hispanics will become the largest ethnic minority group within the U.S. by the year 2050. Approximately 31% of the Latino population will be under the age of 18. This chapter has reviewed many of the issues that are central to the neuropsychological assessment of Latino children. The need to understand the child and his or her family in the context of cultural variables has been underscored. Information on variables such as language use, acculturation experiences, immigration history, family SES, and educational experiences has been described as important for a thorough understanding of the child and any possible neuropsychological deficits that he or she may experience. The neuropsychological evaluation of Latino children is fraught with difficulties stemming from language use (Spanish/English), poorly translated and adapted tests, inadequate normative data, inadequately trained translators, lack of bilingual/bicultural neuropsychologists, and a paucity of research that examines neuropsychological functioning in these children. It was recommended that future research focus on the generation of developmentally appropriate norms across the broad spectrum of Latinos in the U.S. and that new tests be developed, in cooperation with test publishers, that are specific to Latino culture and not simply an adaptation of existing English language tests. Although these may appear to be daunting tasks, it is the responsibility of neuropsychology as a profession to respond to, and provide, appropriate services to a sizable proportion of the U.S. population.

References

Ardila, A., & Roselli, M. (1989). Neuropsychological characteristics of normal aging. *Developmental Neuropsychology, 5*, 307-320.

Ardila, A., & Roselli, M. (1994). Development of language, memory and visuospatial abilities in 5 to 12 year old children using a neuropsychological battery. *Developmental Neuropsychology, 10*, 97-20.

Ardila, A., Rosselli, M., & Ostrosky, F. (1992). Sociocultural factors in neuropsychological assessment. In A.E. Puente & R.J. McCaffrey (Eds.), *Psychobiological factors in clinical neuropsychological assessment* (pp. 181-192). New York: Plenum Press.

Ardila, A., Rosselli, M., & Puente, A.E. (1994). *Neuropsychological evaluation of the Spanish speaker*. New York: Plenum Press.

Ardila, A., Rosselli, M., & Rosas, P. (1989). Neuropsychological assessment in illiterates: Visuospatial and memory abilities. *Brain and Cognition, 11*, 147-166.

Barona, A., & Miller, J.A. (1994). Short acculturation scale for Hispanic youth (SASH-Y): A preliminary report. *Hispanic Journal of the Behavioral Sciences, 16* (2), 155-162.

Bernal, E.M. (1990). Increasing the interpretive validity and diagnostic utility of Hispanic children's scores on tests of achievement and intelligence. In A.S.F.C.

Serafica, R.K. Russell, P.D. Isaac, & L.B. Myers (Eds.), *Mental health of ethnic minorities* (pp. 108-138). New York: Praeger.

Bernal, E.M. (1993). Trends in bilingual special education. *Learning Disability Quarterly, 6*, 424-431.

Berry, J.W., Trimble, J., & Olmedo, E.L. (1988). Assessment of acculturation. In W.J.L. & J.W.Bern (Eds.), *Field methods in cross-cultural research* (pp. 291-324). Beverly Hills, CA: Sage Publications.

Bracken, B., & Barona, A. (1991). State of the art procedures for translating, validating, and using psychoeducational tests in cross-cultural assessment. *School Psychology International, 12* (1-2), 119-132.

Bruner, J.S., Oliver, R.R., & Greenfield, P.M. (1966). *Studies in cognitive growth*. New York: Wiley.

Cuellar, I., Harris, J.G., Lorwen, C., & Jasso, R. (1980). An acculturation scale for Mexican American normal and clinical populations. *Hispanic Journal of Behavioral Sciences, 2*, 199-217.

Cummins, J. (1984). *Bilingualism and special education: Issues in assessment and pedagogy*. Austin: Pro-Ed.

De Lemos, M.M. (1965). The development of conservation in aboriginal children. *International Journal of Psychology, 4*, 2155-2169.

Deosaransingh, K., Moreno, C., Woodruff, S.I., Sallis, J.F., et al. (1995). Acculturation and smoking in Latino youth. *Health Values, 19*, 43-52.

Echemendia, R.J., Harris, J.G., Congett, S.M., Diaz, L.M., & Puente, A.E. (1997). Neuropsychological training and practices with Hispanics: A national survey. *Clinical Neuropsychologist, 11* (3), 229-243.

Epstein, J.A., Botvin, G.J., Dusenbury, L., & Diaz, T. (1996). Validation of an acculturation measure for Hispanic adolescents. *Psychological Reports, 79*, 1075-1079.

Figueroa, R.A. (1990). Assessment of bilingual children. In A. Thomas & J. Grimes (Eds.), *Best practices in school psychology-II* . Washington, D.C.: National Association of School Psychologists.

Geisinger, K. (1994). Cross-cultural normative assessment: Translation and adaptation issues influencing the normative interpretation of assessment instruments. *Psychological Assessment, 6* (4), 304-312.

Golding, J.M., & Burnam, M.A. (1990). Immigration, stress, and depressive symptoms in a Mexican-American community. *Journal of Nervous and Mental Disease, 178* (3), 161-171.

Harris, J.G., Cullum, C.M., & Puente, A.E. (1995). Effects of bilingualism on verbal learning and memory in Hispanic adults. *Journal of the International Neuropsychological Society, 1*, 10-16.

Hickey, T. (1972). Bilingualism and the measurement of intelligence and verbal learning ability. *Exceptional Children, 39*, 24-28.

Kagan, S. (1984). Interpreting Chicano cooperativeness: Methodological and theoretical considerations. In R.H.M.J.L. Martinez (Ed.), *Chicano psychology* (pp. 289-334). Orlando: Academic Press.

Kaufman, A.S. (1979). WISC-R Research: Implications for interpretation. *Journal of School and Psychology Review, 8*, 5-27.

Kaufman, A.S. (1990). *Assessing adolescent and adult intelligence*. Needham: Allyn & Bacon.

Kroll, J., Michael, E. & Sankaranarayanan, A. (1998). A model of bilingual representation and its implications for second language acquisition. In A. Healy & L.E. Bourne (Eds.). *Foreign language learning: Psycholinguistic studies on training and retention* (pp. 365-395). Mahwah: Lawrence Erlbaum Associates.

Lozoff, B., Klein, N., Nelson, E., McClish, D., Manuel, M., & Chacon, M.E. (1998). Behavior of infants with iron-deficiency anemia. *Child Development, 69* (1), 24-36.

Manuel-Dupont, S., Ardila, A., Rosselli, M., & Puente, A. (1992). Bilingualism. In A.E. Puente, & R.J. McCaffrey (Eds.), *Handbook of neuropsychological assessment: A biopsychosocial perspective.* (pp. 193-210). New York: Plenum Press.

Marín, G. (1992). Issues in the measurement of acculturation among Hispanics. In K.F. Geisinger (Ed.), *Psychological testing of Hispanics* (pp. 235-251). Washington, D.C.: American Psychological Associaton.

Marín, G., & Marín, B. VanOss (1991). *Research with Hispanic populations.* Newbury Park, CA: Sage Publications.

Marín, G., Sabogal, F. , Marín, B.V., Otero-Sabogal, R., & Perez-Stable, E.J. (1987). Development of a short acculturation scale for Hispanics. *Hispanic Journal of Behavioral Sciences, 9,* 183-205.

Mendoza, P. (1983). The role of language in psychological assessment of students. *Bilingual Special Education News, 1,* 4-5.

Moore, E.G. (1987). Ethnic social milieu and Black children's intelligence test achievement. *Journal of Negro Education, 56* (1), 44-52.

Ostrosky, F., Canseco, E., Quintanar, L., Navarro, E., Meneses, S., & Ardila, A. (1985). Sociocultural effects in neuropsychological assessment. *International Journal of Neuroscience, 27,* 53-66.

Perez-Arce, P., & Puente, A.E. (1996). Neuropsychological assessment of ethnic minorities: The case of Hispanics living in North America. In R.J. Shorbone, & C.J. Long (Eds.), *Ecological validity of neuropsychological testing* (pp. 283-300). Delray Beach: GR Press/ St. Lucie Press.

Piaget, J. (1928). *Judgment and reasoning in the child.* (Trans. M. Worden). New York: Harcourt, Brace & World.

Politzer, R.L., Shohamy, E. & McGroarty, M. (1983). Validation of linguistic and communicative oral language tests for Spanish-English bilingual programs. *Bilingual Review, 10* (1), 3-20.

Pontón, M.O., Satz., P.., Herrera, L., Urrutia, C.P., Ortiz, F., Young, R., D'Elia, L., Furst, C.J., & Namerow, N. (1996). The Neuropsychological Screening Battery for Hispanics: Initial report. *Journal of the International Neuropsychological Society, 2* (2), 96-104.

Pontón, M.O., & Ardila, A. (1999). The future of neuropsychology with Hispanic populations in the United States. *Archives of Clinical Neuropsychology, 14* (7), 565-580.

Puente, A.E. (1990). Psychological assessment of minority group members. In G. Goldstein & M. Hersen (Eds.), *Handbook of psychological assessment* (pp. 505-520). New York: Pergamon Press.

Puente, A.E., Sol Mora, M., & Munoz-Cespedes, J.M. (1997). Neuropsychological assessment of Spanish-speaking children and youth. In C. R. Reynolds & E. Fletcher-Janzen (Eds.), *Handbook of clinical child neuropsychology* (2nd ed., pp. 371-383). New York: Plenum Press.

Puente, A.E., & Salazar, G.D. (1998). Assessment of minority and culturally diverse children. In A. S. Prifitera, & D. Sahlofsko (Eds.), *WISC-III clinical use and interpretation: Scientist-Practitioner perspectives* (pp. 227-248). San Diego: Academic Press.

Putnam, S.H., & DeLuca, J.W. (1990). The TCN professional practice survey: I. General practices of neuropsychologists in primary employment and private practice settings. *Clinical Neuropsychologist, 4,* 199-243.

Putnam, S.H., & DeLuca, J.W. (1991). The TCN professional practice survey: II. An analysis of the fees of neuropsychologists by practicing demographics. *Clinical Neuropsychologists, 5* (2), 103-124.

Rasch, G. (1960). *Probabilistic models for some intelligence and attainment tests.* Copenhagen: Danish Institute of Educational Research.

Ramirez, A.G., Cousins, J.H., Santos, Y., & Supik, J.D. (1986). A media-based acculturation scale for Mexican-Americans: Application to public health education programs. *Family & Community Health, 9*, 63-71.

Rosselli, M., Ardila, A., & Rosas, P. (1990). Neuropsychological assessment in illiterates II: Language and praxic abilities. *Brain and Cognition, 12*, 281-296.

Rosselli, M. (1993). Neuropsychology of illiteracy. *Behavioral Neurology, 6*, 107-112.

Reynolds, C.R., & Kaiser, S.M. (1990). Test bias in psychological assessment. In T.B. Gutkin, C.R. Reynolds, et al. (Eds.). *The handbook of school psychology* (2nd ed., pp. 487-525). New York: John Wiley & Sons.

The Psychological Corporation (1983). *Escala de inteligencia Wechsler para Niños – Revisada.* San Antonio: The Psychological Corporation.

The Psychological Corporation (1993). *Escala de inteligencia Wechsler para Niños – Revisada de Puerto Rico.* San Antonio: The Psychological Corporation.

Tropp, L.R., Erkut, S., Coll, C.G., Alarcon, O., & Garcia, H.A. Vazquez (1999). Psychological acculturation development of a new measure for Puerto Ricans on the U.S. mainland. *Educational & Psychological Measurement, 59*, 351-367.

United States Census Bureau (2000) Available: www.census.gov/www/projections/natsum-T3.html.

United States Census Bureau (1998) Available: www.census.gov/hhes/income/income98/incxrace.html

Woodcock, R.W., & Johnson, M.B. (1989). *Woodcock-Johnson Tests of Achievement-Revised.* Itasca: Riverside.

Woodcock, R.W., & Muñoz-Sandoval, A.F. (1993a). An IRT approach to cross-language test equating and interpretation. *European Journal of Psychological Assessment, 9* (3), 233-241.

Woodcock, R.W. & Muñoz-Sandoval, A.F. (1993b). *Woodcock-Muñoz Language Survey, English Form.* Itasca: Riverside.

Woodcock, R.W., & Muñoz-Sandoval, A.F. (1993c). *Woodcock-Muñoz Language Survey, Spanish Form.* Itasca: Riverside.

Woodcock, R.W., & Muñoz-Sandoval, A.F. (1996). *Bateria Woodcock-Munoz: Pruebas de habilidad cognitiva-Revisada: Supplemental Manual.* Chicago: Riverside Publishing.

Chapter 11

THE EMPIRICAL DEVELOPMENT OF A NEUROPSYCHOLOGICAL SCREENING INSTRUMENT FOR MEXICAN-AMERICANS

Guadalupe Gutierrez, Ph.D.
Chicano Studies Department, Arizona State University, Tempe, Arizona

Abstract

This chapter will focus on the empirical issues involved in the creation and/or adaptation of tools for use with linguistic minorities, in this case monolingual and bilingual Mexican-Americans. To begin, a brief overview of the available research, addressing instrument adaptation and creation for Spanish speakers, will be provided. The author will then continue by presenting alternative methodology, based on the principles of ethnopsychology, used in the creation of a new tool for neuropsychological screening of brain trauma. This new measure, the Culture-reduced Assessment of Neuro-cognitive Abilities (CANA), will be presented in terms of its development, including item selection, translation and construct validation. The technique and preliminary results regarding norming and standards for Mexican Americans will be discussed. Also, mediating factors (such as acculturation level and language proficiency) and their effects on the measure outcomes will be analyzed. Finally, a self-critique of the CANA's utility as a screener for brain trauma in Mexican Americans (or other Latinos depending on available participants), will be offered.

Introduction

Clinical neuropsychology has long been challenged with the task of appropriately diagnosing and/or addressing issues of neurologic impairment in Spanish speakers. Although several classic neuropsychological tools have been translated (see Ardila, Rosselli, & Puente, 1994) and initial, though limited, norms have been attained, the task of developing appropriate assessment tools for linguistic minorities, in this case Spanish speakers, continues to be in its preliminary stages. As Ardila and his associates have indicated in a previous chapter and in other writings (Ardila et al., 1994; Ardila, 1995), there are several fundamental problems in adapting or creating assessment tools for Spanish speakers. In neuropsychology, these include such issues as language (translation) and moderating factors of age, gender, acculturation, literacy, and education (Ardila, 1995; Butcher, 1996; Ponton & Ardila, 1999; Puente & McCaffrey, 1992). Other literature also brings to light the need to address issues of bilingualism (Harris, Cullum, & Puente, 1995; O'Brien, 1989; Ponton & Ardila, 1999) and cultural differences in cognition (Ardila, 1995; Perez-Arce, 1999). In response to such difficulties, the author, in conjunction with a team of neuropsychologists at a large urban medical campus, embarked upon the task of "building" a neuropsychological screener that can offer a more sensitive set of results for Spanish speakers as compared to the commonly used translation of the Mini-Mental State Examination. (It should be noted that the purpose of a screening tool is to assess general areas of dysfunction and therefore the tool discussed here does not propose to replace the functionality of more specifically oriented assessment tools such as measures of aphasia, specific memory, etc.).

Currently, the standard of practice for the neuropsychological assessment of Spanish speakers is marked by inadequate training and insufficient supervision (Echemendia, Harris, Congett, Diaz, & Puente, 1997). Indeed, in their survey of neuropsychologists (members of the American Psychological Association's Division 40 and the National Academy of Neuropsychologists living in the U.S.; $n = 911$; return rate of 25%), Echemendia and his associates (1997) found that 90% of the sample had no training in providing services to minority populations. Only about 5% (42) of the participants had significant experience in evaluating Latinos. Those who had assessed or treated Spanish speakers reported adequate to fluent bilingualism or used a translator. The respondents also indicated a high rate (41%) of "totally" inadequate supervision, while 52% reported generally adequate supervision in working with Latinos. In general, Echemendia and his associates concluded that competence in the assessment and treatment of Spanish speakers required several improvements in

the training of neuropsychologists, including better supervision, more exposure to cultural issues influencing neuro-cognitive abilities, and more adequate
training regarding cultural influences on assessment measures. These authors
emphasized the need to understand how data provided by neuropsychological
assessment instruments may be altered by the linguistic and cultural qualities
unique to Latinos.

In an effort to contribute to the area of improved neuropsychological
assessment of Latinos, this chapter's goal is to expose the reader to methodology in the development of neuropsychological assessment tools that
are more culturally sensitive to the Spanish speaker, specifically Mexican
Americans. It also exposes the reader to the application of ethnopsychological (emic-based) method and theory in psychometrics. The presentation of instrument development and emic-based theory addresses the questions posed in the introductory paragraphs: how can Spanish speakers be
accurately assessed for neuro-cognitive functioning and how might cultural
issues be integrated into the assessment tools so as to reduce the skewing
of data? The chapter has five major sections, which fundamentally follow
the initial four stages of instrument adaptation, as presented by Geisinger
(1994). (Geisinger's work will be elaborated shortly.) First, there is a brief
introduction to the psychometric considerations involved in the adaptation
and/or development of measures for use on linguistic minorities. This is
followed by a presentation of how the author and her associates have
incorporated the previously presented considerations into the building of
a new tool (the CANA-Culturally-sensitive Assessment of Neuro-cognitive
Abilities). The reader will also, within the discussion of how the CANA is
being developed, be introduced to the use of ethnopsychological method
in regards to norming and standardization. The subsequent two sections
focus on the methods and preliminary statistical analyses of the empirical
pilot study exploring aspects of construct validity in the CANA, including
a comparison with the MMSE. Finally, the last section, the discussion,
centers on analyzing these initial results of the pilot study and providing a
self-critique of the CANA in its current form.

Psychometric Considerations

According to Anastasi and Urbina (1997), there are three basic approaches
to cross-cultural testing. The first approach involves choosing several "universal" (common among many cultures) items to test a construct and then
validating the resulting test per local criteria. This is the basic principle of
"culture-free" or "culture-fair" measures which are premised on repeated
validation in different cultures. Culture-free or culture-fair measures tend
to be non-verbal task tools requiring minimal, if any, language interaction
between the tester and the person being tested (Anastasi, 1976, pp. 287-298).
Cronbach (1990) cautioned, however, that "no method of item selection

yields 'culture free' tests" (p. 339) because even these measures depend on behavioral evidence that is culturally influenced. Indeed, Cronbach cautions that the best one can hope for is a culture-reduced measure. These culture-reduced measures, theoretically, emphasize and incorporate cultural information into the assessment tool as opposed to the "culture-free" or "culture-fair" tests that focus on universals.

A second approach to cross-cultural testing involves developing a test within one culture and administering it to persons of different cultural backgrounds. This method is among the most traditional in the U.S. and is well exemplified by classic intelligence and personality measures. The results provided by such measures should not be confused as providing appropriate universal measures of a given construct (such as intelligence or psychopathology) but rather serve to examine or ascertain the cultural distance between cultural groups. For example, classic tests of intelligence as developed in the U.S. can, at best, only describe the degree to which an ethnic (or linguistic) minority has acculturated or been exposed to U.S. education or educational values. The construct of interest, in this case intelligence, cannot be assumed to be measured accurately because it (intelligence) was defined according to the values of an external group and therefore may not represent the construct as defined within the minority group.

A third approach to cross-cultural testing promotes the use of different tests, or substantial adaptations of existing tests, to be developed within a given culture. Each test may measure a similar or the same construct, but the construct is defined and the test is only applied within the culture in which it was developed for use. No cross-cultural comparisons are made—as the criteria being tested are solely constructed per intra-cultural norms. This third approach is similar to the idea proposed by Cronbach (1990) of culture-reduced tests that incorporate cultural values rather than ignore or overgeneralize these in the adaptation of a measure. The CANA (Culturally-sensitive Assessment of Neurological Abilities) Test, which will be presented in more detail later in this chapter, serves as an example of this approach. The stimuli of the CANA were developed with special attention to Latino cultural experience, social norms, and values. The tool was also adapted linguistically to emphasize the appropriate dialect and vocabulary of Mexican-descendent people (on whom it will be piloted and normed). Furthermore, in keeping with this third approach to cross-cultural testing, norming is being done in an ethnopsychological fashion, with a focus on within-group comparisons only, not between-group comparatives. Such an approach provides the opportunity for a culturally specific and bias-reduced tool.

As the reader may imagine, validation of a tool within a culture makes it necessary to assure that the tool is properly developed or adapted for the cultural group of interest. Geisinger (1994) provided a thorough and extensive list of guidelines for adapting or creating cross-cultural assessment tools. Specifically, Geisinger described ten procedures/stages to be considered in the cross-cultural adaptation of a tool. In brief, these guidelines included:

(1) The translation of measure including back-translation
(2) Review of the translated version by a group of bilingual individuals for content and construct quality
(3) Adoption of a draft of the measure incorporating comments from the reviewer
(4) Piloting the instrument to learn of potential problems in the administration and patient response to the tool
(5) Field testing the instrument (with revisions from the pilot study); administering the instrument to a large sample and complete initial analyses for internal consistency and item analysis
(6) Standardizing the scores
(7) Performing validation research as appropriate
(8) Developing a manual
(9) Training users
(10) Collecting reactions from users of the instrument for subsequent refinement and revision.

As indicated by Geisinger, the above guidelines are recommended but may not all be necessary. In some cases more steps may be necessary, or the guidelines may require application in a different order than listed above depending on the particular qualities of the measure being adapted or developed. Nevertheless, the steps presented by Geisinger provide cross-cultural psychometricians with a common set of approaches for adapting a measure to a new target population.

According to Dana (1993), measure adaptations should also account for functional equivalence, metric equivalence, and construct equivalence (also see Butcher & Han, 1996). Functional equivalence pertains to different behaviors developed in different cultures to cope with similar problems. That is, a similar stimulus can provoke different reactions but these reactions are equally culturally effective in dealing with the stimulus. For example, in the case of stress, Anglo culture may typically engage a very active and overtly interventive coping style (more person over nature, and internal locus of control; see Carter, 1991 for review of cultural values). Meanwhile, in traditional Mexican culture the activity of coping may center on acceptance and "waiting" to see how the situation settles out on its own (nature over person and external locus of control; see Carter, 1991; Diaz-Guerrero, 1989; Diaz-Loving & Andrade-Palos, 1984). Metric equivalence refers to the presentation formats of scales, questionnaires, and personality measures. Cross-culturally the question of metric equivalence centers on the idea of "distance" between responses. That is, does the difference between "somewhat satisfied" and "satisfied" on a likert-type scale have the same meaning in another cultural context? Construct equivalence centers on the meaning of items within a measure. Does the item have the same meaning or purpose in the culture for which it is being adapted? Closely linked to construct equivalence is linguistic equivalence which includes not literal translation but construct-relevant translation incorporating culturally appropriate value and affect responses.

Associated with the above issues of equivalence (functional, metric, and construct) is the issue of validity. Any adaptation or development of a tool requires careful attention to the validity of the "new" measure. Validation of a tool can come from three sources: content-related, criterion-related and construct-related (Geisinger, 1994; Kaplan & Saccuzzo, 1997). Content validity refers to how well the items of a measure are an adequate representation of the conceptual domain that is being evaluated. Criterion-related validity is based on the principle of predictability—how well does the measure (predictor variable) forecast the quality being assessed (criterion). Criterion validity serves as a primary technique for evaluating measure usefulness (predictive ability) but is not generally the most useful approach in answering questions of interest to cross-cultural research (such as equivalence of item meaning) (Geisinger, 1994). The third form of validation, construct-related validity, refers to a construct being defined as part of a tool and being meaningfully measured. For example, if the construct of attention is being measured, not only is it desirable to have items that seem to cover that domain (content validity) and items that seem predictive (e.g., digit span--criterion validity) but also to make sure the items are meaningful in assessing the construct across cases (thus, items that assess the same construct should be closely interrelated in meaning, even cross-culturally).

Construct-related validity is arguably the most useful form of validity in the evaluation of measures cross-culturally because it attests to the general stability of the tool. That is, content and criterion can often change cross-culturally but construct meaning should remain the same. Geisinger (1994) illustrated how content- and criterion-related validity might differ cross-culturally. Imagine if a measure had been constructed to measure a given school subject (e.g., the content area of reading), it is not likely that the domain for the school subject would be the same cross-culturally because of differences in teaching style, language, and educational values. Similarly, with criterion-related validity, the criterion (e.g., scholastic success) may be differentially defined across cultures. One culture may value a concrete measure of success such as grades, while another may value more inter-personal properties such as communication abilities and manners. Thus, even when using the same measure, the criterion for prediction may vary.

Empirical Development of a Neurological Screening Tool

When considering neuropsychological abilities it is important to note that the issue of interest is not whether the brain injury will manifest differently in a member of a linguistic minority (content), but rather if the measure is accurately assessing the impairment in a meaningful manner (construct). For example, when assessing basic frontal-lobe abilities such as simple language abilities and short-term memory a client may be asked to repeat a common phrase. However, it may be the case that the phrase is "common" in one language but not in another. Thus, when presented as a literal translation to a linguistic minority the phrase is unfamiliar (i.e., no longer considered common) and requires more complex language processing than was originally intended. In such instances, linguistic minorities may be inappropriately assessed with greater frontal lobe deficit than is actually present. Traditional screening tools such as the Mini-Mental State Examination (MMSE) have not accounted for the psychometric considerations denoted by Dana (1993). For example, the MMSE has been adapted for functional equivalence and metric equivalence, but construct equivalence is assumed, not tested, across cultural and linguistic groups. In an effort to improve the service and diagnostic screening available to the fastest increasing minority in the U.S., the current author and her colleagues have begun an empirical endeavor to develop a Spanish-language neurological screening tool for Mexican-American monolinguals. This investigative effort led to the development of the Culturally-sensitive Assessment of Neurocognitive Abilities Test (CANA). (The content make-up of the CANA is detailed in the Methods section of this chapter.)

With the psychometric demands presented in the previous section in mind, the CANA was developed with particular attention to construct equivalence. Functional equivalence was of lesser concern because brain injury in specific parts of the brain has expectable manifestations. (The term "expectable" is used in terms of broad functioning as would be assessed by a screening instrument, and does not indicate specific diagnostic criteria.) The question is not the difference in terms of how, for example, frontal lobe damage would exhibit itself in Spanish-speakers versus English-speakers because it is already neurologically known that, regardless of language, the damage/injury will likely affect certain abilities (e.g., short-term memory, attention, executive functioning). Metric equivalence was minimized in the CANA in that the client is only asked to estimate performance three times during the testing. Furthermore, when asked to estimate a metric, the client is always given a clear idea of the quantification and distance of the scale being used. For instance, the client may be asked "Of the five words on this list (which the client has practiced verbally), how many do you think you will remember in 15 minutes?" The metric, when presented in this manner, is concrete and culturally accessible both in Spanish and in English. All other scales or scoring are relevant only to the examiner, and rely on specific criteria to distinguish between metric values.

Returning to the topic of construct equivalence, this issue was addressed in the CANA through careful, construct-focused translation (and backtranslation) and by providing culturally sensitive stimuli. The CANA Test was originally written in English because of the simple fact that this was the only language shared by all four of the researchers who developed it. The measure was then translated into Spanish by the author of this chapter who is a native Spanish speaker. Backtranslations were provided by three native

Spanish speakers from Texas. Although translation and backtranslation are essential features of construct equivalence, literal translations often do not adequately convey the meaning of a test item. Thus, the CANA was translated not literally but per the intended meaning of the items. In practice, this meant that some sentence structure and organization had to be modified so as to maintain the construct of interest. For example, instead of the literal translation for "What is your age?" (Que es su edad?), the question was translated as "Cuantos anos tiene?" (How many years do you have?). This may seem a simple, almost insignificant change, but the effect is a much more accessible and easily understood item that preserves the construct of interest (orientation of self).

Much of the construct equivalence of the CANA actually occurred prior to full translation into Spanish. The process of construct equivalence was prevalent even at the stage of creating items. For example, the Attention Subscale uses a simple sentence repetition task to assess general issues of aphasia. However, instead of using an U.S.-Anglo-based concept (such as a common saying – "no if, ands, or buts"), a sentence was chosen which incorporated commonly recognized concepts and relationships ("Mother wants chicken and rice from the market."). In another subscale, Reasoning, stimuli were chosen so as to minimize cultural effects. Thus, instead of sequencing drawings that depict an activity such as fishing or buying a candy bar, the client is asked to sequence the rising and setting of the sun (both dawn to dusk and vice-versa are correct responses). Initial efforts early in the formulation of items helped to ensure better and more functional adaptations of the CANA to include important cultural constructs into the tool.

In addition to the structural adaptations within the tool, several steps are being taken to facilitate the cultural applicability of the CANA. (Note that data collection to perform the following analyses is underway but that the author's current sample of Spanish speakers is too small to draw solid results from the data. Thus, this section is focused on future analyses to be completed in order to acquire proper validity with the CANA.) First, in order to validate the CANA in general, statistical analyses of the construct validity both within the tool (i.e., subscale items should cluster together) and of convergence between measures will be performed such that coordinate constructs of the CANA should converge with similar constructs measured by the Spanish MMSE. Second, a divergent analysis should be performed on data from initial cases. This analysis is performed in order to demonstrate the differences between the MMSE and the CANA Test when administered to Spanish-speakers.

Third, and most importantly, as discussed previously, Anastasi and Urbina (1997) describe an approach to cross-cultural testing which involves only intra-group norms and tends to be effective in reducing cultural bias. Given this, the CANA will be normed per ethnopsychological method and theory. Ethnopsychology is based on the fundamental principle that culturally and linguistically different groups, in this case Mexican Americans, are unique, having their own set of beliefs, perceptions, and cognitive patterns (see Diaz-Guerrero, 1992, 1993; Ramirez, 1983). According to the tenets of ethnopsychological theory, culturally and linguistically distinct groups are best served by a psychological theory and application that incorporates the "uniqueness" (values, percepts, cognitive patterns) of the population of interest. Thus, only internal comparisons are considered relevant to creating standards or ranges of performance for the cultural group. This process differs from most other screening tools that rely on general norms without special attention to the specific cultural demands of a Spanish-speaking population. The methods and statistical analyses involved in establishing the preliminary parameters of validity for the CANA in Spanish are discussed in the following sections of this chapter. These methods and analyses basically follow those guidelines suggested by Geisinger (1994) and described earlier in the chapter. For the purposes of the current pilot study the author completed the first four procedures suggested by Geisinger in the adaptation of a tool for cross-cultural use. Only descriptive statistics and initial analyses evaluating the heuristics of convergence and divergence between the measures were included.

Method

Participants. Data for this pilot study were collected from six Spanish monolingual Mexican Americans (Mexican immigrants and U.S. born) living in the metro area of a large southwestern city. Only monolinguals were used for the purposes of this small pilot study because the focus was to explore the use of this tool on Spanish speakers using an ethnopsychological methodology (control of the ethnicities included was necessary in order to be more culturally specific – as warranted by ethnopsychological theory). Subsequent studies on the CANA Test will include bilingual (but Spanish dominant) subjects and will involve an analysis of acculturation, gender, socio-economic status, and education as moderating factors affecting performance on the tool. The participants were recruited by three means. Three were patients undergoing a standard battery assessment upon admission to the neuro-rehabilitation unit of a large medical complex. One was assessed at a nursing home as part of an assessment for a county hospital. The final two patients were assessed by a native Spanish-speaking colleague in private practice. All participants cooperated in the study voluntarily, and were informed that all data would be anonymous.

Participants ranged in age from 21 to 71, with a mean age of 44 years (*SD* = 16.83). Three men and three women participated. The average number of years residing in the U.S. was 16.83 (*SD* = 17.41), with a range from 1 to 50 years. Notice that the outlier of 50 years of residence created a skewed view of the number of years in the U.S. The oldest member in this sample (age 71) had been living in the U.S. for approximately 50 years. However, she resided in a very small town near the border of Mexico with a predominant Mexican immigrant and Mexican-American population. Therefore this patient had never achieved even partial fluency in English. When removed from the sample, the average time in the U.S. was reduced to approximately 12 years. The average level of education for this sample was 8.17 years (SD = 2.71) with a range from 6 to 12 years. All patients included in this sample had damage to the spinal cord, brain, or had a diagnosis of dementia. Type of injury or disorder included: closed head injury; cardiovascular accident; dementia; spinal-cord injury; spinal-cord tumor; and traumatic brain injury. Three of the participants had MRIs within normal limits, one had a left frontal lesion, and one had a right middle cerebral artery clipping. Although the conditions suffered by the participants represent very different afflictions, for the purposes of this initial pilot study the issue of interest was not criterion (prediction) of a particular disorder but rather to explore issues of consistency within the CANA and between the CANA and the MMSE. As the participants were matched with themselves across measures, the broad representation of disorders was not seen as detrimental to the preliminary design of the study.

The sample size was limited by several factors. First only clients with brain injury, spinal cord injury, or dementia were included. No patients with primary affective or personality disorders were included. Second, only monolingual Mexican Americans were asked to participate in this particular study because the research team was interested in evaluating the linguistic and psychometric qualities of the Spanish version of the CANA. (Bilingual persons will be included in later studies of the measure but will need to be evaluated for proficiency in both English and Spanish to account for linguistic anomalies that may emerge in testing.) Third, time constrains for publication from the time of completing and tuning the Spanish translation of the CANA limited the availability of viable participants for inclusion in this study (particularly given the above requirements). Normals were not included at this stage of the study because interest was focused on the CANA's ability to detect broad neurological dysfunction as compared with the MMSE and not necessarily to standardize or norm the tool yet. There are concurrent studies developing norms with English speaking and Spanish speaking normals.

Measures. Two measures were used for data collection in this pilot study. These included: the Spanish translation of the Mini-Mental State Examination (MMSE) (Ardila, et al.,1994) and the Culture-sensitive Assessment of Neuro-cognitive Abilities (CANA) Test.

Mini-Mental Status Examination (MMSE)
The standard version of the Mini-Mental Status Examination was originally presented by Folstein, Folstein, and McHugh (1975). This screening test was devised as a simplified form of the Cognitive Mental Status Examination which required a longer and more tedious administration. The MMSE consisted of 11 items but was later expanded to 20 items worth a total score of 30 points. A score of 23 is usually thought of as indicative of pathology. The MMSE does not include timed items and requires the patient to have

adequate verbal and vision abilities. Folstein et al. (1975) originally normed the tool on 206 patients suffering a variety of trauma including dementia syndromes, affective disorder, affective disorders with cognitive impairment, mania, schizophrenic disorder, and personality disorder. Sixty-three normals were used for comparative purposes in their original between-group norming study.

The MMSE was designed to assess the areas of orientation, registration (immediate memory), attention and calculation, recall, language, and constructional abilities (see Table 1). Orientation refers to the patient's awareness of time and where they are located. Registration requires the learning of a brief list of word for immediate recall. The purpose of testing attention and calculation is to evaluate the patient's ability to organize a concept (i.e., numbers or a word) and then be able to mentally rearrange it (i.e., count backwards or spell backwards). Recall involves memory and the patient's ability to remember a previously learned list of words. The language portion of the MMSE involves naming objects and being able to repeat familiar phrases. Within the four constructional abilities items the patient is asked to follow a verbal command (take a piece of paper in your right hand, fold it in half, and put it on the floor) and a written command (close your eyes – the patient must read this statement first then execute the command). Finally the patient's ability to produce a sentence (language and motor functioning) and to copy a design (visual spatial and motor functioning) are tested.

A standard Spanish translation of the MMSE was provided by Ardila et al. (1994). This translation is based on a literal translation of the original English-language measure. Ardila and his associates normed this translation on 346 neurologically normal subjects who were Spanish speakers with statistical analyses performed to assess the effects of age, gender, and educational level on overall test scores. They found no significant gender differences. However, there was a "mild tendency" to obtain lower scores with increasing age, controlling for educational level. Interestingly, educational level (at the extremes) did have a significant effect on overall scores, with the low-education subjects scoring approximately three points lower on average than the high-education group. The lowest average scores were associated with low-education subjects over 75 years of age.

The Spanish translation of the MMSE used in this study was identical to the Ardila et al. (1994) version except for two item adaptations. Instead of using the attention and calculation task of counting backwards from 100 by 7's, the version used in this study had the client spell a word backwards. Also, instead of using the list of words provided by Ardila et al. (1994) for the retention task (immediate memory) an alternative list was utilized. These changes are consistent with alternate items presented by Folstein et al. originally and by Ardila et al. in their discussions of Spanish versions of the test. These changes were also made in order to coordinate the research data with the standard versions of measures being used by the hospital facility in which the current project is based.

Table 1. MMSE vs. CANA contents.

MMSE (Total pts.=30)	**CANA** (Total pts.=70)
ORIENTATION (10 pts) Que fecha es hoy? En que mes estamos? En que ano estamos? Que dia de la semana es hoy? En que estacion del ano estamos? Me puede decir el nombre de este lugar? En que piso estamos? En que ciudad estamos? En que condado estamos? En que estado estamos	**ORIENTATION (8 pts)** Cuantos anos tiene? Que es la fecha de su nacimiento? En que ciudad esta usted ahora? Que tipo de edificio es este? Que ano es? Que mes es? Que dia de la semana es hoy? Que hora es (+/- ½ hra)?
REGISTR./IMMEDIATE MEMORY (3 pts) Repita las siguientes palabras: pelota, bandera, arbol.	**IMMEDIATE MEMORY (8 pts)** Repita las siguientes palabras: comida, piedra, agua, arbol, mano El/la cliente/a tambien dibuja 3 figuras.
ATTENTION (6 pts) Deletree la palabra MUNDO al revez. Repita la frase "Ni si, ni no, ni pero."	**ATTENTION (8 pts)** Dos reactivos de numeros adelante. Dos reactivos de numeros al revez. Cuente cuantas veces se toca el lapiz contra la mesa. Repita la frase "Mama quiere pollo y arroz del mercado" Cuente de 30 a 1 al revez.
DELAYED MEMORY/RECALL (3 pts) Repita las 3 palabras que memorizo antes (pelota, bandera, arbol)	**DELAYED MEMORY (8 pts)** Repita las palabras que memorizo antes (comida, piedra, agua, arbol, mano) Dibuje las tres figuras que dijujo antes.
LANGUAGE (7 pts) Que es esto? (Mostrando lapiz) Que es esto? (Mostrando reloj) Lea el papel (Cierre los ojos) en voz alta y haga lo que dice la frase. Digale al paciente que tome un pedazo de papel en su mano derecha, que lo doble por la mitad, y que lo ponga en el suelo. Digale al paciente que escriba una frase completa.	**LANGUAGE (8 pts)** Toque un circulo rojo (Mostrando estimulo) Toque un cuadro negro, grande (Mostrando estimulo) Toque el circulo amarillo, pequeno y un cuadro blanco grande (Mostrando estimulo) Que es esto? (Elefante) Como se llama esta parte? (Trompa) Que es esto? (Flores) Nombre todos los animales que pueda en 60"
CONSTR. ABILITIES/VISUOSPATIAL (1 pt) Pidale al paciente que dibuje la figura que se le muestra.	**VISUOSPATIAL (8 pts)** Toque numeros 1-9/Toque numeros 9-1 Resolucion de rompecabezas Completacion de estimulo visual Organizacion de estimulo visual (nido) Calificacion de dibujos hechos anteriormente (3)

Table 1, continued.

MMSE (Total pts.=30)	CANA (Total pts.=70)
	REASONING (8 pts) Dos reactivos de similtudes Dos reactivos de opuestos Organizacion sequencial Organizacion de cuento
	EXECUTIVE FUNCTION (8 pts) Tocando ligeramente con mano Tocando ligeramente en sequencia reversada Laberinto Orden de tocar numeros 1-9/9-1
	PRE-SCREEN/ ALERTNESS AND COMMUNICATION (6 pts) Nivel de Vigilancia (Level of alertness) Nivel de habilidad linguistica (Level of language ability)

Culture-Sensitive Assessment of Neurocognitive Abilities (CANA)
The CANA was originally a 52 item test evaluating ten neurocognitive areas including: Language; Immediate memory; Orientation; Attention; Visual-Spatial abilities; Reasoning; Executive functioning; Delayed memory; Emotional control; and Vigilance (see Table 1). There was also a Pre-screening subscale included as part of the overall scoring, giving a maximum score of 80 points for the test. The CANA was originally written in English, the only shared language of all the research team members. Subsequent to the research team's preliminary experiences with administering the CANA to English and Spanish speakers, the test was modified to exclude the qualitative subscales from the overall score. The qualitative subscales were inconsistent in meaning across subjects and also presented a cultural problem in that most of the Spanish speakers felt too conspicuous and/or embarrassed (verguenza) when asked to emit an emotion upon request. In effect, the test was reduced to look at eight of the ten original cognitive areas (48 items) excluding the Emotional Control and Vigilance subscales. The total of possible points was reduced to seventy. (Initial data on 91 English-speaking normals have indicated that a T-score lower than 40 is associated with moderate neuro-cognitive impairment for ages 18 to 62. A projected goal for subsequent studies is to develop standard scores for Spanish speakers.)

The pre-screen subscale is a simple report of the patient's level of alertness (from conscious and aware to comatose) and his/her level of language capacity (i.e., is s/he able to communicate well and clearly?). The Language subscale consists of eight items. Four of these items measure auditory comprehension and the patient's ability to follow single to multi-step commands (using color and shape stimuli). Three of the items require naming skills, and the last item is a category fluency task. The Immediate Memory subscale is comprised of a verbal portion and a visual portion. The verbal portion requires the immediate recall of a list of words. This list is then repeated several times in order to test delayed memory at a later point in the test. The visual portion of this subscale requires the immediate reproduction of different (and increasingly complex) geometric figures. Again, these same stimuli are used for visual delayed recall and also as part of the Visuospatial subscale (scoring in the Visuospatial subscale is for accuracy of reproduction). The Orientation subscale asks basic questions of age, date of birth, place, city, year, month, day of week, and time. It is very similar to the orientation subscale of the MMSE.

The Attention subscale includes seven items. Four of the items focus on repetition of digits forward and backward. Other items involve listening to taps of a pencil, sentence repetition, and counting backwards (from 30 to 1). The Visuospatial subscale is made up of eight items. Two items are similar to the Trail Making Test (the patient need only touch each number regardless of order). These items later serve as part of the Executive Functioning subscale with the criteria of proper order being added for credit in scoring (the items are NOT re-administered). The patient is also given a puzzle to solve, a picture completion task (saw), and a picture organization task (nest) as part of the Visuospatial subscale. The final three items of this subtest include the reproduction of several drawings. These three figures are the same as those administered during the Immediate Memory subscale and are scored for accuracy in reproduction in the Visuospatial subscale. The Reasoning subscale includes six items having to do with naming categories of similarities, opposites, and sequencing stimuli (arranging a picture to tell of a sunrise/sunset).

The Executive Function subscale contains five items. In two of the items the patient is asked to repeat a tapping sequence as quickly as they can within a ten-second period. The three remaining items include the completion of a maze and a re-scoring of earlier items administered on the Visuospatial subscale (touching numbers 1-9). These latter items are not re-administered but are scored here for accuracy in the order in which the numbers were touched (ascending or descending). The final subscale, Delayed Memory, occurs fifteen minutes after the stimuli were originally presented. The stimuli include the word list and drawings presented during the Immediate Memory subscale.

Norms for the CANA on Spanish-speakers were unavailable at the time of writing the current chapter. The data presented at this time represent a small exploratory study based on a limited sample of Mexican-American (including Mexican immigrants and U.S. born) Spanish monolinguals.

Procedure
All participants were approached by the author or an other bilingual research team member directly upon delivery of assessment services. The participants

were asked to participate in a research project that involved a neuro-cognitive screening tool for Spanish-speakers. They were informed that their participation was voluntary, that their anonymity was secured by the researchers, and that they could discontinue at any time in the administration of the tools. They were informed that the data collection would not take more than thirty minutes total. Of course, all of this information was presented to the client in Spanish. The client was then asked to sign a release form for the use of the data. The results of the testing were not released as part of any official diagnostic report, and were only described as experimental in the patient interview summaries.

Results

This section includes three sets of statistical analyses. The first group of analyses are descriptive statistics regarding test subscale scores and how these differ across the measures. The subsequent analyses represent a preliminary attempt to address the following issues: (A) the convergence between constructs of the CANA and the MMSE, and (B) the divergence between the constructs of the CANA and the MMSE. For the first question, a correlation matrix was used to evaluate how the individual items of each subscale of the CANA held together. These analyses involved the use of a correlation matrix with the subscale summary scores of the CANA and the MMSE to test for convergence and divergence. A simple matrix was used due to the limited sample size. (The small sample size also made it difficult to examine within-measure item clustering in the CANA, therefore the analyses have focused on comparisons of convergence with the MMSE.)

Descriptive statistics
The subscale average scores for the CANA and MMSE are presented in Tables 2 and 3.

Table 2 shows subscale averages and ranges on the CANA. Although the sample size was small, there seemed to be sufficient scatter (superficially) to support the idea that the individual subscales are able to detect differences in performance within the subscales. Table 3 shows subscale averages and ranges for the MMSE. Most noticeable is the restricted range of scores on the subscales, especially on the immediate memory scale that indicated no scatter at all. Also, the scatter within the subscales of the MMSE, in general, was less than that shown on the corresponding subscales of the CANA.

Convergence and divergence
The results of the correlation matrix comparing the subscale scores of the Spanish-language MMSE and the CANA should be viewed with caution given the small sample size. However, for the purposes of seeking heuristic patterns of relationships between the constructs on the two measures, these initial

Table 2. CANA subscale scores (*n* = 6).

Subscale Name	Max. Score	Mean (SD)	Range (Max-Min)
Pre-screen	6.0	5.50 (.84)	4-6
Language	8.0	5.67 (1.37)	4-8
Immediate Memory	8.0	6.33 (1.37)	4-8
Orientation	8.0	6.67 (2.80)	1-8
Attention	8.0	5.00 (2.53)	2-8
Visuospatial	8.0	4.83 (1.83)	2-7
Reasoning	8.0	4.67 (1.37)	3-6
Executive Functioning	8.0	4.00 (2.61)	1-8
Delayed Memory	8.0	4.33 (1.75)	3-7
Total Score	70.0	47.00 (13.80)	24-65

Table 3. MMSE subscale scores (*n* = 6).

Subscale Name	Max. Score	Mean (SD)	Range Min-Max
Orientation	10.0	8.17 (2.64)	3-10
Registration/Immediate Memory	3.0	3.00 (0.00)	3-3
Attention	6.0	4.17 (2.56)	0-6
Delayed Memory	3.0	2.33 (0.82)	1-3
Language	7.0	6.67 (0.52)	6-7
Construction Abilities/Visuospatial	1.0	0.67 (0.52)	0-1
Total Score	30.00	25.00 (6.69)	13-29

results may indicate directions for future analyses with increased sampling.

In terms of convergence, only one subscale of the MMSE showed significant correlation with the corresponding subscale of the CANA. The Orientation subscale of the MMSE indicated a .98 correlation with the Orientation subscale of the CANA ($p < .01$). There was also a trend toward significance in the association between the total score on the MMSE and the total on the CANA ($r = .78$; $p < .10$). See correlation matrix, Table 4.

In terms of divergence, in general, the subscales of the CANA showed some relationship to several of the subscales of the MMSE but not exclusively with a given corresponding construct subscale (see Table 4). The Pre-screen subscale correlated significantly with the Delayed Memory subscale of the MMSE ($r = .88$; $p < .05$). The Immediate Memory subscale of the CANA was associated with several subscales of the MMSE, including: Orientation ($r = .87$; $p < .05$); Attention ($r = .84$; $p < .05$); and the MMSE total score ($r = .88$; $p < .05$). The Orientation subscale, in addition to being associated with the corresponding subscale on the MMSE as noted above, was significantly related to the Attention ($r = .83$; $p < .05$), Delayed Memory ($r = .84$;

Table 4. Subtest correlations for MMSE and CANA.

	MMSE Lang.	MMSE Immed. Mem.	MMSE Orient.	MMSE Atten.	MMSE Visuo-spatl.	MMSE Delay. Mem.	MMSE Total
CANA Pre-scrn.	.463	----	.770	.606	.463	.878**	.714
CANA Lang.	.378	----	.518	.476	.378	.657	.525
CANA Immed.Mem.	.756*	----	.869**	.838**	.756*	.777*	.875**
CANA Orient.	.736*	----	.982***	.827**	.736*	.844**	.938***
CANA Atten.	.306	----	.569	.370	.306	.484	.472
CANA Visuospatl.	.352	----	.709	.432	.352	.712	.586
CANA Reas.	.378	----	.518	.419	.378	.837**	.525
CANA Exec.Funct.	.594	----	.552	.599	.594	.845**	.642
CANA Delay.Mem.	.590	----	.332	.654	.590	.606	.546
CANA Total	.617	----	.780*	.707	.617	.870**	.780*

$* \ p < .10; ** \ p < .05; *** \ p < .01.$

$p < .05)$ and the total MMSE score ($r = .94; p < .01$). Results indicated that the Reasoning subscale was significantly correlated with Delayed Memory on the MMSE ($r = .85; p < .05$). The Executive Functioning subscale of the CANA was significantly related with the Delayed Memory subscale of the MMSE ($r = .85; p < .05$). The total score of the CANA showed relatedness to the Delayed Memory subscale of the MMSE as well ($r = .87; p < .05$).

Discussion

Given the limited generalizability of this exploratory study due to a small sample size, the results will be discussed in terms of broad issues of method, convergence, and divergence that may arise in the comparison of tools. In regards to the convergence between the Orientation subscale of the CANA and the corresponding subscale of the MMSE, this seems a natural relationship because both contain very similar questions (see Table 1). It would seem unlikely that if the patient were able to answer the questions appropriately on one measure that they would not do so on the other test. The trend toward significant relatedness between the total scores of the CANA and the MMSE may be important to examine more closely with increased sample sizes. That is, the overall scores may ultimately prove to be correspondent or may show a general divergence indicating that the tools are either measuring different constructs or are differentially sensitive to the same constructs.

When evaluating the divergence of constructs (subscales) between measures several issues need to be considered. In the case of the current study, one major issue was sample size. For example, the lack of convergence between the Immediate Memory subscales of the two measures may have been compromised because of the difference in how the construct is measured. On the

MMSE, Immediate Memory was measured by a single item that evaluated verbal immediate memory only. The CANA uses several items to evaluate the same construct both verbally and visually. Thus, on the MMSE, with only one item, there was not sufficient scatter in the scores to create viable statistical analyses for comparison with the CANA. The scores for the MMSE on this construct were read as a constant because all six participants had a score of one (full points on that item). Meanwhile, the CANA used a greater number of items to evaluate immediate memory, therefore allowing for more variability of scores. These statistical qualities may change with increased sample sizes to give better indication of correlations that exist between the subscales of the measures.

A second consideration, as alluded to above and in Table 1, is that the CANA may measure a broader domain within a given construct than does the MMSE. For example, in the CANA Immediate Memory subscale both verbal and visual memory is tested. In the MMSE only verbal memory is measured. This qualitative difference may lead to interesting results in future statistical analyses between measures. In essence, it may be that the MMSE and the CANA measure similar constructs but the CANA provides information about the construct domains that is more inclusive and generalizable. The broadening of the domain being measured is important, especially with linguistic minorities, given that what may not be understood through one medium may be accessible through another (i.e., providing both verbal AND visual stimuli may provide a better indication of actual ability after injury rather than drawing from only one source of information).

Third, it is important to recognize, in general, when examining construct issues within or between measures that these constructs (in this case neuro-cognitive abilities) are not independent. All the cognitive functions of the brain can be seen as overlapping. For example, attention affects immediate memory, orientation may affect one's performance on language tasks, and so forth. Therefore, the idea of multiple intercorrelations between the subscales within and between the measures is expectable. However, it is important to determine that the relationship of items *within* subscales is stronger than between subscales in order to establish construct/subscale intra-reliability. Such analyses as this will be the focus of future studies on the CANA.

Despite the limitations of the current study, the author and her research team have found the CANA can be very helpful in clinical practice. This is best exemplified through a clinical case. Mrs. S was 71 years at the time of her participation in this pilot study. She had resided in a small border town for 50 years but had not learned English (there was no functional need to do so in her town). She had attended primary school in Mexico, was classified in the lowest socio-economic category (< $ 5,000), and had never worked outside her home. At the time of her testing, she was interned at a nursing home for dementia and several physical problems. Her score of 29 out of 30 points on the MMSE indicated no general neuro-cognitive impairment. However, her CANA showed quite a different picture. Although she was well oriented in terms of time, space, and self, Mrs. S showed severe limitations in her performance of reasoning tasks (abstraction and sequencing; scored 3 of 8 pts.), visuospatial abilities (4 of 8 pts.), and executive functioning (2 of 8 pts.). Her attention (5 of 8 pts.) and language (5 of 8 pts.) abilities were also somewhat compromised per the CANA results. Such findings raise two important issues: (1) are the standard neurocognitive evaluation tools overlooking deficits (or strengths) in Spanish speakers; and (2) the need to not only evaluate existing tools, but also develop new instruments (such as the CANA) that may be more accurate in the evaluation of this population by incorporating linguistically and culturally consistent stimuli.

Conclusions

The study presented in this chapter is a preliminary work that serves, primarily, as an initiative for future research. The need for an adequate neuropsychological screening tool for Spanish speakers is growing rapidly and with greater urgency in the Western and Southwestern US, especially at the rate which the Latino population is growing in these areas. The CANA, given the qualities of its construction to be culture-specific and bias-reduced for Spanish speakers, presents a viable alternative to the simple translations of traditional measures without attention to construct equivalence. Furthermore, the method by which the CANA is being validated and normed (i.e., per the standards of ethnopsychology) provides an opportunity to produce internal norms for Spanish-speaking groups, in this case Mexican Americans. Nonetheless, much research remains to be done to evaluate the construct validity of the CANA, as well as the factors within the target sample that may affect performance. Specifically, future research should focus not only on validity issues but also on the effects and interactions of important factors that may influence neurocognitive performance such as acculturation level, bilingualism, socio-economic status, and education level. Of course, gender issues should be considered as well. Overall, the current study represents only a minute exploration of the psychometric topics to be examined in the development of a neurocognitive abilities measure for Spanish speakers.

References

Anastasi, A. (1976). *Psychological testing*. New York: Collier Macmillan Publishers.

Anastasi, A., & Urbina, S. (1997). *Psychological testing*. Upper Saddle River: Prentice Hall.

Ardila, A. (1995). Directions of research in cross-cultural neuropsychology. *Journal of Clinical and Experimental Neuropsychology, 17*, 143-150.

Ardila, A., Rosselli, M., & Puente, A.E. (1994). *Neuropsychological evaluation of the Spanish speaker*. New York: Plenum Press.

Butcher, J.N. (1996). Translation and adaptation of the MMPI-2 for international use. In J.N. Butcher (Ed.), *International adaptations of the MMPI-2, research and clinical applications* (pp. 27-43). Minneapolis: University of Minnesota Press.

Butcher, J.N., & Han, K. (1996). Methods of establishing cross-cultural equivalence. In J.N. Butcher (Ed.), *International adaptations of the MMPI-2, research and clinical applications* (pp.27-43). Minneapolis: University of Minnesota Press.

Carter, R.T. (1991). Cultural values: A review of empirical research and implications for counseling. *Journal of Counseling and Development, 70,* 164-170.

Cronbach, L.J. (1990). *Essentials of psychological testing.* New York: Harper & Row Publishers.

Dana, R.H. (1993). *Multicultural assessment perspectives for professional psychology.* Boston: Allyn & Bacon Publishers.

Diaz-Guerrero, R. (1989). *Los primos y nosotros, la personalidad de los Mexicanos y los Norteamericanos: Partes uno a ocho* [Our cousins and ourselves, personality of Mexicans and Northamericans: Parts one to eight]. Unpublished manuscript.

Diaz-Guerrero, R. (1992). The need for an ethnopsychology of cognition and personality. *Psychology: A Journal of Human Behavior, 29,* 19-26.

Diaz-Guerrero, R. (1993). Mexican ethnopsychology. In U. Kim and J.W. Berry (Eds.), *Indigenous psychologies: Research and experience in cultural context* (pp. 44-55). Newbury Park: Sage Publications.

Diaz-Loving, R., & Andrade-Palos, P. (1984). Una escala de locus de control para ninos Mexicanos [A locus of control scale for Mexican children]. *Revista Interamericana de Psicologia, 18,* 21-33.

Echemendia, R.J., Harris, J.G., Congett, S.M., Diaz, M.L., & Puente, A.M. (1997). Neuropsychological training and practices with Hispanics: A national survey. *The Clinical Neuropsychologist, 11,* 229-243.

Folstein, M.F., Folstein, S.E., & McHugh, P.R. (1975). Mini-mental state: A practical method for grading the cognitive state of patients for the clinician. *Journal of Psychiatric Research, 12,* 189-198.

Geisinger, K.F. (1994). Cross-cultural normative assessment: Translation and adaptation issues influencing the normative interpretation of assessment instruments. *Psychological Assessment, 6,* 304-312.

Harris, J.G., Cullum, C.M., & Puente, A.E. (1995). Effects of bilingualism on verbal learning and memory in Hispanic adults. *Journal of the International Neuropsychological Society, 1,* 10-16.

Kaplan, R.M., & Saccuzzo, D.P. (1997). *Psychological testing.* Pacific Grove: Brooks/Cole Publishing Company.

O'Brien, M.L. (1989). Psychometric issues relevant to selecting items and assembling parallel forms of language proficiency instruments. *Educational and Psychological Measurement, 49,* 347-353.

Perez-Arce, P. (1999). The influence of culture on cognition. *Archives of Clinical Neuropsychology, 14,* 581-592.

Ponton, M.O., & Ardila, A. (1999). The future of neuropsychology with Hispanic populations in the United States. *Archives of Clinical Neuropsychology, 14,* 565-580.

Puente, A.E., & McCaffrey, R.J. (1992). *Handbook of neuropsychological assessment.* New York: Plenum Press.

Ramirez, M. (1983). *Psychology of the Americas: Mestizo perspectives on personality and mental health.* New York: Pergamon Press.

PART V

NATIVE AMERICANS

Chapter 12

PRELIMINARY NORMATIVE DATA FROM A BRIEF NEUROPSYCHOLOGICAL TEST BATTERY IN A SAMPLE OF NATIVE AMERICAN ELDERLY

F. Richard Ferraro, Brian J. Bercier,
Jeffrey Holm and J. Douglas McDonald
Department of Psychology, University of North Dakota,
Grand Forks, North Dakota

Abstract

The present chapter summarizes our attempt at collecting preliminary normative data from Native American elderly adults on a brief neuropsychological test battery. To this end we tested approximately 51 enrolled members of a tribe in North-Central North Dakota (M age = 69 years) and 30 non-Native American elderly adults (M age = 72 years). The brief neuropsychological test battery was taken from Hill and Storandt (1989). In general, the Native American elderly performed as well as the non-Native American elderly. Results are discussed in relationship to the development and standardization of neuropsychological tests and test batteries for Native Americans.

Introduction

In the current neuropsychological literature there seems to be much more aging and dementia research directed toward minority cultures with larger populations, rather than the Native American cultures (Adebimpe, 1981; Ardila, 1995; Baker, 1988; Chee & Kane, 1993). This relative absence of research may in part be attributed to the fact that the Native American population is significantly lower in actual numbers than the other minority cultures (Norton & Manson, 1996). This relative lack of research may also be because Native Americans may distrust Non-Native researchers, particularly Caucasian researchers, because of poorly recognized differences between cultures. Caucasian people are often seen as greedy by Native Americans, thus Native Americans may be suspicious of researchers' motives (Arean & Gallagher-Thompson, 1996; Schneider, 1994; Welsh, Ballard, Nash, Raiford, & Harrell, 1994).

The omission of Native Americans is critical, however, because as a group, Native Americans are an extremely diverse population, with over 200 federally recognized tribes (and many not recognized). Likewise, there are over 2 million Native American and Alaska Natives currently, according to the most recent (1990) Census (Norton & Manson, 1996; Stenger, 1994). Despite these numbers, there has been relatively little in the way of careful, empirical research reports (especially dealing with neuropsychological issues) with Native American elderly adults (although see Cooley, Ostendorf, & Bickerton, 1979; Kramer, 1991, 1992; Lowe, Tranel, Wallace, & Welty, 1994; Manson, 1989; Novak, 1974; Strong, 1984). Furthermore, Indian Health Services (IHS) provides a disproportionate amount of health care services to Native elders, although this group only makes up approximately 5.8% of the total IHS population (Stenger, 1994). Thus, there appears to be a need for an increase in such research activities.

Why examine the Native American?

The Native American minority group has been called the fastest-growing culture in the United States (McDonald et al., 1992). This observation, coupled with the scarcity of the information available about Native Americans in general on a wide array of topics, would thus dictate the need for investigation into all aspects of the Native American culture, as well as on topics that relate most particularly to neuropsychological assessment and neuropsychology test battery development.

This area of study may be of importance due to the rising life expectancies of this particular minority group over the last few decades (Schneider, 1994). This greater life expectancy may be attributed to improved medical care on the reservation. Thus, with the advent of modern medicine as well as the comforts of modern technology, native people are presumably living longer than they did before the advent of modern technology. This may then open the door for research in areas concerning the Native American aged, or

Native elders. It offers many possibilities to do research on aging that before may not have been possible, or practical due to longevity issues.

One other issue relates to the relationship of Alzheimer's disease (AD) and Native American elderly. The greatest predictor of AD is advancing age and there is now some preliminary evidence that in some tribes AD is relatively rare (Hendrie et al., 1993) and virtually non-existent due to genetic influence (Rosenberg, Richter, Risser et al. (1996). Thus, any new information regarding neuropsychological assessment and normative data collection/ neuropsychological test battery test construction is critical, as these would have an impact on dementia screening and dementia prevalence issues.

Problems to overcome when studying Native Americans

The biggest hurdle that faces the prospective researcher is one that may be unique to that of the Native American people of this country (see also Norton & Manson, 1996). When dealing with issues in "Indian Country", there are several considerations that one must keep in mind. These include, but are not limited to, political and cultural issues. Tribal governments have limited sovereignty, meaning that they are free to establish their own policies, rules and regulations that are implemented within the boundaries of reservation and tribal lands (Schneider, 1994). Other things to be aware of are: in some Native cultures it is considered disrespectful to look someone in the eyes. It is also customary when asking for something, whether it be information or whatever, to offer a gift of some kind (usually tobacco), to the person that one asks. There are also geographic issues, there can be differences within reservations regarding dialects, and even customs.

For example, on the reservation that participated in the present experiment, there is some variation in one of the Native languages spoken there (Michif) depending on where the particular person lives on the 6 mile x 12 mile reservation. Many Native Americans also may have an inherent distrust of people conducting research. This distrust may stem from past experience in dealing with the "white world". These experiences may include, but are not limited to, broken treaties, promises, and experiences with prejudice.

There are also problems with issues related to acculturation. Acculturation (Padilla, 1980) can be viewed as a point on a continuum (see also Serpell & Boykin, 1994). At one point is total immersion in the dominant culture (totally acculturated), at the other point is the total immersion in the traditional culture (totally unacculturated). Native People may be at any point along this continuum.

On the reservation that participated in the present experiment, for instance, there are two distinct cultures. The predominant culture is the "Michif" (a Native American version of the French word "Metis", which means mixed blood) culture who are of mixed Native American and French ancestry. These people have a distinct language that is made up of French and Cree languages. They have also adopted various aspects of both the French and Native American cultural traditions. The other group of people are the more traditionally Chippewa. This group practices more traditionally Native American ways, and speaks the Chippewa language. Both groups have varying levels of acculturation with respect to the dominant culture. Both groups speak English as either a first or second language. In both cases there may be a limited English vocabulary in contrast to the majority population. Thus words that may be common in the majority culture may not be used in this culture. If you asked someone from this reservation, what the word "diminutive" meant they would probably not know what it meant, but would assuredly know the meaning of small. Also, certain things that Native Americans believe in may be misconstrued as abnormal in the majority culture. For example in many native cultures it may be ordinary for one to say that a spirit spoke with them. There is a belief in many Native cultures (including the more traditionally Chippewa of the reservation that participated in the present study) that all things have spirits, and that if one would, for example, chop down a tree, one would talk to the spirit thanking that tree for the warmth it gave or for the shelter it provides. This would indeed be considered by the majority culture to be aberrant behavior. There are others of the Reservation that are devout Christians, and their beliefs parallel that of the majority cultures.

Families may also be located in a particular area of a reservation. Thus if one restricts her research to a particular area of the reservation one will probably get many of the same family members, rather than a more representative sample of the whole tribe. In the Turtle Mountain Reservation there are three areas of more traditional tribal members all located in different sections of the reservation. One group is located in an area north of Dunseith, another in an area by where Greatwalker school used to be (this area is around the North Western boundaries of the reservation) and the third group is located in the North East area of the reservation. These three areas are all located by where the Traditional Chippewa of the reservation, hold or used to hold Sun dances.

Other considerations that one must kept in mind are that there are different ways of approaching the elders of the tribe. If the Elder is a more traditional Native American then one should offer him a gift of tobacco, for example, then and only then respectfully ask for his participation. More non-traditional members and the more traditional Michif may be approached in a more direct manner, but should always be treated with the respect due to them because of their age. One important thing to keep in mind when utilizing standardized tests on minority populations is that minorities tend to score lower on these tests than do their "Euro-American" counterparts (Ferraro & Bercier, 1996).

Depending on how "traditional" the subject is, one problem that may arise is one of language: words that are used in particular tests may not have any utility or purpose in a Native American community, (McDonald et al., 1992). Thus when interpreting any results involving Native Americans one needs to remain aware of these differences and adjust the interpretation accordingly.

Thus far we have seen that the Native American culture is one of the least-studied minority cultures in the United States, especially from a cognitive and neuropsychological perspective. This may be because of cultural differences that have seemed to place white researchers in an adversarial role in the eyes of many Native Americans. This is somewhat ironic, as there are several published reports in the literature dealing with a variety of other cultures and minority groups as they relate to neuropsychological test performance. These include, but are not limited to Hispanics (Ponton & Ardila, 1999), rural populations (Blazer et al., 1985), AfricanAmericans (Fillenbaum, Huber, & Taussig, 1997), and Japanese (Sugishita, Otomo, Kabe, & Yunoki, 1992). Growing native populations, however, along with higher life spans, may be ample justification for more studies. Furthermore, it is imperative that this neglected cultural group be included, especially as there is ample evidence that culture and cognitive performance are not only related to each other but influence each other (Helms, 1992; Lee, 1994; Perez-Arce, 1999). This added emphasis may, in turn, result in information that may help their culture deal with age-related problems such as memory impairment and dementia.

Hypothesis for the present study

We were concerned with how the elderly of the Turtle Mountain tribe compare on a brief neuropsychological test battery, in relation to the majority culture. This is important because of the rising age of the Native American elderly population. Similarly, this study represents one of the first (as far as the authors can tell) to begin construction on a short neurpopsychological test battery.

It is important to keep in mind that the present study intends to gather preliminary normative neuropsychological test data from Native American elderly adults using a brief neuropsychological testing battery. The tests to be used have been shown to delineate a characteristic pattern of cognitive deficit in patients with very mild dementia of the Alzheimer type versus normal aging. However, the tests used in the present experiment do not specifically test for competencies such as problem-solving, judgment, abstraction, and spatial orientation. Likewise, these four tests do not tap directly into functions related to visual construction, motor functions, and attentional capacities. Thus, the present study does not allow for making differential dementia diagnoses. Perhaps inclusion of the Mini-Mental Status Examination in future studies would satisfy some of these short-comings. However, use of these four tests in a preliminary neuropsychology test battery, and the results obtained by Hill and Storandt (1989) regarding the sensitivity of these tests in differentiating very mild senile dementia of the Alzheimer type from normal aging, are a first step in the right direction.

Additionally, no such normative data exist for elderly Native Americans on the tests that comprise this test battery. Thus, making any clear diagnoses or attempting to detect dementia in this sample of Native American elders would be premature and unjustified. The present study, by examining two ethnic groups and various age groups, will result in a way of validating these various neuropsychological tests.

Methods

Subjects
Subjects in this study included 51 enrolled members of a North-Central North Dakota tribe and 30 non-tribal members. Subjects were divided by culture (native, non-native) and age (60-69, 70-79, 80-89). The non-native control group consisted of Euro-American male and female aged, randomly selected from areas from surrounding communities adjacent to the Reservation in question. Matching of subjects was attempted on sex and age. The Native American sample was not stratified by acculturation level.

Materials
A four-battery series of psychometric tests was employed. Hill and Storandt (1989) found three of these particular tests to be of significant value in assessing for very mild and questionable forms of Senile Dementia of the Alzheimer type from normal healthy aging. They include: 1) The Boston Naming Test, 15-item version. This shortened version was found to be useful in screening for Alzheimer's disease (Mack et al., 1992); 2) The Logical Memory Test (immediate and delayed); 3) The Wechsler Adult Intelligence Scale - Revised (WAIS-R) Vocabulary Subscale (Wechsler, 1981) and 4) the WAIS-R Digit Symbol Subscale.

Apparatus
The apparatus used for administering these protocols consisted of a stop watch to measure the protocols that are timed, and one cassette player used to play prerecorded stories.

Procedure
Prospective participants were solicited on a door-to-door basis by the second author. A representative sample from both the Michif and the more traditional people was sought. Subjects were solicited from all areas of the reservation to satisfy any differences that may be due to geographic location, although this factor was not systematically varied. These include two cultures living within the reservation, and both live in various part of the reservation.

The second author and one or two research assistants (who also lived on the reservation) were responsible for administering all tests and gathering all data. An effort was made to reduce any experimenter bias by having all instructions presented in a standardized format (typed out and spoken). The second author was aware of the hypotheses in question (as this project represented his Master of Arts Thesis project) but the research assistants were unaware of the hypotheses being tested. At the conclusion of the study, all research assistants were told of the various hypotheses under investigation.

Design
The design is a 2 (Group: Native American, Non-Native American) × 3 (Age: 60-69, 70-79, 80-89) between-subjects design. This design resulted in 29, 12, and 10 Native American subjects across the three age ranges, respectively, and 11, 10, and 9 non-Native Americans across the three age ranges, respectively. Although an attempt was made to examine gender differences, some of the resulting cells contained five or less individuals and analyses with gender are not reported.

Results and Discussion

Table 1 lists mean, standard deviation and range scores for all demographic and neuropsychological variables as a function of Group and Age. Next, several 2 (Group) × 3 (Age) ANOVAs were performed across many of the variables presented in Table 1. For these analyses, the Group main effect had 1 and 75 degrees of freedom, and the main effect for Age and the Group x Age interaction had 2 and 75 degrees of freedom. All p values are at $p < .05$ or less, unless otherwise stated. These ANOVA results can be grouped into two categories, Demographic Information and Neuropsychological Test Battery Performance.

Demographic Information
For Education, there was no main effect of Group ($F = .76$) a marginal main effect of Age ($F = 2.86$, $p = .063$) and a significant interaction ($F = 4.68$, $p < .02$). This interaction revealed that whereas the 60-69 and 70-79 year old Non-Natives had significantly ($p < .05$) more education than their Native counterparts, the reverse was true for 80-89 year-old Natives, who possessed significantly ($p < .01$) more education than their non-Native counterparts.

For Self-Rated Health, no main or interaction effects were present ($F < 3.00$, $p > .06$).

For Number of Medications Currently Taken, no main or interaction effects were present ($F < 2.00$, $p > .16$).

For Geriatric Depression Scale-Short Form scores, there was a main effect for Group ($F = 6.84$, $p < .02$), as well as for Age ($F = 6.79$, $p = .002$). There was no interaction between these variables ($F = 1.37$, $p = .26$). The Native Group reported less overall probable depression ($M = 4.36$) than the non-Native group ($M = 6.21$). Also, as both groups age, there was an increase in self-reported probable depression ($M = 4.32$, 4.34, 7.21, respectively).

For WAIS-R performance, there was no main effect of Group ($F = .86$) but there was a main effect for Age ($F = 4.10$, $p = .02$). This main effect

Table 1. Mean and standard deviation performance as a function of Group (Native, Non-Native) and Age (60-69, 70-79, 80-89).

		Native			Non-Native		
		60-69	70-79	80-89	60-69	70-79	80-89
Age	M	62.00	74.17	84.90	62.91	73.40	83.44
	SD	5.67	2.91	2.84	4.50	2.80	2.92
Educ.	M	10.55	9.17	10.60	12.36	12.40	7.67
	SD	3.49	5.27	1.90	2.46	3.37	.87
Health	M	2.59	2.58	2.80	2.64	2.60	3.67
	SD	1.15	.79	.79	.81	1.07	.71
Meds.	M	1.31	1.61	1.40	.54	1.80	1.22
	SD	1.85	1.56	1.26	.52	1.40	.97
GDS-SF	M	2.72	4.08	6.30	5.91	4.60	8.11
	SD	2.84	2.23	2.16	3.36	3.75	3.14
WAIS-R	M	40.69	41.92	32.70	37.36	42.40	25.33
	SD	14.39	19.92	11.60	14.94	20.26	4.85
BNT	M	13.38	12.67	13.40	12.91	13.30	13.00
	SD	1.61	3.39	1.84	2.26	1.49	1.32
LogM-I	M	8.69	10.25	4.30	7.55	10.50	4.56
	SD	4.94	6.74	2.50	4.84	6.50	1.67
LogM-D	M	8.00	10.25	5.50	9.54	8.80	6.56
	SD	4.35	6.74	3.57	5.05	4.29	3.24
Digit	M	21.41	18.50	20.80	18.73	24.70	16.56
	SD	11.83	10.53	9.33	15.89	10.04	8.19

Notes: GDS-SF indicates Geriatric Depression Scale-Short Form; WAIS-R indicates Wechsler Adult Intelligence Scale-Revised; BNT indicates Boston Naming Test (15-item version); LogM indicates Logical Memory; I indicates Immediate; D indicates Delayed; Digit indicates Digit Symbol.

indicated that vocabulary ability increased across the 60-69 and 70-79 year-olds ($M = 39.03, 42.16$, respectively) then decreased in the 80-89 year-olds ($M = 29.02$). No interaction resulted ($F = .34$).

Neuropsychological Test Battery Performance
Boston Naming Test performance resulted in no main effects for either Group ($F = .03$) or Age ($F = .06$). There was also no interaction ($F = .53$).

Logical Memory (Immediate) performance resulted in no main effect for Group ($F = .03$), but a significant main effect of Age ($F = 8.06, p < .01$), in which performance increased, then decreased as age increased ($M = 8.12$, 10.38, 4.43, respectively). There was no interaction ($F = .19$).

Logical Memory (Delayed) performance mirrored Immediate performance with no main effect for Group ($F = .12$) and a significant main effect of Age ($F = 3.13, p = .05$). With advancing age, there was evidenced of an increase, then a decrease, in performance ($M = 8.77, 9.53, 6.03$, respectively). There was no interaction ($F = .19$).

Digit Symbol performance resulted in no main effects for Group ($F = .01$) or Age ($F = .33$) and no interaction ($F = 1.32$).

Correlational Analyses

In addition to the ANOVA results reported above, correlation coefficients were also calculated. Tables 2, 3, and 4 present correlational results for the various demographic and neuropsychological variables for all subjects (Table 2), non-Native Americans (Table 3) and Native Americans (Table 4).

The present experiment was an attempt to begin the process of attaining preliminary normative data on a brief neuropsychological test battery in Native American elderly adults. To this end, a neuropsychological test battery, patterned after Hill and Storandt (1989) was given to 51 Native American elderly adults and 30 non-Native American elderly adults. For the most

Table 2. Correlation table for all subjects.

	1	2	3	4	5	6	7	8	9	10	11
1 Year	–										
2 Age	.91**	–									
3 Educ.	–.20	–.19	–								
4 Hlth	.22*	.20	–.20	–							
5 Meds	.09	.17	–.10	.25**	–						
6 GDS-SF	.41**	.39**	–.32**	.40**	.10	–					
7 WAISR	–.23**	–.19	.67**	.10	.10	–.47**	–				
8 BNT	–.02	–.04	.32**	.05	–.02	–.26**	.51**	–			
9 LMI	–.25**	–.22*	.55**	–.26**	.02	–.56**	.62**	.18	–		
10 LMD	–.16	.16	.35**	–.25**	.08	–.31**	.55**	.36**	.62**	–	
11 Dig	–.06	–.14	.41**	–.08	–.11	–.38**	.36**	.31**	.43**	24**	–

Notes: Hlth indicates Self-Rated Health; GDS-SF indicates Geriatric Depression Scale-Short Form; WAISR indicates Wechsler Adult Intelligence Scale-Revised; BNT indicates Boston Naming Test; LMI indicates Logical Memory-Immediate; LMD indicates Logical Memory Delayed; Dig indicates Digit Symbol; *significant correlations at $p < .05$; **significant correlations at $p < .01$ (significance varies across tables due to N differences).

Table 3. Correlation table for non-Natives only.

	1	2	3	4	5	6	7	8	9	10	11
1 Year	–										
2 Age	.93**	–									
3 Educ.	–.58**	–.52**	–								
4 Hlth	.42*	.42*	–.53**	–							
5 Meds	.27	.31	.10	.16	–						
6 GDS-SF	.23	.15	.70**	.42*	–.38*	–					
7 WIASR	–.29	–.26	.80**	–.23	.43*	–.70**	–				
8 BNT	.03	.03	.18	–.02	.12	–.30	.38*	–			
9 LMI	–.21	–.17	.80**	–.42	.37*	–.77**	.85**	.26	–		
10 LMD	–.28	–.27	.38*	–.31	.17	.46*	.49**	.48**	.47**	–	
11 Dig	–.06	–.07	.50**	–.59**	.55	.34	.57**	.21	.24	.27	–

Notes: See Table 2.

Table 4. Correlation table for Native Americans only.

	1	2	3	4	5	6	7	8	9	10	11
1 Year	–										
2 Age	.89**	–									
3 Educ.	-.04	-.07	–								
4 Hlth	.07	.07	-.06	–							
5 Meds	.04	.15	-.16	.31*	–						
6 GDS-SF	.48**	.51**	-.18	.35*	.41**	–					
7 WAISR	-.17	-.13	.64**	.00	-.05	-.28*	–				
8 BNT	-.03	-.06	.39**	.08	-.06	-.25	.58**	–			
9 LMI	-.27	-.25	.43**	-.16	-.13	-.43**	.47**	.15	–		
10 LMD	-.12	-.12	.33*	-.24	-.16	-.28*	.61**	.31*	.71**	–	
11 Dig	-.05	-.18	.37**	-.15	-.30**	-.23	.24	.30*	.34*	.25	–

Notes: See Table 2.

part, the Native elderly and the non-Native elderly performed very similarly. That is, in only one instance (for GDS-SF performance) was there significant main effect for Group and in only one instance (for Education level) was there an interaction involving Group. For all intents and purposes, and across all remaining neuropsychological tests used in the present study, the Native elderly performed as well as the non-Native elderly. While this pattern of results is encouraging, there are several caveats that must be made regarding the present study and the results obtained.

While the results provide a valuable information resource about a Native American group where little such data has existed (Ferraro & Bercier, 1996), it should be stressed that there are many different Native American cultures or tribes. Our results cannot be assumed to be valid for any other Native American tribe except the one under investigation in the present study. Although there are similarities between tribes, they are different cultures, each distinct and each unique. Ardila (1999) makes this point quite nicely in his article on intelligence and neuropsychology. Specifically, he states that "cultural and linguistic diversity is an enormously, but frequently overlooked, moderating variable" (p. 132). One future direction would be to compare and contrast performance across different cultures, or tribes on various neuropsychological tests.

The elderly Native Americans that took part in the present experiment may have been the most appropriate sample of Native Americans for the present project. This is because many of these people, due to the influence of early French traders intermarrying with the Native Chippewa women, already show a significant amount of acculturation. This study included a majority of the population of "Michif" people, a culture that has the influence of both the Native, and French customs and spirituality. Also included in the sample were a smaller proportion of more "traditional" people. Thus, this unintentional confounding of cultures may have produced some of the obtained results. Valle (1994) discusses ways of differentiating such confounds when performing research as detailed in the present chapter, and these include socioeconomic status versus cultural variables, literacy levels and cultural factors, and race, racism, and the gene pool and the possibility of shared gene pools. His point is that if these factors are taken into account, it is possible to construct a culture-fair behavioral assessment and intervention model. His model relates specifically to dementing illnesses. However, given that one of the fastest-growing populations presently (in Native Americans as well as non-Native Americans) is adults over the age of 60, then this model becomes relevant for issues associated with the factors of age as well as neuropsychological assessment.

It may be possible that specific intervention strategies that have proven useful in the Non-native culture may have some use in the Native communities as well. One very interesting finding from the present study is that the Non-Native culture had a significant amount of more self-reported depression than the Native culture. One may speculate that in the Native cultures, the continued reliance on the elderly as wise and knowledgeable, and as useful and productive members of the community, may have a beneficial effect on degree of self-reported depression. Thus the Non-native community may learn from this and implement more programs that utilize the knowledge and wisdom that their elderly have acquired over the course of the years. This would perhaps have a twofold benefit. The communities would benefit from the knowledge of the elderly, and the elderly, finding more purpose to their existence, would possibly show a decrease in their level of depression. This is especially relevant, given the recent data to suggest that there may be some biases present in the belief systems of some Native Americans (Lightdale, Oken, Klein, Landrigan, & Welty, 1997) as well as the importance of education programs (based on information gathered from specific research projects) as ways of enhancing community healing processes (McShane, 1987).

Summary

The information found in the present study represents the first (to the author knowledge) attempt to collect preliminary normative data on tests that tap into neuropsychological performance. The development and standardization of neuropsychological tests suitable for Native American populations have long been overdue. These results represent one of the few studies aimed at achieving these goals. Of course, there are some caveats that need to be discussed. First, although the four tests used have been shown to delineate and classify very mild senile dementia of the Alzheimer type from normal aging, these tests do not specifically tap into problem-solving, abstraction, judgement, spatial orientation, multiple-trial memory tests, motor function, and attention. The inclusion of the Mini-Mental Status Examination could accommodate these requirements, and should be used in future studies. Furthermore, additional tests as those described above would also assist in determining and classifying different forms of dementia, such as vascular dementia and subcortical dementia. Second, level of acculturation was not measured in the present study, but such information would be important regarding how acculturation affects neuropsychological test performance. Different levels of acculturation might lead to differing levels of performance. Third, since the individual in charge of data collection was an enrolled member of the tribe who participated, the issues of experimenter bias cannot be totally discarded. However, the research assistants were blind to the purposes and hypotheses of the present study, which may have reduced this possible experimenter bias. It must also be made clear that data collection was made much easier by the fact that one of the authors was from this particular tribe. As always, though, there are costs and benefits to any research project and the same is true in the case of the present study. Despite these caveats, the present study and the results obtained are clearly a step in the direction of developing and standardizing neuropsychological tests for Native American populations, especially older populations. Additionally, these results can be used in future validation studies to see whether or not specific neuropsychological tests are suitable for Native American populations. The present results are encouraging, although extensive additional work is needed in this very slim research area (Jackson et al., 1990; Moody, 1994).

References

Ardila, A. (1995). Directions of research in cross-cultural neuropsychology. *Journal of Clinical and Experimental Neuropsychology, 17*, 143-150

Ardila, A. (1999). A neuropsychological approach to intelligence. *Neuropsychology Review, 9*, 117-136.

Adebimpe, V. R. (1981). Overview: White norms and psychiatric diagnosis of Black patients. *American Journal of Psychiatry, 138*, 278-285.

Arean, P. A., & Gallagher-Thompson, D. (1996). Issues and recommendations for the recruitment and retention of older ethnic minority adults into clinical research. *Journal of Consulting and Clinical Psychology, 64*, 875-880.

Baker, F. M. (1988). Dementing illness and Black Americans. In J. Jackson (Ed.), *Black American elderly* (pp. 215-233). New York: Springer.

Baker, F. M., Espino, D. V., Robinson, B. H., & Stewart, B., (1993). Assessment of ethnic minorities. *Ethnic, Psychiatric, and Societal Minorities, 2*, 15-29.

Blazer, D., George, L. K., Landerman, R., Pennybacker, M., Melville, M. L., Woodbury, M., Manton, K. G., Jordan, K., & Locke, B. (1985). Psychiatric disorders: A rural/urban comparison. *Archives of General Psychiatry, 42*, 651-656.

Chee, P., & Kane, R. (1983). Cultural factors affecting nursing home care for minorities: A study of Black American and Japanese American groups. *Journal of the American Geriatric Society, 31*, 109-112.

Cooley, R. C., Ostendorf, D., & Brikerton, D. (1979). Outreach services for elderly Native Americans. *Social Work, 28*, 151-153.

Ferraro, F. R., & Bercier, B. (1996). Boston Naming Test performance in a sample of Native American elderly adults. *Clinical Gerontologist, 17*, 60-63.

Fillenbaum, G. G., Huber, M., & Taussig, I. M. (1997). Performance of elderly white and African-American community residents on the abbreviated CERAD Boston Naming Test. *Journal of Clinical and Experimental Neuropsychology, 19*, 204-210.

Helms, J. F. (1992). Why is there no study of cultural equivalence in standardized cognitive testing? *American Psychologist, 47*, 1083-1101.

Hill, R. D. & Storandt, M. (1989). Very mild senile dementia of the Alzheimer type. *Archives of Neurology, 46*, 383-386

Hendrie, H. C., Hall, K. S., Pillay, N., Rodgers, D., Prince, C., Norton, J., Brittain, H., Nath, A., Blue, A., Kaufert, J., Shelton, P., Postl, B. & Osunkotun, B. (1993). Alzheimer's disease is rare in the Cree. *Research and Reviews: International Psychogeriatrics, 5*, 5-15

Jackson, J. S., Antonucci, T.C., & Gibson, R. C. (1990). *Cultural, racial, and ethnic minority influences on aging.* Handbook of the psychology of Aging (3rd ed). New York: Academic Press.

Kramer, J. B. (1991). Urban American Indian aging. *Journal of Cross-Cultural Gerontology, 6*, 205-217.

Kramer, J. B. (1992). Health and aging of urban American Indians. *Western Journal of Medicine, 157*, 281-285.

Lee, Y.-T., (1994). Why does American psychology have cultural limitations? *American Psychologist, 49*, 524.

Lightdale, J. R., Oken, E., Klein, W. M., Landrigan, P. J., & Welty, T. K. (1997). Psychosocial barriers to health promotion in an American Indian population. *American Indian and Alaskan Native American Mental Health Research, 7*, 34-49.

Lowe, L. P., Tranel, D., Wallace, R. B., & Welty, T. K. (1994). Type II diabetes and cognitive function: A population-based study of Native Americans. *Diabetes Care, 17*, 891-896.

Mack, W. J., Freed, D. M., Williams, B., & Henderson, V. W. (1992). Boston Naming Test: Shortened versions for use in Alzheimer's disease. *Journal of Gerontology: Psychological Sciences, 47*, 154-158.

Manson, S. M. (1989). Provider assumptions about long-term care in American Indian communities. *Gerontologist, 29*, 355-358.

McDonald, J. D., Morton, R. & Stewart, C. (1992) Clinical concerns with American Indian patients. *Innovations in Clinical Practice, 12*, 437-454.

McShane, D. (1987). Mental health and North American Indian/Native communities: Cultural transactions, education and regulation. *American Journal of Community Psychology, 15*, 95-116.

Moody, H. R. (1994). *Aging: Concepts and controversies.* Thousand Oaks: Pine Forge Press.

Norton, I. M., & Manson, S. M. (1996). Research in American Indian and Alaska Native communities: Navigating the cultural universe of values and process. *Journal of Consulting and Clinical Psychology, 64*, 856-860.

Novak, F. (1974). Home nursing care programs on an Indian reservation. *Public Health Reports, 89*, 545-550.

Padilla, A. M. (1980). *Acculturation: Theory, models, and some new findings.* Boulder: Westview Press.

Perez-Arce, P. (1999). The influence of culture on cognition. *Archives of Clinical Neuropsychology, 14*, 581-592.

Ponton, M. O., & Ardila, A. (1999). The future of neuropsychology with Hispanic populations in the United States. *Archives of Clinical Neuropsychology, 14*, 565-580.

Rosenberg, R. N., Richter, R. W., Risser, R. C., Taubman, K., Prado-Farmer. I., Elabo, E., Posey, J., Kingfisher, D., Dean, D., Weiner, M. F., Svetlik, D.,

Adams, P., Honig, L. S., Cullum, C. M., Schafer, F. V., & Schellenberg, G. D. (1996). Genetic factors for the development of Alzheimer disease in the Cherokee Indian. *Archives of Neurology, 53,* 997-1000.

Schneider, M. J. (1994). *North Dakota Indians: An introduction* (2nd ed.), Dubuque: Kendall Hunt.

Serpell, R., & Boykin, A. W. (1994). Cultural dimensions of cognition: A multiplex, dynamic system of constraints and possibilities. In R. J. Sternberg (Ed.), *Thinking and problem solving.* New York: Academic Press.

Stenger, P. W. (1994). *The data base of aging and health in Native Americans.* Presented at the annual meeting of the Gerontological Association of American.

Strong, C. (1984). Stress and caring for elderly relatives: Interpretations and coping strategies in an American Indian and white sample. *Gerontologist, 24,* 251-256.

Sugishita, M., Otomo, K., Kabe, S., & Yunoki, K. (1992). A critical appraisal of neuropsychological correlates of Japanese ideogram (kanji) and phonogram (kana) reading. *Brain, 115,* 1563-1585.

Taussig, M. I., Henderson, V. W., & Mack. W. (1992). Spanish translation and validation of neuropsychological battery: Performance of Spanish and English speaking Alzheimer's disease patients and normal comparison subjects. *Clinical Gerontologist, 2,* 95-107.

Valle, R. (1994). Culture-fair behavioral symptom differential assessment and intervention in dementing illness. *Alzheimer Disease and Associated Disorders, 8,* 21-45.

Wechsler, D. (1981). *Wechsler Adult Intelligence Scale – Revised.* New York: The Psychological Corporation.

Welsh, K. A., Ballard, E., Nash, F., Raiford, K., & Harrell, L. (1994). Issues affecting minority participation in research studies of Alzheimer disease. *Alzheimer Disease and Associated Disorders, 8,* 38-48.

Chapter 13

NATIVE AMERICANS:
FUTURE DIRECTIONS[1]

James C Gardiner and Dennis P. Tansley
Department of Veteran Affairs, Fort Meade, South
Dakota

Dewey J. Ertz
Manlove Psychiatric Group, Rapid City, South Dakota

PROLOGUE (By the senior author)

It has always been an honor to assess American Indians. I grew up in a rural South Dakota county surrounded by the Pine Ridge and Rosebud Indian Reservations. The Indian population was a high percentage of my neighborhood. As the only Caucasian in my one-room country school, I discovered what it was like to be in a minority group. Fortunately, I was always treated well by my Indian friends, and did not have to suffer as many of them did when they were outside our mutually supportive environment.

Years later, after my neuropsychological training was completed, I found a special thrill working with American Indian clients, particularly when I encountered those who, like me, had migrated from our South Dakota home. I returned to South Dakota in 1984 to work in a community mental health center. As the newcomer, I was given the assignment of assessing the American Indian clients from the local Indian Health Services (IHS) hospital. The standard practice for assessing American Indians at the mental health center at that time was to administer a computerized battery consisting of the Multidimensional Aptitude Battery {roughly equivalent to the verbal subtests of

---

[1]   The opinions expressed in this chapter are those of the authors and do not necessarily reflect the views of the IHS.

the Wechsler Adult Intelligence Scale – Revised (WAIS-R)} and the Minnesota Multiphasic Personality Inventory (MMPI). The interpretive printout far too often mislabeled the client as mentally retarded and schizophrenic. Had that practice continued, the IHS hospital and the local tribal officials would have likely teamed up to cancel our contract.

The distinguished neuropsychologist Charles Matthews, reflecting on his days as a student attempting to apply Caucasian neuropsychological tests to Indian clients on the Pine Ridge Reservation, feared that his efforts would result in being "tied down on an anthill somewhere between Broken Bow and Wounded Knee." I also reflected that continuing our American Indian assessment practices at the mental health center would have dire consequences, not only for us, but for the Indian clients who were the recipients of our shortsighted efforts.

After fifteen years and conducting more than 1000 psychological evaluations of American Indians, my assessment work has explored and found several appropriate tests that provide helpful psychological information for American Indian clients, their helpers, and their families. I have accumulated a data base of more than 350 neuropsychological assessments along with a wealth of experience. I appreciate the opportunity to share these with you, the reader.

Abstract

The contents of this chapter will be based on approximately 365 neuropsychological evaluations of American Plains Indians conducted in various South Dakota locations by the senior author from 1984 to the present. All test results have been saved on a computer database and include demographic (age, sex, marital status, educational level, handedness, occupation, diagnosis and location of the evaluation) as well as raw scores and scaled scores for all tests administered to each person. The primary focus of this chapter will be to present the findings of our analysis of these 365 evaluations. The first profile will include the entire sample, including demographics. Then, the sample will be presented according to age, education level, and diagnoses represented in the sample. The diagnoses will include brain injury, substance abuse, depression, schizophrenia, anxiety, PTSD, dementia, mental retardation, and medical problems. In the closing section of the chapter, guidance will be presented for future neuropsychological evaluations of American Indians.

Introduction

This chapter aims to accomplish two overall goals. The first is to provide neuropsychological data for comparison with future assessments on American Indians. Profiles of evaluation results are presented from clients with traumatic brain injuries, substance abuse, depression, other psychiatric disorders, and other neurological disorders. The second goal is to provide guidance for neuropsychological evaluations with American Indian clients, so that future assessments results can be accurate, meaningful, and beneficial.

Table 1.Demographic characteristics of American Indian clients evaluated.

Number		371
Age range		13 to 82
Mean age		38.11
Percent female		33.15
Percent male		66.85
Education in years		11.33
Marital status in percentages:	Single	42.59
	Married	29.65
	Divorced	19.68
	Widowed	4.58
	Unknown	3.50
Diagnoses represented in the sample:		
	Adjustment Disorder	
	AIDS/HIV	
	Alcoholism	
	Alzheimer's Disease	
	Anoxia	
	Anxiety Disorder	
	Attention Deficit Disorder	
	Bipolar Disorder	
	Brain Infection	
	Brain Tumor	
	Cerebrovascular Accident	
	Conduct Disorder	
	Conversion Disorder	
	Depression	
	Dissociative Disorder	
	Drug Abuse	
	Explosive Disorder	
	Fetal Alcohol Syndrome	
	Huntington's Disease	
	Hypochondriasis	
	Inhalant Abuse	
	Learning Disability	
	Mental Retardation	
	Pain Disorder	
	Personality Disorder	
	Posttraumatic Stress Disorder	
	Schizophrenia	
	Seizure Disorder	
	Toxic Exposure	
	Traumatic Brain Injury	

Methodology

The neuropsychological evaluation results presented in this chapter were from assessments conducted between 1984 and 1998 by the senior author at various locations in the upper plains of the United States. Included are several IHS Hospitals, a mental health center, a rehabilitation hospital, a medical hospital, several medical clinics, a sheltered workshop, and a Veterans Affairs medical center. The clients assessed were primarily from Northern Plains states, including South Dakota, North Dakota, Wyoming, Nebraska, Minnesota, and Montana. They were both inpatients and outpatients and were referred for neuropsychological evaluations by physicians, counselors, attorneys, vocational rehabilitation counselors, social service agencies, and other sources. Table 1 shows the demographic characteristics of the clients, including a listing of the various diagnoses. The tests administered varied with each evaluation. Not every client was administered every test, and the tests chosen depended on the referral question, the amount of time available for the assessment and the stamina and abilities of each client. The norms chosen to interpret the test results were carefully selected from those that stood the test of time, experience, clinical judgment, and goodness of fit. Table 2 presents a list of the tests and the norms used to provide interpretation of the test results.

Table 2. Neuropsychological tests and norms used with American Indian clients.

Test	Norms
Beck Depression Inventory (BDI)	Beck (1967)
Category Test (CT)	Heaton et al. (1991)
Finger Tapping Test (FTT)	Heaton et al. (1991)
Grip Strength (GS)	Heaton et al. (1991)
Grooved Pegboard	Heaton et al. (1991)
Hooper Visual Organization Test (HVOT)	Hooper (1983)
Minnesota Multiphasic Personality Inventory-2 (MMPI2)	Hathaway & McKinley (1989)
Multilingual Aphasia Examination (MAE):	Benton, et al. (1994)
Aural Comprehension	
Controlled Oral Word Association Test (COWAT)	
Reading Comprehension	
Sentence Repetition Test	
Visual Naming Test	
Porteus Mazes	Porteus (1965)
Rey Auditory Verbal Learning Test (RAVLT)	Geffen, et al. (1990)
Trail Making Test	Heaton et al. (1991)
Wechsler Adult Intelligence Scale-Revised (WAIS-R)	Wechsler (1981)
Wechsler Adult Intelligence Scale-III (WAIS-III)	Wechsler (1997)
Wechsler Memory Scale-Revised (WMS-R)	Wechsler (1987)
Wechsler Memory Scale-III (WMS-III)	Wechsler (1997)
Wide Range Achievement Test-3 (WRAT3)	Wilkinson (1993)
Wisconsin Card Sorting Test (WCST)	Heaton et al. (1993)

Findings of the Neuropsychological Evaluations

The neuropsychological evaluation results from the entire group of clients are presented in the last column of Table 3. It is necessary to use caution in examining these overall results, as the interpretation of the scores will be limited due to the mixture of diagnoses, age, sex, and educational level. By examining the Ns in the table, it can be noted that the tests most commonly administered were the Wechsler Adult Intelligence Scale-Revised (with Vocabulary, Similarities, Arithmetic, and Block Design given most frequently), Wechsler Memory Scale-Revised (Logical Memory I & II, Visual Reproduction I & II and Digit Span), Rey Auditory Verbal Learning Test, Sentence Repetition Test and Controlled Oral Word Association Test. Table 3 also presents the test results categorized into various diagnoses, including traumatic brain injury, a mixture of neurological disorders, substance abuse, depression and a variety of other psychiatric disorders. The results are presented in this manner so that the reader can have a basis for comparison with neuropsychological evaluations conducted on American Indian clients with those disorders. Figures 1 through 5 display in bar graph form, the results of the five most common diagnoses from the client group: traumatic brain injury, substance abuse, depression, other psychiatric disorders and other neurological disorders. Each of the graphs in Figures 1 through 5 presents the results in percentiles, based on the norms for each test.

Future Directions for the Assessment Process

The following remarks are presented to help the reader develop a philosophy of assessment that will facilitate successful neuropsychological examinations of American Indian clients. Areas to be discussed include necessary preliminary information, the initial contact, the preliminaries, seating arrangement, interviewing, test selection/administration and a list of recommended tests.

Preliminary questions

The assessment process begins when the first information from the referral reaches the evaluator. Important questions that need to be asked by the examiner include: What was the intent of the referral source in asking for an evaluation? How will the information from the evaluation be used? Who will stand to benefit from the assessment process? What possible harm can be caused by the evaluation?

The initial contact

The first half-second of contact with each client is vital. It is important to carefully observe the cues surrounding that event. Does the person establish eye contact? If not, he or she may be highly traditional in lifestyle. The absence of eye contact may be a sign of respect, not avoidance or opposi-

Table 3. Neuropsychological test results for various diagnoses and total sample.

Cognitive Skill	Test and Scale	Brain Injury			Other Neur	
		Mean	*SD*	*N*	*Mean*	*SD*
Demographics:	Age	40.25			39.95	
	Education	11.64			11.76	
	% Female	32			33	
Attention						
Auditory attention	WMS-R, DSF	6.37	1.61	19		
Auditory concentration	WMS-R, DSB	4.50	1.34	18		
Tracking & sequencing	Trails A	41.95	21.97	57	34.44	20.92
Alternating attention	Trails B	138.25	116.67	57	98.40	62.50
Memory and Learning						
Auditory-immediate	WMS-R, LM I	14.52	4.92	21		
Auditory-delayed	WMS-R, LM II	8.86	5.62	20		
Visual-immediate	WMS-R, VR I	31.70	6.78	20		
Visual-delayed	WMS-R, VR II	21.25	11.29	20		
Verbal learning	RAVLT, Total	34.85	11.72	34	34.46	11.49
Verbal recall	RAVLT, 20min	6.34	4.16	32	5.92	3.82
Verbal recognition	RAVLT, Recog	11.13	3.27	30	10.00	3.51
Verbal & Academic						
Vocabulary	WAIS-R, Voc	7.92	2.20	36	8.00	2.18
Abstract reasoning	WAIS-R, Sim	10.23	2.00	39	8.22	2.65
Judgment knowledge	WAIS-R, Com	7.06	2.11	32	6.75	1.06
General information store	WAIS-R, Infor	7.17	2.15	30	7.56	2.28
Oral arithmetic problem solving	WAIS-R, Ari	6.03	2.00	40	8.17	2.04
Verbal expression	Sentence Repetition	9.79	2.71	28	10.00	2.08
Word fluency	COWAT	31.78	11.30	32	23.33	11.93
Visuospatial						
Visual detail perception	WAIS-R, PC	8.29	2.84	34	8.31	2.55
Social sequencing	WAIS-R, PA	8.59	2.93	32	5.81	2.18
Visuospatial construction	WAIS-R, BD	8.64	2.66	39	10.88	3.43
Visuospatial reasoning	WAIS-R, OA	8.79	2.22	33	8.54	3.36
Visuospatial learning	WAIS-R, Dsy	7.13	2.25	31	9.69	3.50
Visual organization	Hooper VOT	24.56	4.33	18		
Intellectual						
Verbal intelligence	WAIS-R, VIQ	82.74	7.59	34	86.38	6.97
Performance intelligence	WAIS-R, PIQ	88.71	11.57	34	95.44	14.99
Full scale intelligence	WAIS-R, FSIQ	84.44	8.21	34	89.06	8.67
Motor						
Speed, dominant	FTT, dom	45.51	11.10	39	51.09	8.23
Speed, nondominant	FTT, nondom	44.78	8.48	41	49.45	8.47
Executive Control						
Planning & foresight	Porteus Mazes	14.37	2.11	19	14.64	2.67
Cognitive flexibility	WCST, pers resp	32.86	20.96	21	24.78	16.97
Problem solving errors	WCST, errors	45.73	21.92	22	33.56	20.14
Problem solving accuracy	WCST, categories	3.82	1.94	22	4.11	2.26

	Diagnosis											
Substance Abuse			Depression			Other Psychiatric			Total Sample			
ean	SD	N	Mean	SD	N	Mean	SD	N	Mean	SD	N	
.56			37.91			33.15			38.11			
).53			12.28			12.46			11.33			
26			44			46			33			
.00	2.42	14	6.69	1.93	13	7.44	2.13	16	6.46	1.99	105	
.64	3.03	14	5.17	1.27	12	6.38	3.01	16	5.07	2.24	103	
.44	32.33	36	32.89	15.13	19	32.32	15.38	25	40.73	25.90	226	
.25	75.09	32	76.11	37.13	18	113.12	92.81	25	121.34	88.22	215	
.05	9.25	21	16.79	6.42	14	18.38	7.68	16	14.83	7.53	127	
.67	2.52	21	12.93	5.36	14	8.40	8.66	16	10.60	8.02	124	
.47	6.81	17	32.62	5.81	13	33.50	6.46	16	31.98	6.95	118	
.06	6.08	17	28.23	9.98	13	27.81	9.76	16	24.21	11.44	115	
.22	12.13	19	40.63	6.41	8	41.00	11.72	12	36.68	11.38	121	
.21	3.74	19	8.75	2.25	8	9.00	3.72	12	6.97	3.96	115	
.11	2.92	19	13.50	1.20	8	12.33	2.67	12	10.98	3.50	111	
.84	1.89	32	8.47	3.84	17	8.45	2.93	20	7.37	2.77	221	
.03	2.60	34	9.11	3.77	19	9.09	3.01	23	7.51	3.00	242	
.41	2.21	27	8.09	4.32	11	8.36	2.92	14	6.98	2.85	175	
.33	1.68	21	7.17	3.10	12	7.83	2.37	12	6.77	2.83	153	
.09	1.68	34	6.94	2.41	17	8.38	2.94	21	6.59	2.47	229	
).33	1.97	12	10.60	2.32	10				10.56	6.78	104	
.64	6.65	11	36.55	12.40	11	42.58	9.38	12	33.90	10.60	108	
.35	2.54	26	10.00	3.63	11	10.38	3.48	13	8.13	2.91	176	
.11	2.36	27	8.56	2.96	9	8.54	2.50	13	8.16	2.78	171	
.29	2.73	35	9.94	3.02	18	10.27	3.07	22	9.09	3.04	233	
.50	2.27	28	9.54	2.15	13	9.84	2.67	19	8.68	2.82	192	
.26	2.28	31	8.50	2.88	14	8.64	2.95	14	7.53	2.69	195	
									25.34	3.23	53	
.29	7.71	28	89.17	19.52	12	88.69	12.31	13	82.03	12.96	178	
.32	10.56	28	96.91	16.53	11	96.69	14.30	13	88.68	13.61	176	
.68	7.84	28	93.18	18.72	11	91.62	14.04	13	84.03	12.49	175	
.45	7.88	20	53.25	12.70	8				47.23	10.22	130	
.80	6.53	20	48.75	12.46	8				45.05	8.50	133	
.19	2.91	13	15.50	1.07	8				14.11	2.52	92	
.00	18.48	10	21.18	19.23	11	20.10	14.41	10	39.28	18.17	86	
.18	13.73	11	35.73	22.88	11	33.70	23.31	10	39.28	20.85	93	
.73	1.49	11	4.45	1.75	11	4.30	2.21	10	4.09	1.94	93	

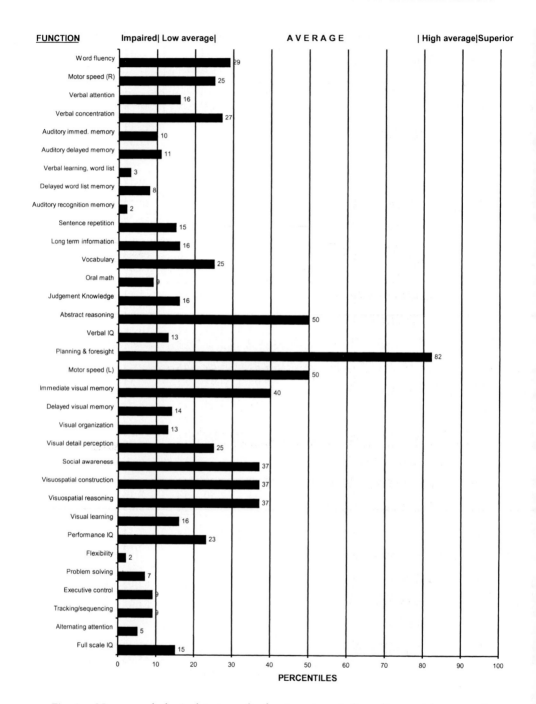

Fig. 1.   Neuropsychological test results for American Indian clients with traumatic brain injuries.

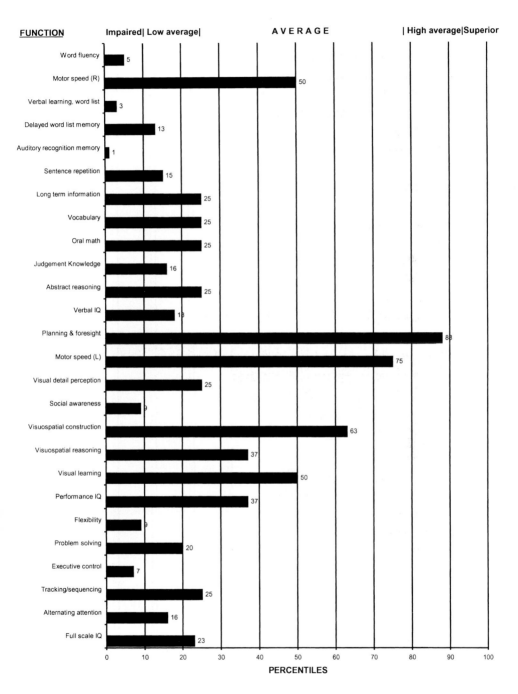

Fig. 2.   Neuropsychological test results for American Indian clients with various neurological disorders.

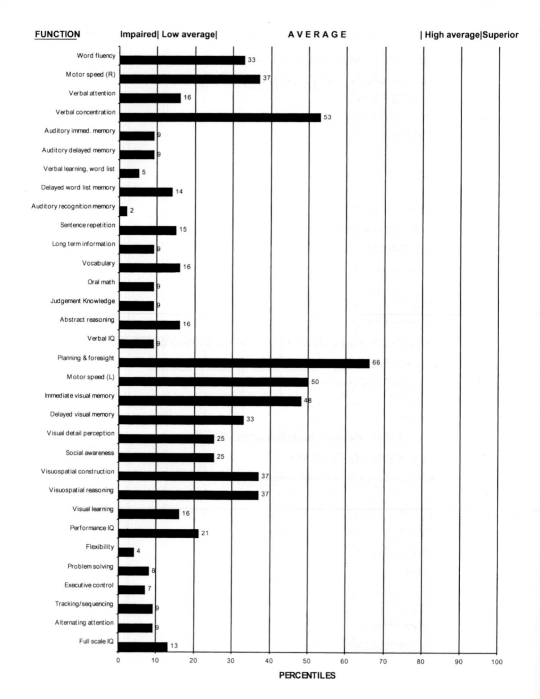

Fig. 3.   Neuropsychological test results for American Indian clients with substance abuse problems.

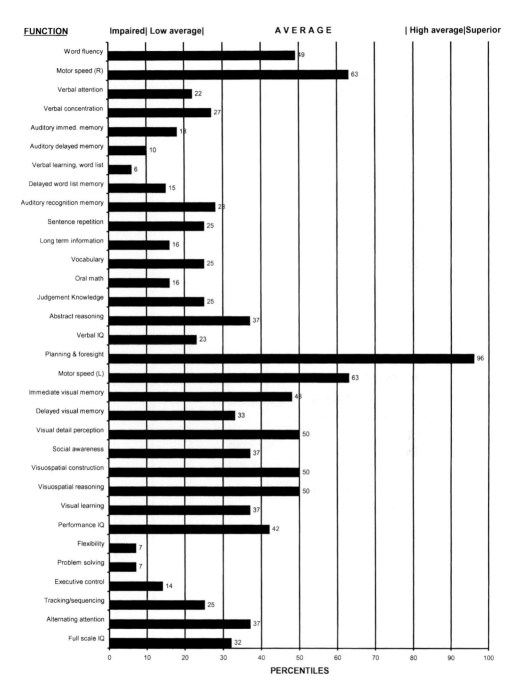

Fig. 4. Neuropsychological test results for American Indian clients with depresseion.

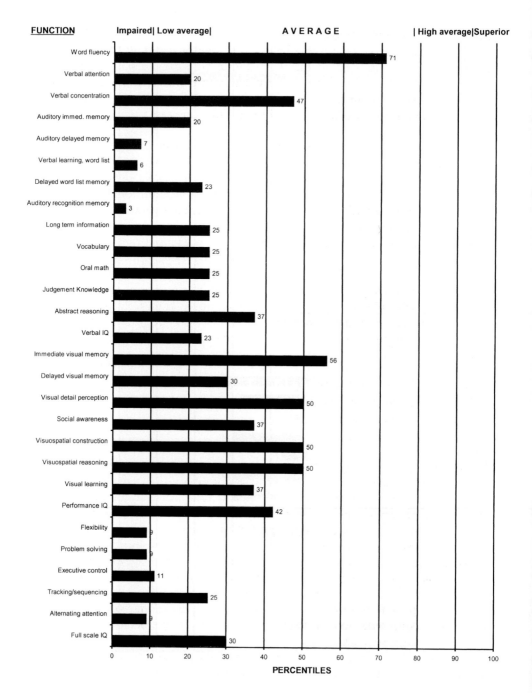

Fig. 5.   Neuropsychological test results for American Indian clients with other psychiatric conditions.

tion. Is a handshake offered? If so, is it a soft or tentative grip? If so, it can be another sign of traditional beliefs. Then extra time will be needed in establishing a relationship so that the examination can be successful. The behaviors observed during the early moments of the initial meeting with the clients tell a story about their background, their degree of comfort with the meeting between the two of you, and their willingness to participate in the assessment.

Another helpful area to understand and question during the initial contact is how persons identify with their Indian heritage. This is an ethnic variable rather than viewing the person from a racial perspective. This identification is generally viewed on a continuum from contemporary to traditional. Individuals who identify themselves as traditional often practice ceremonies such as the sweat lodge and have leisure or family activities that involve established tribal beliefs. They are more likely to speak or understand their native language and to have knowledge of their tribal history. Contemporary individuals are identified with the broader American culture and value system. Individuals may identify at any point along this continuum, or they may not identify with either contemporary or traditional values. Such individuals have been referred to as marginally identified. May (1989) has reported that American Indians with marginal identification have an increased risk to develop emotional and substance use problems.

One possible instrument to use for measuring identification with cultural norms is the Northern Plains Bicultural Inventory (NPBI) (Allen & French, 1996). It employs a Likert-type response to questions that focus on traditional Indian practices.

The preliminaries
It is important to clearly establish with the client the nature and purpose of your meeting. The person may come to the appointment expecting everything from a CT Scan to paper and pencil tests. The query of who sent them, what they were informed about the examination, what they expect to happen in the evaluation, and what they anticipate will take place as a result of the assessment is vital to the success of the evaluation. This process is particularly important because many American Indians will not be outspoken or aggressively inquire about why you are examining them. It is thus helpful to be clear about the purpose of the evaluation, to give the person plenty of time to think over the situation and to encourage them to respond with any objections or questions. If the person has highly traditional Indian beliefs, the responses may come slowly. That will not signal oppositional behavior, but rather a careful consideration of the implications and possible outcomes of their participation in the examination. Allowing this time and respecting the needs of the person to be examined will strengthen the examiner/examinee relationship and improve the validity of the assessment.

Seating

The seating arrangement of the assessment is extremely important. Custom-ary seating across a table where the examiner and examinee face each other can create an uncomfortable atmosphere. This likely stems from the unfamiliar stimuli that are created when having to face a stranger in a con-strained environment. The most comfortable position for most examinees in an examination setting is across the corner of a table from the examiner. With this arrangement the client can have the freedom to gaze around the room without frequently meeting the eyes of the examiner. If the testing table is rectangular, the client can be invited to sit at the narrow end of the table. It is possible to present the place of seating as an honor and say: "I want you to sit at the head of the table." The neuropsychologist should convey to the client that the examiner is there to honor their strengths and to examine their weaknesses and not to demean their abilities in any way. The client should be seated where there is a clear and easy access to the door. That will help avoid all feelings of entrapment and give the client the freedom to leave at any time.

The interview

The successful neuropsychological evaluation begins with a thorough clinical interview. The importance of the interview is clearly illustrated through an experience early in the senior author's career. Faced with a severe time con-straint when testing a client, it was decided that there was time for only a few tests. The interview was dispensed with. After the exchange of a few pleasant-ries and an explanation of the purpose of the testing, the examination began. The results were disastrous, in that the client held back and cooperated to a minimal degree. That experience illustrated that the interview not only yields important information, but it mentally prepares the client for the testing as well. The interview content needs to be as comprehensive as possible, yet respectful of the client's need for privacy and degree of willingness for self-disclosure. The interview is normally begun with safe subjects such as where and when the client was born and raised, a description of their family, and where they attended school. As the client becomes more comfortable with the interview, more delicate subjects such as substance abuse, memory failings, and spirituality can be approached. Important information to be gleaned from the interview includes: (a) the degree to which the client's family practiced American Indian traditions; (b) the language(s) spoken in their home; (c) the nature, location, and extent of the client's education; (d) her or his vocational background, and (e) primary places of residence during their lifetime. While it may be tempting for an examiner to stereotype American Indians as coming from a poverty-stricken background, it is highly important to carefully exam-ine each person's background, which can range from lifelong residence on a reservation to living in a major city while pursuing a professional career.

An interview of this nature is not complete without considering the trauma history of the person being evaluated. The effect of trauma is a complex issue, as only a percentage of individuals exposed to traumatic events suffer adverse reactions. Sameroff, Garbarino, and their colleagues have documented that early traumas may have a greater influence based on a relationship between lower intelligence and adaptive abilities in young children as risk factors such as troubled families, hostile communities and impaired functioning increase (Sameroff, Siefer, Barocas, Zax, & Greenspan, 1987; Garbarino, Dubrow, Kostelny, & Pardo, 1992). The histories of many American Indian Tribes and families often show an accumulation of such risks. It is recommended that the interview always question sources of trauma. An extensive trauma history of the person and his or her family is recommended when the person to be evaluated presents severe behavioral and cognitive difficulties without a definitive history of injury or illness. Many professionals working with American Indians have employed the Trauma Symptom Inventory (TSI) (Briere, 1995) to objectively assess the extent of a person's traumatic experience. Another source of trauma that many American Indians experience is living in an alcoholic environment. That possibility needs to be explored in each interview.

Designing the test battery

It is vital that a unique set of tests be selected for each client in each evaluation setting. The tests need to be based on the question to be answered, the makeup of the client, the time constraints, and the degree to which a comprehensive examination is desired. According to Lezak (1995), important areas that need to be addressed in a comprehensive neuropsychological evaluation include: attention, memory and learning, verbal and academic, visuospatial, motor, executive control, intellectual, and emotional status.

Test selection

After the purpose and scope of the examination have been established, the next important determination should be to decide which tests the client will be comfortable taking. The following guidelines are offered in each major area of neuropsychological assessment:

Attention

Digit span forward and backward have proven to be effective measures of auditory attention and concentration, respectively. In the author's experience, most American Indian clients have been comfortable dealing with numbers. In addition, the Trail Making Test, parts A and B have been helpful in measuring tracking, sequencing, and alternating attention, provided the client is comfortable with the English alphabet.

Memory and learning

Logical Memory I & II as well as Visual Reproduction I & II from the Wechsler Memory Scale-Revised had been effective in assessing auditory and visual recall. The Rey Auditory Verbal Learning Test is particularly effective in assessment of verbal learning. The words on the Rey test are compatible with rural life and are meaningful to most American Indians. In addition, there is a recognition memory component to the test.

Verbal and academic

Test selection in this area needs to be done with great caution. Compatibility with cultural background needs to be carefully considered when assessing vocabulary, judgment knowledge, general information store, reading recognition, reading comprehension, spelling, object naming, and verbal fluency. Tests in this area that have found to be generally effective for use with American Indians include the Vocabulary, Similarities and Arithmetic subtests of the WAIS-III, along with the Sentence Repetition Test of the Multilingual Aphasia Examination.

Visual spatial

Tests in this area have been generally compatible with the experiences of most American Indians and are suitable for use in assessment. Those most effective include the Block Design, Object Assembly, and Matrix Reasoning from the Wechsler Intelligence Scales. The Hooper Visual Organization Test is appropriate for assessing perceptual accuracy. The Picture Completion and Picture Arrangement subtests of the Wechsler scales need to be used with caution, since the contents of those tests have a cultural context that may not be compatible with the client being assessed.

Motor

Most motor tests of strength, speed, and dexterity are not culturally biased and can be given without reservation except for the usual considerations of peripheral neurological damage.

Executive control

Several tests of cognitive flexibility, problem solving, planning, and foresight are useful and appropriate to utilize with American Indians. The Wisconsin Card Sorting Test, which emphasizes color, shape, and number in its measurement of executive control, has proven to be effective. In addition, the Porteus Mazes, Category Test, and mazes from the Wechsler Intelligence Scale for Children have proven effective as measures of executive control.

Intellectual

Measures of intelligence need to be used with extreme caution with American Indians subjects. The validity of verbal intelligence scales with American Indians is highly questionable, given the large number of questions on the Information, Vocabulary, and Comprehension subtests that are unfamiliar to the cultural background of many American Indians. While many psychologists consider the performance intelligence valid for measuring most Indian clients, the contents of both Picture Completion and Picture Arrangement can be culturally biased. Given these limitations associated with intellectual assessment, it is inadvisable to administer a complete intelligence test to an American Indian client with a traditional background. When requested by a referring agency, or when needed for classification purposes, the use of complete intellectual assessment with American Indians must be carefully presented in the report by highlighting possible sources of bias and cultural unfairness from the tests administered. The recently released Wechsler Abbreviated Scale of Intelligence (Wechsler, 1999) has good potential for accurately assessing intellectual capacity with American Indians. The two performance subtests included in the scale, Block Design and Matrix Reasoning, will likely prove to be valid measures of visuospatial skills with American Indian clients. The two verbal measures, Vocabulary and Similarities, are also relatively free of cultural bias and have good potential for assessing the verbal skills of Indian clients. Another type of instrument to consider using in evaluation of intellectual potential is an adaptive behavioral scale. Good information is often yielded from comparing intellectual and adaptive abilities as adaptive behaviors are less influenced by cultural background. An added advantage of an adaptive behavioral scale is that administrating the scale involves interviewing collateral sources which frequently adds to the validity of the information collected.

Emotional status
The assessment of emotional status among American Indians is a delicate issue. Many standardized objective tests of personality are highly inappropriate to use with this population. The Minnesota Multiphasic Personality Inventory, for example, has not been effective with Plains American Indians, at least in the experience of the authors. Too often the test results indicate the diagnosis of schizophrenia, when the clinical data and behaviors of the person do not support that diagnosis. When the first revision of the Minnesota Multiphasic Personality Inventory appeared in 1989, it was encouraging to learn that American Indians had been included in the standardization sample. At that time it was decided to try the new MMPI on the psychiatric patients at an Indian Health Services Hospital in South Dakota. The test was administered to ten consecutive admissions to the psychiatric unit and the results were interpreted with no knowledge of the patient and then presented to the psychiatric staff. The psychiatric staff determined that nine of the ten blind interpretations were accurate. It was concluded that the MMPI –2 had excellent potential for the personality assessment of American Indians in the upper Plains area, when used in connection with clinical findings, collateral data, behavioral observations, and other appropriate test results.

Also helpful in the assessment of personality among American Indians are several of the projective personality tests. The House-Tree-Person drawings (Wenck, 1977), Thematic Apperception Test (Murray, 1943), and Rorschach Inkblot Technique (Exner, 1986) have been effective. Again, care must be taken in the interpretation of the projective tests. All drawings, stories and responses to the Rorschach Inkblot cards need to be interpreted in light of the person's cultural background and experiences. The stories from the Thematic Apperception Test have been helpful in assessing the thought patterns, motivations, emotional states, and lifestyle themes of the person being assessed.

Fixed neuropsychological test batteries
Subjecting American Indian clients to a fixed battery of tests is a practice to be avoided. There have been projects in American Indian settings where fixed batteries were purchased for the purpose of wholesale neuropsychological assessment of all referrals from the Indian population by unqualified examiners without adequate supervision. Some of these tests appropriately remain in storage beside antiquated biofeedback equipment and outdated craft supplies. Other such tests, due to American Indian ingenuity, have found a useful place in the children's play area of the clinic or as a lamp stand in a waiting room.

Similarly, computerized batteries need to be avoided for general use with Native American populations. Unless the client is a regular and comfortable computer user, the experience of sitting at a computer for an assessment can be anxiety-provoking and will likely produce invalid results.

Future Directions in Neuropsychological Assessment with American Indians

The ideal future world of neuropsychological assessment with American Indians will unite the experience gained from past assessments with the best technology available now and in the future. The following list of tests is offered for neuropsychological testing with American Indians:

Attention:
  Digits forward and backward, Wechsler Memory Scale-III
  Trail Making Test

Memory and learning:
  Auditory: Logical Memory I & II, Wechsler Memory Scale-III
  Visual: Visual Reproduction I & II, Wechsler Memory Scale-III
  Learning: Word Lists I & II, Wechsler Memory Scale-III

Verbal and academic:
  Wechsler Adult Intelligence Scale-III, Arithmetic
  Wechsler Abbreviated Scale of Intelligence, Vocabulary and Similarities
  Wide Range Achievement Test 3, Spelling, Reading, and Arithmetic

Visuospatial:
  Visuospatial organization: Hooper Visual Organization Test
  Visuospatial construction: Block Design from the Wechsler Abbreviated Scale of Intelligence

Visual spatial reasoning: Matrix Reasoning from the Wechsler Abbreviated Scale of Intelligence

Motor:
Finger Tapping Test, Grip Strength, and Grooved Pegboard

Executive control:
Mazes from the Wechsler Intelligence Scale for Children-III
Wisconsin Card Sorting Test

Intellectual:
Wechsler Abbreviated Scale of Intelligence

Emotional status:
Minnesota Multiphasic Personality Inventory-2
Thematic Apperception Test
House-Tree-Person Drawings
Rorschach Inkblot Technique

The test battery proposed above will need to be normed carefully with various American Indian populations. The norms will also need to be localized. Norms developed for one tribe will not be valid with others. Thus, one cannot establish norms for Navaho tribes and expect them to apply to the Lakota or Hopi. It is proposed that neuropsychologists who are working with American Indians in various regions of North America begin norming the tests listed above on persons with no known brain dysfunction or psychiatric illness. A site on the World Wide Web or a section at an existing American Indian research center needs to be established to serve as a gathering place for the normative data gathered by neuropsychologists throughout North America. As the norms accumulate, they can be communicated back to local practitioners through the Internet, journal articles, or other forms of neuropsychological literature.

Conclusions

As with any neuropsychological examination, the evaluation of an American Indian client requires close attention to the purpose of the encounter, the perception of the encounter by the client, and the possible benefit or harm that may result from the examination. Because of the lack of adequate norms for American Indian populations and the lack of established procedures for performing valid assessments on persons from the population, it is very likely that the field of neuropsychology has poorly served many American Indians. The time has come to establish a standardized practice of neuropsychological assessment with American Indians. This effort should begin with a focus on appropriate norms and selection of tests that reduce the potential for cultural variables to negatively influence test results.

This chapter has offered a starting point to provide neuropsychological data for comparison with future assessments of American Indians from various locations in the Northern Plains. Evaluation results were presented from clients with traumatic brain injuries, substance abuse, depression, other psychiatric disorders, and other neurological disorders. This effort needs to be continued by other neuropsychologists who are working with American Indians in other regions of North America including norming tests on persons with no known brain dysfunction or psychiatric illness. It is hoped that these norms will be localized and combined into a data base that is accessible to individuals who have the qualifications to interpret and use the data to enhance neuropsychological assessment.

Besides norming and test selection there are three additional areas where neuropsychological assessment with American Indians can be improved to produce accurate, meaningful, and beneficial results. These areas include expanding interviews to specifically address areas of Indian identity, considering and documenting the potential risk factors or effects of trauma, and employing alternative methods to understand each person's functioning such as adaptive behavioral scales or collateral contacts. Neuropsychologists completing assessments with American Indian clients can meet this complex challenge by implementing the above recommendations, expanding current assessment procedures, employing other professionals in the assessment process to help gather necessary information, and gaining additional training. Hopefully the greatest reward for all these efforts will come to American Indian clients and their families, who will benefit from well-administered, accurate neuropsychological assessments.

References

Allen, J., & French, C. (1996). *Northern Plains Bicultural Inventory*. Vermillion, SD: University of South Dakota.

Benton, A.L., Hamsher, K. deS., & Sivan, A.B. (1994). *Multilingual Aphasia Examination*, 3rd Ed. Iowa City: AJA Associates.

Briere, J. (1995). *Trauma symptom inventory*. Odessa: Psychological Assessment Resources, Inc.

Exner, J.E. (1986). *The Rorschach: A comprehensive system*, (vol, 1 2nd ed.). New York: Wiley-InterScience.

Garbarino, J., Dubrow, N., Kostelny K., & Pardo, C. (1992). *Children in Danger: Coping with the consequences of community violence*. San Francisco: Jossey-Bass.

Geffen, G., Moar, K.J., O'Hanlon, A.P., Clark, C.R., & Geffen, L.B. (1990). Performance measures of 16 to 86 year old males and females on the Auditory Verbal Learning Test. *The Clinical Neuropsychologist, 4*, 45-63.

Hathaway, S.R., & McKinley, J.C. (1989). *The Minnesota Multiphasic Personality Inventory-2*. Minneapolis: University of Minnesota Press.

Heaton, R.K., Chelune, G.J., Talley, J.L., Kay, G.G., & Curtiss, G. (1993). *Wisconsin Card Sorting Test. Manual.* Odessa: Psychological Assessment Resources.

Heaton, R.K., Grant, I., & Matthews, C.G. (1991). *Comprehensive norms for an expanded Halstead-Reitan battery: Demographic corrections, research findings, and clinical applications.* Odessa: Psychological Assessment Resources.

Hooper, H.E. (1983) *Hooper Visual Organization Test (VOT).* Los Angeles: Western Psychological Services.

Lezak, M.D. (1995) *Neuropsychological assessment,* 3rd Ed. New York: Oxford University Press.

May, P.A. (1989). Alcohol abuse and alcoholism among American Indians: An overview. In T.D. Watts & R. Wight (Eds.), *Alcoholism in minority populations* (pp. 96-119). Springfield: Charles C. Thomas.

Murray, H.A. (1943). *Thematic Apperception Test.* Pictures and manual. Cambridge: Harvard University Press.

Porteus, S.D. (1965). *Porteus Maze Test: Fifty years application.* Palo Alto: Pacific Books.

Reitan, R.M., & Wolfson, D. (1993). *The Halstead-Reitan Neuropsychological Test Battery: Theory and clinical interpretation.* Tucson: Neuropsychology Press.

Sameroff, A., Seifer, R., Barocas,R., Zax, M., & Greenspan, S. (1987). Intelligence quotient scores of 4-year-old children: Social-environmental risk factors. *Pediatrics, 79,* 343-350.

Wechsler, D. (1999). *Wechsler Abbreviated Scale of Intelligence Manual.* San Antonio: The Psychological Corporation.

Wechsler, D. (1981). *Wechsler Adult Intelligence Scale-Revised Manual.* San Antonio: The Psychological Corporation.

Wechsler, D. (1997). *Wechsler Adult Intelligence Scale-3rd Ed. Administration and Scoring Manual.* San Antonio: The Psychological Corporation.

Wechsler, D. (1991). *Wechsler Intelligence Scale for Children-3rd Ed. Manual.* San Antonio: The Psychological Corporation.

Wechsler, D. (1987). *Wechsler Memory Scale-Revised Manual.* San Antonio: The Psychological Corporation.

Wechsler, D. (1997). *Wechsler Memory Scale-3rd Ed. Administration and Scoring Manual.* San Antonio, TX: The Psychological Corporation.

Wenck, L.S. (1977). *House-Tree-Person drawings: An illustrated diagnostic handbook.* Los Angeles: Western Psychological Services.

Wilkinson, G.S. (1993). *Wide Range Achievement Test* 3rd ed. Wilmington: Wide Range, Inc.

PART VI

RURAL POPULATIONS/ ELDERLY/ SAUDI ARABIAN

Chapter 14

CURRENT ISSUES IN NEUROPSYCHOLOGICAL ASSESSMENT WITH RURAL POPULATIONS

Richard W. Williams, Ph.D., and
Michelle L. Bowman
State University of New York at Potsdam, Potsdam,
New York

Abstract

Are there differences in neuropsychological or intellectual test performance for people who live in rural areas as compared to those living in urban environments? Early studies showed that people in urban settings performed better on some intellectual skills. More current research finds that test performance differences are minimal, with the possible exception of young children. Research on mental health issues indicates that some disorders are more likely in rural settings. We discuss conceptual issues concerning the study of the urban-rural factor. Problems with defining "rural" settings are outlined, and we argue that the definition should include measured aspects of the environment rather than just the number of people who live in that environment. Implications of this review include that neuropsychological testing can be done with rural residents without too much concern about the validity of the test results, but more normative data are needed for most tests that are used.

Introduction

As neuropsychologists learn more about target populations and particular disorders, they are able to focus their evaluations and modify their interpretations. In this chapter, we will examine the literature related to urban versus rural place of residence and whether there is an impact of geographical residence upon cognitive functioning. We will address the question of whether people in rural settings perform differentially on intellectual and neuropsychological tests.

The focus of the chapter will be on studies that compare urban and rural people on intelligence, memory, language, and other cognitive processes. We will review the research concerning the mental health problems and needs of rural people and the availability of services in rural settings. We will address the commonly used definition of "rural" and its limitations, and will discuss alternative ways of studying rural people. The implications of the research for conducting neuropsychological assessments in rural settings will be outlined. First, we begin by examining the interest in urban/rural factors in the psychological literature.

Increased Interest in Urban/Rural Factors

We conducted a literature search of articles in English that contained reference to urban/rural content (PsycINFO, 1999). We made no attempt to verify the content of the publications; rather, we searched for any reference to the words urban or rural. The search was done in 10-year blocks beginning with 1901.

We found one article between 1901 and 1910, and another in the next decade. After the 1920's, the number of records began nearly doubling as the decades progressed. As of March 1999, there were 3,174 publications in the 1990's that examined some aspect of urban and rural issues. A subset of the publications in the 1990's was selected by searching for articles that included urban and rural in the article abstract. A total of 815 articles met this criterion. Of these, 22 were related to psychometric testing/assessment, although they did not always include a comparison of urban and rural groups. Most of the 22 concerned the Wechsler scales, while the remaining articles focused on personality, emotions, and other psychological issues.

These numbers show an increased interest in urban and rural research. Whether this increase is due to sensitivity to cultural/environmental factors, or whether it is just associated with the overall increase in the scientific productivity in psychology is unclear.

Psychological and Neuropsychological Tests

Comparisons between urban and rural test performance on intellectual tasks have been conducted for decades (e.g., Smiley, 1910). Evidence for reliable differences between urban and rural people would have implications for test interpretation. We will examine the findings related to residence on psychological and neuropsychological tests.

Research on intelligence

Studies of Children

The early data in the United States showed that urban children performed better on intelligence tests than did rural children. McNemar (1942) showed that urban children scored 6 to 12 points higher on the Stanford-Binet at various ages (2-18). Seashore, Wesman, and Doppelt (1950) found that urban children scored an average of 5.5 points higher than rural children did on the Full Scale IQ of the Wechsler Intelligence Scale for Children (WISC). More recent studies found that urban children scored about two points higher on Full Scale IQ (Kaufman & Doppelt, 1976). Reschly and Jipson (1976) found no differences in the prevalence of childhood mental retardation based upon urban-rural residence.

What are the findings in other countries? Alexopoulos (1997) found that urban students in Greece performed significantly better on intelligence testing (the AH4: Heim, 1970) than did rural children. The urban children's mean Total IQ score was six points higher. This partially replicated the earlier results by the same author (Alexopoulos, 1979, as cited in Alexopoulos, 1997) that found even greater differences (10-13 points for Full Scale IQ) between urban and rural children in Greece using the WISC-R. Alexopoulos (1997) stated that the group differences might have been due to the fact that Greece is a developing country, and that the rural areas have less educational opportunities. Thus, these findings are similar to those found in the early studies conducted in the United States (e.g., Seashore et al., 1950) with urban children performing better on intelligence tests.

There was, however, one important difference between the Alexopoulos (1997) and Seashore et al. (1950) findings. The Seashore et al. data showed that the difference between urban and rural children in the United States was primarily on Verbal IQ, while the verbal and performance scores were both higher for the urban children in Alexopoulos (1997). The difference may be due to the different tests used in each study. The AH4 used by Alexopoulos (1997) is a group test of intelligence which is divided into two parts (Heim, 1970). Part I consists of verbal and numerical questions (verbal analogies, verbal opposites, synonyms, arithmetic computations), while Part II consists of items involving spatial relationships (analogies, similarity, series, superimposition, computations). Thus, although similar to the Wechsler scales in that Part II of the AH4 consists of non-verbal items, the types of items are considerably different. Therefore, whether the conflicting results are due to the particular samples, the use of different tests, to random variability, or to other factors is not known.

The evidence of decreasing urban/rural differences on intelligence testing in the U.S. suggests that some factor(s) may be responsible. Later, we will discuss the interpretation of these findings.

Studies of Adults
Reynolds, Chastain, Kaufman, and McLean (1987) pointed out that the 1955 Wechsler Adult Intelligence Scale (WAIS) was never analyzed as systematically as were the Wechsler scales for children in terms of demographic characteristics such as place of residence. Thus, there is limited data about the urban/rural variable for the first half of this century. Studies conducted in the 1980s found that there were no differences between rural and urban adults on overall Wechsler Adult Intelligence Scale – Revised (WAIS-R) performance (e.g., Matarazzo & Herman, 1984; Reynolds et al., 1987). Rural and urban people did not differ on their Verbal IQ, Performance IQ, or Full Scale IQ performance on the WAIS-R.

Kaufman, McLean, and Reynolds (1988) compared urban and rural residents on the 11 subtests of the WAIS-R. The results showed that there were no differences between urban and rural groups (taken from the WAIS-R standardization sample) on any of the subscales except for the oldest group (ages 55-74). The urban examinees in the oldest group showed significantly better performance than the rural examinees of the same age group on Information, Digit Span, Vocabulary, and Arithmetic. Those authors noted that three of the four subtests (all but Digit Span) measure school-acquired skills. They argued that the educational opportunity differences for this oldest group (raised and educated before World War II) were likely to be the reason for these differences. They also believed that the lack of differences for the younger groups was due to mass media, television, and educational differences after World War II. They state: "Our interpretation of the WAIS-R residence data, therefore, attributes the significant urban superiority, notably on achievement-oriented subtests, to *when* the 55-74-year-olds were raised and not to their age per se" (p. 238, emphasis in original).

Recent Work on the WAIS-R
We recently conducted a study (Williams, Bowman, & Narloch, 1999) comparing two samples of adult cases that completed a Wechsler Adult Intelligence Scale - Revised (WAIS-R) as part of a disability evaluation. The urban sample consisted of 25 cases evaluated in a metropolitan statistical area (U.S. Census Bureau, 1990) of more than 150,000 inhabitants inside the urbanized area, while the rural sample consisted of 23 cases evaluated in a geographically isolated area in a small village of less than 11,000 people. The cases in the urban group all lived within 30 miles of the metropolitan area, while the cases in the rural group all lived within 60 miles of the village (many in

much smaller towns and rural areas). All cases were referred for known or suspected intellectual deficits.

The results of the Williams et al. (1999) study showed that both groups were similar in mean age (41.72 vs. 39.57), gender proportion (17 males/6 females vs. 21 males/4 females), mean years of education (11.08 vs. 11.39), and mean length of disability in months (46.64 vs. 50.74; urban vs. rural, respectively). The mean WAIS-R Full Scale IQ scores did not differ (Urban = 82.44, Rural = 84.00, ns.), nor did the Verbal or Performance IQ scores (Verbal IQ = 83.32 vs. 84.39; Performance IQ = 84.00 vs. 85.65, urban and rural, respectively). There were also no differences found on any of the subtest scores. These results showed that two samples of adults applying for disability did not differ based on whether they lived in a rural or urban setting. Note that both groups had equal levels of education (at least to the extent that can be shown by years of education). Also, the results were consistent with the Kaufman et al. (1988) study that found no differences in WAIS-R performance for this age group.

Research on memory
Two studies (Kagan, Klein, Haith, & Morrison, 1973; Kagan, Klein, Finley, Rogoff, & Nolan, 1979) found that memory functioning was significantly better for urban children than rural children at younger ages (ages 5-7) but not later ages (10-11). These authors suggested that rural children are slower to acquire these skills but schooling may eliminate the group differences. These studies show that rural children may obtain concepts at a later age, but there are no differences by age eleven.

Macoby and Modiano (1969) found that urban children in Mexico were significantly better at abstractions while rural children were significantly better at concrete responses. They argued that these results reflected the skills that were needed in the respective environments. We will further address this issue in the section on interpretations of urban/rural differences.

Wagner (1974) assessed the development of short-term and incidental memory among Mayan children in Yucatan. The results showed that rural children performed more poorly on short-term and incidental memory than urban children, while overall recall improved as a function of number of years of education and not as a function of age. Wagner interpreted the results in terms of the impact of schooling on learning mnemonic strategies (i.e., the rural children had less education than did the urban children and thus did not have as much opportunity to learn mnemonic strategies).

Stevenson, Parker, Wilkinson, Bonnevaux, and Gonzalez (1978) compared 5- and 6-year-old children on memory and other cognitive skills. They showed that rural children performed worse on most tasks except for perceptual learning, and single and double seriation. School children performed better than did the children who were not in school. The authors stated that the results were attributable to the differences in environmental stimulation. The rural children's environments were ranked as having less verbal stimulation and more perceptual stimulation.

Research on language

Studies have shown that the development of language skills for rural children lags behind that of urban children (e.g., Entwistle, 1966). This difference appears to disappear as children receive education. For example, in the Entwistle (1966) study, rural Maryland and Amish groups (both considered to be environmentally deprived in early years) both caught up to the urban children by the sixth grade. These findings appear to be similar to those cited above on memory.

Other cognitive abilities

A small number of studies have examined other cognitive variables. Majeed and Ghosh (1983) conducted two studies comparing college freshmen attending an urban university in India who were raised either in the city since birth or in a rural setting. The first study (45 participants, ages 15-16) found that the students with rural backgrounds showed significantly lower cognitive differentiation on the Witkin's Embedded Figures Test, than did the urban students. These results were interpreted as due to rural settings being more homogeneous and traditional in terms of interpersonal relations and individual functioning. However, the results of their second study indicated that social class was an important variable in cognitive differentiation that may have at least partially accounted for the differences found in their prior study. In this second study, 60 college freshmen from three ethnic groups were broken into high and low socioeconomic status (SES) groups. The results showed a main effect of social class, and no significant effect of ethnicity and no interaction effect upon the Witkin's Embedded Figures Test performance. The higher SES group was significantly higher in cognitive differentiation. Two limitations for the generalizability of these studies are small sample size, and the failure to use other, more commonly used, cognitive measures.

Okonji (1969) showed evidence that college students raised in rural, illiterate homes were significantly more field-dependent than those raised in urban, literate homes (using Witkin's Rod and Frame Test). Tharakan (1987) studied 40 urban and 40 rural Nigerian students (ages 16 - 20) who were matched for educational background and intelligence. As the author predicted, the rural group showed a more field-dependent cognitive style than did the urban group. These two studies may have limited applicability for neuropsychologists due to the limitations in the construct investigated. However, they at least suggest that there may be some differences in the way urban and rural people perceive their environment.

An interesting study was conducted by Taylor, Sternberg, and Partenio (1986) that compared urban and rural children on their performance on the System of Multicultural Pluralistic Assessment (SOMPA). The SOMPA consists of the WISC-R, Bender Gestalt, Weight-by-Height, Physical Dexterity Tasks, adaptive behavior scales, and sociocultural scales (the latter being administered to the child's parent). The urban group performed significantly better on 27 of the 47 measures. The superior performance for the urban children included the Performance IQ, Full Scale IQ, Arithmetic, all WISC-R Performance subtests, and the Bender Gestalt (errors and physical dexterity). There were also significant differences in socioeconomic status and family size. The authors noted that 14 of the 27 variables on which there were group differences require motor or physical performance, suggesting the urban-rural differences are largely performance-oriented. This is similar to the results noted above by Alexopoulos (1997) but it runs counter to our common conception that urban dwellers are superior in verbal and school-related skills. It should be noted that the children in Taylor et al. (1986) ranged in age from 5 – 11. As we noted above, maximum differences in intellectual performance may be seen in children below age eleven.

Normative data on tests

Lezak (1995) addressed the growing awareness of the need for adequate norms, and the concern that many neuropsychological tests have inadequate norms. In addition, there are limited data available on the neuropsychological test performance of rural inhabitants, either for normal or clinical groups.

For example, most tests do not provide a breakdown between urban and rural people in the standardization data in their manuals. For example, the norms used for the Halstead-Reitan Neuropsychological Test Battery are 50 pairs of brain-damaged and non-brain-damaged individuals matched on sex, age, and education (Reitan & Wolfson, 1985). These authors stated that "regional normative differences may exist" (p. 99), but provided no further information. Similarly, the original Luria-Nebraska Neuropsychological Battery was normed on 50 hospitalized normal patients (Golden, Hammeke, & Purisch, 1978).

Lacks (1984) combined, from a number of studies, the normative data on 495 non-patients who completed the Bender Gestalt. Lacks (1984) noted that almost all of the people in their sample were urban, and only about 15% were described as living in a small town or rural area. However, the data were not analyzed separately for urban and rural groups. More recently, Viljoen, Levett, Tredoux, and Anderson (1994) provided normative data on the Bender Gestalt for Zulu-speaking children.

The limited data available on urban/rural samples is of concern, especially since subject characteristics can lead to the biased diagnosis of neurological conditions (Adams, Boake, & Crain, 1982). These authors showed that increased age, low education, and nonmajority ethnicity all led to misclassification of examinees as brain damaged using the Bender Gestalt Test. Similarly, Fox (1994) showed that the standard norms for the Wechsler Memory Scale were inadequate and served to classify worker's compensation cases as having a neuropsychological problem when they did not. Earlier, Prigatano (1978) argued that the Wechsler Memory Scale was poorly standardized (200 normal individuals, ages 25 to 50 from New York City: Wechsler, 1945) and required additional improvement.

The effects of education and age can vary depending upon the test used. Ivnik, Malec, Smith, Tangalos, and Petersen (1996) studied a large sample

(750) of normal older persons (ages 56 to 97). They found that age was most strongly associated with performance on some tests (Stroop, Trail Making Test, and Boston Naming Test), while education level was most strongly associated with performance on other tests (Controlled Oral Word Association Test, Token Test, reading test from the Wide Range Achievement Test – Revised, and the American version of the National Adult Reading Test). These results provide at least partial support for the notion that specific tests are more affected by educational experiences. These data help explain the results discussed earlier by Kaufman et al. (1988) that found that only the oldest group from the WAIS-R standardization sample showed urban/rural differences, presumably because of education differences.

The studies cited point out that we have limited normative data available and that there are problems with using norms that do not take subject characteristics into account. The education and age variables have been shown to be important, but urban/rural test performance norms are lacking. For those readers interested in summarized data on test administration and test norms, see the thorough works of Lezak (1995) and Spreen and Strauss (1991).

Summary of interpretations of urban/rural differences in test performance
Various interpretations of differences between urban and rural test performance have been offered including: (a) cultural or social class differences (Alexopoulos, 1997; Okonji, 1969; Tharakan, 1987); (b) test bias (Taylor et al., 1986); and (c) educational opportunity differences (Alexopoulos, 1997; Majeed & Ghosh, 1983).

The interpretation of poorer educational opportunities has been most often cited in the literature. The assumption has been that people in rural settings have poorer quality schools, have parents who place less value on formal education, and that the rural environment does not offer the same number of educational opportunities such as museums, plays, etc. While this may have intuitive appeal, the data to support this assumption are lacking.

Hollos (1983) argued that the interpretation of urban/rural differences in terms of "deprivation" in rural settings was flawed. Hollos stated that the apparent developmental "lag" of rural children in many studies might have been due to a biased definition of the rural environment, a lack of knowledge about the cognitive skills needed in rural environments, and a lack of relevance of some tests for rural examinees. Hollos' work (reviewed in Hollos, 1983), tested the hypothesis that role-taking during verbal communication (Flavell, 1968), and logical operations on physical objects (e.g., class inclusion, multiplication of classes, multiplication of relations, and conservation) would show differences between urban and rural children. Hollos predicted that rural children would show poorer role-taking but similar logical operations as would urban children. In one study (done in Norway), the results supported this hypothesis: rural children performed as well on the logical operations tasks but not as well on the role-taking tasks as did the urban children.

Importantly, Hollos (1983) did not just assume environmental differences among urban and rural settings, but rather measured differences on such variables as verbal interaction with adults, time spent exploring the physical environment, and time spent playing with peers. Rural children were found to have fewer verbal interactions and spent more time with their mothers than did their more urban peers. These results were replicated in Hungary (Hollos, 1975). Hollos (1983) summarized this line of research and stated that rural environments are not necessarily impoverished, but rather are simply different from urban environments in terms of the type of stimulation children receive and the specific cognitive skills fostered.

Thus, the work by Hollos (1983) shows that differences between urban and rural children are not necessarily due to limited stimulation and less parental emphasis on educational pursuits in rural settings (i.e., deprivation), but rather are due to different environmental factors. This work has significant implications for future studies.

Others have argued that any urban/rural differences found in some studies have been confounded by racial and social differences between the urban and rural samples (Conley, 1973). This latter interpretation was supported by the data from Reschly and Jipson (1976) that did not show urban-rural differences in their uncontaminated samples in terms of ethnicity.

While the literature cited earlier showed mixed results in terms of differences between urban and rural people, there is rather convincing evidence for significant effects of education (e.g., Reynolds et al., 1987; Majeed & Ghosh, 1983). As Kaufman and Doppelt (1976) pointed out, it may be reasonable to assume that the small differences sometimes found between urban and rural individuals may be due to factors other than residence per se (such as education or socioeconomic status).

Summary of findings

As can be seen, much of the work has been done with intelligence scales, while little has been done with neuropsychological tests. Although this state of affairs is a cause for concern, there is some reason to not be alarmed. The Wechsler scales are among the most frequently used test instruments by both psychologists and neuropsychologists (Butler, Retzlaff, & Vanderploeg, 1991; Sullivan & Bowden, 1997). Thus, it is reasonable to assume that the majority of neuropsychological evaluations include these tests.

However, the Wechsler subscales are not statistically independent and measure overlapping intellectual skills. Thus, while this makes them very useful as measures of intelligence, they alone do not provide the information about many of the specific skills and cognitive functions (Silverstein, 1982) that are usually desired in a neuropsychological evaluation.

What we currently know is this: there may be differences in cognitive functioning between urban and rural children, but these differences may not persist after children go to school. It appears that adults in industrial societies may not differ based upon their place of residence.

Mental Health Concerns in Rural Settings

Neuropsychologists in rural or urban settings often evaluate individuals with multiple conditions or diagnoses. We will briefly review the literature on the comparison between urban and rural settings in terms of mental health problems.

Rural residents show higher rates of alcohol abuse/dependence (Blazer et al., 1985), but lower rates of agoraphobia and panic disorder (George, Hughes, & Blazer, 1986), and depression (Crowell, George, Blazer, & Landerman, 1986) than do their urban counterparts. Individuals from rural settings who suffer from severe mental illness show fewer vocational activities, and more severe symptoms than do urban patients (Dottl & Greenley, 1997). A higher proportion of mentally ill in rural settings are older women who are or were married, while a higher proportion of urban counterparts are young, unmarried males (Greenley & Dottl, 1997).

One important impact on rural mental health may be the erratic nature of the rural economy. Rural economies have a tendency to vary between economically stable and unstable conditions in short periods of time. The stress caused by this rapidly changing financial stability can result in an increased need for specialized mental health professionals in these areas (Human & Wasem, 1991). The specific effects of this stress may not be much different for rural residents. For example, Hagen (1987) stated that research has not borne out the assumption that rural youth have unique mental health problems.

While these findings suggest some overall group differences, the applicability for a given examinee may be minimal. Thus, the neuropsychological evaluation of rural people may not vary from that of urban people with regards to the presence of mental illness.

Rural and Urban Availability of Services

Efforts have been made in the past to bring more health care professionals to rural areas (Human & Wasem, 1991). Psychologists to a large extent are concentrated in and around urban areas, mostly due to higher demand. Yet there still exists a demand for psychology professionals in rural areas. Additionally, these professionals may need to be specially trained in dealing with the unique issues that face rural residents. Some authors suggest that psychologists need to study the intricacies of rural life (Murray & Keller, 1991).

Along with this increased need for mental health care in rural areas is the need for these services to be accessible. Many rural areas are plagued with weather conditions that make building, maintenance, and repair costly. This may be a contributing factor to the inaccessibility of mental health care (Murray & Keller, 1991). Elderly rural inhabitants especially can benefit from improved accessibility to health-care. Many elderly people cannot drive or do not have access to transportation to health care facilities. This is an even larger problem in rural areas than in urban (Dibner, 1983).

What is Urban and What is Rural?

The definition of urban and rural geographic locations has varied in the studies cited which makes interpretation more difficult. The definition used in many studies is one based upon the population of a geographic area. One of the U.S. Census Bureau definitions states that an "urban" area consists of a minimum of 2,500 persons, and all areas not defined as urban are considered "rural" areas (U.S. Census Bureau, 1995a). This <2,500 definition has been used in test standardization (e.g., Wechsler, 1981, 1997), and in some of the research studies cited above.

An alternative Census Bureau statistical definition divides areas into Metropolitan and Non-Metropolitan categories (U.S. Census Bureau, 1999). A Metropolitan area consists of a minimum of 50,000 persons. Melton and Hargrove (1987) suggested that Metropolitan and Non-Metropolitan statistical areas may be more easily applied for research, but that definitions based upon census are limited because they are unidimensional (just based upon population numbers) and have no conceptual basis.

Melton (1983) noted that many of the early researchers used the <2,500 definition. Some authors have used other definitions (e.g., rural <2,000 in Alexopoulos, 1997; rural classified by school psychologist, social worker, and school principal in Taylor, Sternberg, & Partenio, 1986; rural defined as 25 or more miles from Tucson in Rechsly and Jipson, 1976). A considerable number of studies do not specifically state their definition of rural or urban.

Statistical definitions based upon population have major limitations (e.g., Hewitt, 1992; Melton & Hargrove, 1987). One limitation is that the numerical cut-off appears to be arbitrary and not based upon any research data. Second, statistical definitions may not be good indicators of a given area's rurality (Melton, 1983). Melton argues that percentages and population numbers do little to assist our understanding of the concepts of rural people and places versus urban people and places. For example, assuming that all places under 2,500 people are the same (e.g., have limited access to information, limited educational opportunities, and are geographically isolated) is incorrect. In addition, statistical definitions do not examine both the negative and the positive effects of living in rural settings (or the negative and positive effects of living in urban settings). For example, the physical isolation of rural areas may result in both increased stress, and stronger familial and societal ties (Melton, 1983). Some authors have suggested that rurality may appear to be an explanatory factor affecting intelligence only as a "proxy variable" for racial and social class differences (e.g., Conley, 1973; Reschly & Jipson, 1976). Others have stated a similar notion in terms of educational differences.

The limitations in the statistical definition suggest that it may be more beneficial for researchers to define rural in terms of a psychological construct. Melton and Hargrove (1987) examined students from five different colleges in the U.S., and asked them about their hometowns. Most of the participants viewed the concept of ruralness and urbanness in terms of population numbers (consistent with the census definition). However, many that perceived their hometowns as rural did not rate themselves as being rural. Thus, this suggests that the ruralness of a person can not be inferred from the ruralness of their environment. This study gives further support to the notion that ruralness may be best viewed in terms of the perceptions and identification of the individual (Melton & Hargrove, 1987).

The studies cited earlier (including Hollos, 1975) show that rural environments are not necessarily impoverished, but rather are simply different from urban environments in terms of the type of stimulation children receive and the specific cognitive skills fostered. Environmental demands may work to accentuate or devaluate specific skills. Demonstrated differences in skills or cognitive abilities would thus be more likely to be based upon environmental factors other than just population. Thus, this further argues for a definition based upon psychological, rather than population factors.

The foregoing shows that there are some good arguments for modifying or expanding our definition of rural. One of the biggest limitations at this time is that people can live in a town of 2,000 and be near a metropolitan area. The impact of living and working near a metropolitan area could certainly lead to a different life experience than living in a small, isolated area. The research on such comparisons is lacking.

It may be that the original definition (population < 2,500) was more appropriate at one time but is no longer. For example, the educational and cultural opportunities available 50 to 70 years ago may have been distinctly different for people in communities of less than 2,500. In this era of mass communication, it is unlikely that such a distinction still holds.

Neuropsychological Practice

Neuropsychological test practice, among other things, involves the interpretation of test-score patterns (e.g., Lezak, 1991). Test-score variability and deviation from normative patterns are both crucial for neuropsychological interpretation (e.g., Ryan & Bohac, 1994). Practicing in rural settings may bring the additional issue of considering the implications of the rural environment. We will examine some of the major issues involved in test interpretation.

Test-score variability
An important principle underlying the concept of ability assessment is individual variability (Laoso, 1977). Some variability is expected and over-inter-

pretation is always a risk. Thus, any interpretation of test-score patterns must take normative variability into account.

Some studies have found that rural children show greater within-group variability on cognitive skills than urban groups do (Entwistle, 1966; Stevenson, Parker, Wilkinson, Bonnevaux, & Gonzalez, 1978). These results suggest that the interpretation of variability in a particular assessment protocol may be different depending upon the residence of the examinee.

However, one of the difficulties for practitioners is that inter-test scatter is often large among normal examinees. For example, Matarazzo, Daniel, Prifitera, and Herman (1988) used WAIS-R subtest score ranges (difference between the highest and lowest scaled scores for each examinee) as a measure of scatter. These authors found that scatter ranged between 2 and 16 points. The average scatter was 4.7 points on Verbal IQ, and 4.7 points on Performance IQ. Importantly, they also found that the average amount of scatter was not related to demographic variables (gender, age, race, and education level), but was positively correlated with IQ level. Individuals with higher IQ scores showed more inter-test scatter.

There are two other issues important in the interpretation of test-score scatter (Silverstein, 1982; Atkinson, 1992). First, there is the issue of regression towards the mean (the probability that if an individual obtains a score on a less than perfectly reliable scale, they would perform closer to the mean if administered multiple, randomly parallel scales). Second, the problem of inflated Type I error rate (e.g., the 11 subtests of the WAIS-R permit 55 comparisons).

Atkinson (1992) provided a method of correcting for Type I error by computing reliability estimates for the difference between a single WAIS-R subtest and the mean of all subtests. Similarly, Silverstein (1982) recommended a comparison between single subtests and their respective Verbal or Performance subtest mean scores. Both approaches attempt to minimize the chances of interpreting differences among subtests as significant when they may be reasonably attributed to chance. The Silverstein (1982) approach may be more practical for practitioners.

Deviation from normative profiles
Recent efforts to improve our ability to compare test scores to normative profiles have shown interesting results. McDermott, Glutting, Jones, and Noonan (1989) found a nine-cluster solution (i.e., nine profiles) for the WAIS-R, using the standardization sample. In their study, only one significant difference in profiles was found between urban and rural people. There was a higher proportion of urban residents in the Above Average Profile With VIQ > PIQ. This shows an interaction effect such that urban residents showed higher verbal ability only if they were above average in intelligence. However, to make this finding even more limited in it's applicability, there was no difference found between urban and rural groups for the most intelligent profile (labeled "High" by McDermott et al., 1989). Thus, the

expectation that urban residents have proportionally higher verbal intelligence received only partial support.

Crockett (1993) conducted another study that examined the McDermott et al. (1989) profiles. In that study, more than 90% of a large clinical sample (consisting of cases with either neurological or psychiatric diagnoses) were found to "fit" into one of the nine McDermott et al. (1989) profile types. Interestingly, although the pattern of performance was similar for these patients and those from the standardization sample in McDermott et al. (1989), the proportion of cases falling into each profile was not the same. The Crockett (1993) sample was over-represented in the lower functioning profiles as would be expected given their clinical status. Thus, this study suggests that there may not necessarily be a unique "impaired" profile pattern of performance for patient samples; but rather, the consequence of disorders may be to produce an increased frequency of patterns in the lower functioning range. Such findings of pattern differences need to be addressed further. For example, it may be that differences between urban and rural populations will show up in pattern analysis more than in analysis of group means.

Deviation from clinical profiles

Test interpretation includes an analysis of patterns (e.g., how do the Vocabulary and Digit Span scores compare?) in comparison to clinical groups. We were unable to find any studies that examined the urban/rural variable for specific clinical groups.

Our field needs a considerable increase in normative data for clinical populations and demographic groups, including urban and rural residents. Future studies replicating the findings mentioned above of increased group variability in rural populations, or of proportional changes from expected groups, would shed light on the urban/rural issue.

Is the Urban/Rural Designation Needed?

Our review of the literature has indicated that early studies showed significant differences between urban and rural children in cognitive performance, but the more recent studies have shown small or no differences. Many of the cognitive performance differences in young children appear to occur in early ages and disappear by age 11. This would suggest that educational opportunities allow rural children to "catch up" with their more urban peers.

In addition, Reynolds et al. (1987) stated that "the impact of mass media and improved educational facilities and opportunities has led to an elimination of any advantage that urban children experienced" (pp. 331-332). Kaufman and Doppelt (1976) made a similar argument a decade earlier.

However, evidence of the factors cited is seldom, if ever, given. Assumptions about improved educational opportunities, while intuitively appealing, need to be addressed empirically. For example, the authors wonder how this proposed improvement in educational opportunities for rural residents relates to data on increasing IQ scores and decreased achievement scores over the years (Flynn, 1984; Murphy & Davidshofer, 1998). A large increase in the numbers of people who take achievement tests could explain the decrease in those scores, but would not explain the increase in IQ scores.

As Reschly and Jipson (1976) pointed out, most of the studies showing urban-rural differences were conducted at a time when the population of the United States was more rural (proportion of 58:42, urban and rural, respectively), while the current proportions have shifted (70:30, urban to rural, respectively). As of the latest census in 1990, about 24.8% of Americans are considered to be rural (U.S. Census Bureau, 1995). Why this change would necessarily bring about fewer differences between urban and rural people is not clear. In fact, it could be argued that we should be finding greater differences in the most recent studies if geographic location, per se, was the causal factor.

Interestingly, although Alexopoulos (1997) found decreasing urban/rural differences, the argument was made that both environmental and genetic factors may be responsible for the differences between urban and rural children. The reasoning goes like this: the intellectually superior leave rural areas in higher proportion than the less intelligent which compounds the differences between urban and rural children. This argument would suggest that there should be increasing differences in intelligence between urban and rural as more people leave rural settings. However, the opposite pattern has been shown rather consistently.

The most compelling interpretation of decreasing differences is that exposure to information (via television, radio, Internet, etc.) reduces or eliminates the differences between urban and rural people. The studies which show that rural children catch up by about age 11, if they are in school, strongly supports the idea that learning and experience are the key factors.

The brief review of the mental health problems of rural people showed that they may not be much different from those of urban people. This, taken together with the findings on cognitive performance, suggests that the urban/rural variable, per se, may not be critical when evaluating rural people and interpreting their test performance. Consideration of educational and vocational background, and other specific factors for each individual should suffice. This of course does not mean that the urban/rural variable is not still a viable one for research or that there are no differences in health care accessibility, etc.

Summary

The current review indicates that some differences in cognitive performance have been shown between urban and rural people on various intellectual tests. In general, earlier studies found rural people to perform worse on intellectual tasks than did urban people. The more recent studies have found urban/rural differences primarily for children under age eleven. We discussed the findings and the major conceptualizations about urban/rural differences. We argued that statistical definitions of rural are too limited and do not correspond to modern society. Defining rural in terms of access to and isolation from information is one alternative. A second alternative is measuring environments in terms of specific characteristics (as suggested by Hollos, 1983). This latter approach would broaden the scientific investigation of environmental factors beyond the urban/rural distinction to include a larger realm of issues that might be relevant for other geographical and cultural comparisons.

We believe that there are some positive implications of the current review. One implication is that the interpretation of the test scores of rural residents can be done as is typical for all examinees, with a focus on individual factors. This review showed that most of the differences (if any) between urban and rural residents are small. The between-group differences (and variability) that have been found between urban and rural people, while sometimes significant in large group studies, do not usually approach even one-half of a standard deviation. The IQ score differences for rural children in the U.S. are typically only a couple of points in the most recent studies.

Therefore, conducting evaluations of rural people with an analysis of test-score variability and comparison to normative groups should be adequate at the present time. The assessment of children under age 11 in rural settings may be an exception. The current limitation in normative data for demographic and clinical group variables holds for both rural and urban people.

A second implication is that the types of disorders seen in rural settings are very similar to those in urban settings. While there are small differences in large group studies that suggest proportional differences in diagnostic groups, the implications for working with a given individual appear to be minor.

A third implication is that researchers have many opportunities to add to our knowledge. The impact of specific environments upon cognitive functioning is just one of the areas which holds promise. Such research could help build upon our basic research on cognitive development, and assist clinicians in understanding individual test performance.

While the current review shows that only minor differences exist between urban and rural people, this may not be the case in all areas of the world (particularly under-developed countries). Countries in which a large percentage of the rural citizens does not receive formal education would likely show test-performance differences.

The lack of normative data for many tests makes the conclusion of minor differences between urban and rural people very tentative. Our field needs a significant increase in research studies that provide normative data before we can make definitive statements about urban and rural performance.

References

Adams, R. L., Boake, C., & Crain, C. (1982). Bias in a neuropsychological test classification related to education, age, and ethnicity. *Journal of Consulting and Clinical Psychology, 50,* 143-145.

Alexopoulos, D. (1979). *Revision and standardization of the WISC-R for the age range 13-15 years in Greece.* Unpublished doctoral dissertation, University of Wales, Great Britain.

Alexopoulos, D. (1997). Urban versus rural residence and IQ. *Psychological Reports, 80,* 851-860.

Atkinson, L. (1992). Mental retardation and the WAIS-R scatter analysis. *Journal of Intellectual Disability Research, 36,* 443-448.

Blazer, D., George, L. K., Landerman, R., Pennybacker, M., Melville, M. L., Woodbury, M., Manton, K. G., Jordan, K., & Locke, B. (1985). Psychiatric disorders: A rural/urban comparison. *Archives of General Psychiatry, 42,* 651-656.

Butler, M., Retzlaff, P., & Vanderploeg, R. (1991). Neuropsychological test usage. *Professional Psychology: Research and Practice, 22,* 510-512.

Conley, R. (1973). *The economics of mental retardation.* Baltimore: Johns Hopkins University Press.

Crockett, D. J. (1993). Cross-validation of WAIS-R prototypical patterns of intellectual functioning using neuropsychological test scores. *Journal of Clinical and Experimental Neuropsychology, 15,* 903-920.

Crowell, B. A., Jr., George, L. K., Blazer, D., & Landerman. R. (1986). Psychosocial risk factors and urban/rural differences in the prevalence of major depression. *British Journal of Psychiatry, 149,* 307-314.

Dibner, A. S. (1983). Is there a psychology of the rural aged? In A. W. Childs & G. B. Melton (Eds.), *Rural psychology* (pp. 95-112). New York: Plenum Press.

Dottl, S. L., & Greenley, J. R. (1997). Rural-urban differences in psychiatric functioning among clients with severe mental illness. *Community Mental Health Journal, 33,* 311-321.

Entwistle, D. R. (1966). Developmental sociolinguistics: A comparative study of four sub-cultural settings. *Sociometry, 29,* 67-84.

Flavell, J. F. (1968). *The development or role-taking and communication skills in children.* New York: Wiley.

Flynn, J. R. (1984). The mean IQ of Americans: Massive gains 1932 to 1978. *Psychological Bulletin, 101,* 29-51.

Fox, D. D. (1994). Normative problems for the Wechsler Memory Scale – Revised Logical Memory Test when used in litigation. *Archives of Clinical Neuropsychology, 9,* 211-214.

George, L. K., Hughes, D. C., & Blazer, D. C. (1986). Urban/rural differences in the prevalence of anxiety disorders. *The American Journal of Social Psychiatry, 1,* 249-258.

Golden, C. J., Hammeke, T. A., & Purisch, A. D. (1978). Diagnostic validity of a standardized neuropsychological battery derived from Luria's neuropsychological tests. *Journal of Consulting and Clinical Psychology, 46,* 1258-1265.

Greenley, J. R., & Dottl, S. L. (1997). Sociodemographic characteristics of severely mentally ill clients in rural and urban counties. *Community Mental Health Journal, 33,* 545-551.

Hagen, B. H. (1987). Rural adolescents and mental health: Growing up in the rural community. *Human Services in the Rural Environment, 11,* 23-28.

Heim, A. W. (1970). *AH4 Group Test of General Intelligence, manual* (rev. ed.). Windsor: NFER-Nelson.

Hewitt, M. (1992). Defining "rural" areas: Impact on health care policy and research. In W. M. Gesler & T. C. Ricketts (Eds.). *Health in rural North America: The geography of health care services and delivery* (pp. 25-54). New Brunswick: Rutgers University Press.

Hollos, M. (1983). Cross-cultural research in psychological development in rural communities. In A. W. Childs & G. B. Melton (Eds.). *Rural psychology* (pp. 45-73). New York: Plenum.

Hollos, M. (1975). Logical operations and role-taking abilities in two cultures: Norway and Hungary, *Child Development, 46,* 639-649.

Human, J., & Wasem, C. (1991). Rural mental health in America. *American Psychologist, 46,* 232-239.

Ivnik, R. J., Malec, J. F., Smith, G. E., Tangalos, E. G., & Petersen, R. C. (1996). Neuropsychological tests' norms above age 55: COWAT, BNT, MAE Token, WRAT-R Reading, AMNART, STROOP, TMT, and JLO. *The Clinical Neuropsychologist, 10,* 262-278.

Kagan, J., Klein, R. E., Finley, G., Rogoff, B., & Nolan, E. (1979). A cross-cultural study of cognitive development. *Monographs of the Society for Research in Child Development, 44* (5).

Kagan, J., Klein, R. E., Haith, M. M., & Morrison, F. J. (1973). Memory and meaning in two cultures. *Child Development, 44,* 221-223.

Kaufman, A. S., & Doppelt, J. E. (1976). Analysis of WISC-R standardization data in terms of stratification variables. *Child Development, 47,* 165-171.

Kaufman, A. S., McLean, J. E., & Reynolds, C. R. (1988). Sex, race, residence, region, and education differences on the 11 WAIS-R subtests. *Journal of Clinical Psychology, 44,* 231-248.

Lacks, P. (1984). *Bender Gestalt Screening for Brain Dysfunction.* New York: Wiley.

Laoso, L. M. (1977). Nonbiased assessment of children's abilities: Historical antecedents and current issues. In T. Oakland (Ed.), *Psychological and educational assessment of minority children* (pp. 1-20), New York: Brunner/Mazel.

Lezak, M. D. (1991). Identifying neuropsychological deficits. In R. G. Lister & H. J. Weingartner (Eds.). *Perspectives on cognitive neuroscience* (pp. 357-367). New York: Oxford University Press.

Lezak, M.D. (1995). *Neuropsychological assessment* (3rd ed.). New York: Oxford University Press.

Macoby, M., & Modiano, N. (1969). Cognitive style in rural and urban Mexico. *Human Development, 12,* 22-33.

Majeed, A., & Ghosh, E. S. K. (1983). Effects of ethnicity, social class, and residential background on cognitive differentiation. *Psychological Studies, 28,* 13-17.

Matarazzo, J. D., Daniel, M. H., Prifitera, A., & Herman, D. O. (1988). Inter-subtest scatter in the WAIS-R standardization sample. *Journal of Clinical Psychology, 44,* 940-950.

Matarazzo, J. D., & Herman, D. O. (1984). Relationship of education and IQ in the WAIS-R standardization sample. *Journal of Consulting and Clinical Psychology, 52,* 631-634.

McDermott, P. A., Jones, J. N., Glutting, J. J., & Noonan, J. V. (1989). Typology and prevailing composition of core profiles in the WAIS-R standardization sample. *Psychological Assessment, 1,* 118-125.

McNemar, Q. (1942). *The revision of the Stanford-Binet scale.* Boston: Houghton-Mifflin.

Melton, G. B. (1983). Ruralness as a psychological construct. In A. W. Childs & G. B. Melton (Eds.). *Rural psychology* (pp. 1-13). New York: Plenum Press.

Melton, G. B., & Hargrove, D. S. (1987). Perceptions of rural and urban communities. *Journal of Rural Community Psychology, 8,* 3-13.

Murphy, K. R., & Davidshofer, C. O. (1998). *Psychological testing: Principles and practice* (4th ed.). Upper Saddle River: Prentice Hall.

Murray, D. & Keller, P. K. (1991). Psychology and rural America: Current status and future directions. *American Psychologist, 46*, 220-231.

Okonji, M. O. (1969). The differential effects if rural and urban upbringing on the development of cognitive styles. *International Journal of Psychology, 4*, 293-305.

Prigatano, G. P. (1978). Wechsler Memory Scale: A selective review of the literature. *Journal of Clinical Psychology, 34*, 816-832.

PsycINFO [Bibliographic Database] (1999). American Psychological Association (Producer). Available: http://www.apa.org/psycinfo/ [Accessed March 1999].

Reitan, R. M., & Wolfson, D. (1985). *The Halstead-Reitan neuropsychological test battery: Theory and clinical interpretation.* Tucson: Neuropsychology Press.

Reschly, D. J., & Jipson, F. J. (1976). Ethnicity, geographic locale, age, sex, and urban-rural residence as variables in the prevalence of mild mental retardation. *American Journal of Mental Deficiency, 81*, 154-161.

Reynolds, C. R., Chastain, R. L., Kaufman, A. S., & McLean, J. E. (1987). Demographic characteristics and IQ among adults: Analysis of the WAIS-R standardization sample as a function of the stratification variables. *Journal of School Psychology, 25*, 323-342.

Ryan, J. J., & Bohac, D. L. (1994). Neurodiagnostic implications of unique profiles of the Wechsler Adult Intelligence Scale – Revised. *Psychological Assessment, 6*, 360-363.

Seashore, H. G., Wesman, A., & Doppelt, J. (1950). The standardization of the Wechsler Intelligence Scale for Children. *Journal of Consulting Psychology, 14*, 99-110.

Silverstein, A. B. (1982). Factor structure of the Wechsler Adult Intelligence Scale – Revised. *Journal of Consulting and Clinical Psychology, 50*, 661-664.

Smiley, W. S. (1910). A comparative study of the results obtained in the elementary branches of graded and rural schools. *The Journal of Educational Psychology, 1*, 538-539.

Spreen, O, & Strauss, E. (1991). *A compendium of neuropsychological tests.* New York: Oxford University Press.

Stevenson, H. W., Parker, T., Wilkinson, A., Bonnevaux, B., & Gonzalez, M. (1978). Schooling, environment, and cognitive development: A cross-cultural study. *Monographs of the Society for Research in Child Development, 43(3)*, 1-92.

Sullivan, K., & Bowden, S. C. (1997). Which tests do neuropsychologists use? *Journal of Clinical Psychology, 53*, 657-661.

Taylor, R. L., Sternberg, L. & Partenio, I. (1986). Performance of urban and rural children on the SOMPA: Preliminary investigation. *Perceptual and Motor Skills, 63*, 1219-1223.

Tharakan, P. N. O. (1987). The effect of rural and urban upbringing on cognitive styles. *Psychological Studies, 32*, 119-122.

U. S. Census Bureau (1995a). *Urban and rural definitions.* Available: http//:www.census.gov/population/censusdata/urdef.txt.

U. S. Census Bureau (1995b). *U. S. Census summary tape file 3C – part 1: Nation and state totals, Metropolitan Statistical Areas (MSA's).* Available: http://www.census.gov/population/censusdata/urpop0090.txt. (Accessed 24 January 1999).

U. S. Census Bureau (1999). *About metropolitan areas.* Available: http//:www.census.gov/population/www/estimates/aboutmetro.html. (Accessed 24 January 1999).

Viljoen, G., Levett, A., Tredoux, C. & Anderson, S. (1994). Using the Bender Gestalt in South Africa: Some normative data for Zulu-speaking children. *South African Journal of Psychology, 24*, 145-151.

Wagenfeld, M. O., Goldsmith, H. F., Stiles, D., & Manderscheid, R. W. (1993). Inpatient mental health services in rural areas: An interregional comparison. *Journal of Rural Community Psychology, 12,* 3-19.

Wagner, D. (1974). The development of short-term and incidental memory: A cross-cultural study. *Child Development, 45,* 389-396.

Wechsler, D. (1945). A standardized memory scale for clinical use. *Journal of Psychology, 19,* 87-95.

Wechsler, D. (1981). *Manual for the Wechsler Adult Intelligence Scale - Revised.* New York: Psychological Corporation.

Wechsler, D. (1997). *Manual for the Wechsler Adult Intelligence Scale-Third Edition.* New York: Psychological Corporation.

Williams, R. W., Bowman, M. L., & Narloch, R. (1999). *Rural versus urban IQ scores of disability applicants.* Poster presented at the meeting of the American Psychological Association, Boston, MA.

Chapter 15

CROSS-CULTURAL NEUROPSYCHOLOGY OF AGING AND DEMENTIA:
AN UPDATE

Nicola Wolfe, Ph.D.
California School of Professional Psychology (CSPP),
Alliant University, Alameda, California

Abstract

This chapter is an update of the field of cross-cultural neuropsychology of aging and dementia. Recent advances in the cross-cultural area have been driven by the surge in demand for neuropsychological instruments for many ethnic/racial groups and for cross-national studies of aging. Recently developed cross-cultural cognitive screening instruments aim to overcome the shortcomings of earlier instruments, specifically their documented education and culture biases. Three newer cross-cultural cognitive screening instruments are briefly described. These are: the Cognitive Abilities Screening Instrument (CASI) (Teng et al., 1994), the Cross-Cultural Cognitive Examination (CCCE) (Glosser et al., 1993) and the Community Screening Instrument for Dementia (CSID) (Hall et al., 1996). Some methods for cross-cultural test construction are reviewed. These include: selection and adaptation of individual test items, item analysis, defining item bias, psychometric methods to reduce bias, specific adaptations to instruments to 'control' for education differences, validity and reliability studies. The chapter concludes with a discussion of future directions in cross-cultural neuropsychology.

Introduction

As the population of the United States ages, and regional demographics change, neuropsychologists have been challenged to adapt to a range of different clinical populations. Cross-cultural approaches to the neuropsychology of aging are in increasing demand for two major applications. First, the ethnic, racial, linguistic, cultural and urban/rural differences within the United States have been posing a need for tools of assessment and research that are appropriate for each of these groups of differing backgrounds. Second, research on aging and dementia has increasingly moved toward epidemiological studies which compare rates and expression of illness across nations, rural versus urban settings, or between ethnic groups with different linguistic, racial or socio-cultural identities.

A Recent Historical Perspective

The need for a cross-cultural approach to neuropsychology has been increasingly recognized over the past few years. In 1992, Matthews' Presidential address to the International Neuropsychological Society (INS) called for increasing the "international" role of the INS (Matthews, 1992, p. 421). In 1993, the first INS symposium on "Cross-cultural Neuropsychology" was held at the annual INS meeting in Galveston, Texas. Interest among professionals was growing and several instruments were already developed specifically designed for cross-cultural use. By 1995, Ardila pointed to the need for a new field called "cross-cultural neuropsychology" He described this as a "critical new direction of research" for the 21st century (Ardila, 1995). There has been a surge in interest in comparative rates of dementing illnesses for example in the U.S. and Asia (Graves et al., 1996; White et al., 1996) or in the U.S. and East African populations (Friedland & Kalaria, 1998). Key to this process is development of standardized diagnostic methods.

Historically, until the past few years, neuropsychologists have generally relied on standard normative data obtained from a cross-section of the American population, and extrapolated to the individual, knowing only limited information about a client's culture and language. With non-English speakers, neuropsychologists relied on simple translation of items, assuming that the test instruments administered in an individual's own language would still yield valid information in spite of the lack of norms based on that client's cultural or linguistic group.

Limitations of Existing Instruments

However, in neuropsychological assessment, as has occurred in the field of educational assessment, many of the existing neuropsychological instruments used to evaluate neuropsychological functioning in the elderly have been demonstrated to have limitations in cross-cultural use. For example, the Mini-Mental State Exam (MMSE), a standard instrument for screening for cognitive decline and dementia, has been reported to be biased by education level (Escobar et al., 1986; Anthony et al., 1982) and culture (Katzman et al., 1988). Gurland et al. (1992) applied a compendium of five widely used screening scales in cross-cultural application. The five scales examined were: CARE Diagnostic (Golden et al., 1983), Kahn-Goldfarb Mental Status Questionnaire (Kahn et al., 1960), Short Portable Mental Status Questionnaire (Pfeiffer, 1975), Blessed Memory Information Concentration (Blessed et al., 1968), Mini-Mental State Exam (MMSE) (Folstein et al., 1975). In application with Black, Hispanic, and White groups they found drastic, conflicting, results for absolute and culturally relative rates of cognitive impairment. They concluded that differences between the scales were mostly due to their varying sensitivities, but that socio-cultural bias also played a role. Education bias has also been reported on many other neuropsychological instruments such as the Wisconsin Card Sort Test (WCST) (Rosselli & Ardila 1993).

Advances in the cross-cultural neuropsychology of aging can be grouped into three general areas.

1. Modification of existing tests: Translation and adaptation of existing instrument for different linguistic and socio-cultural groups.

2. "De- Novo" Tests construction: Construction of totally new tests specifically designed for cross-cultural use using individual items and neuropsychological constructs (including item selection, item analysis, pilot studies, normative studies, validity and reliability studies)

3. Norm development: Developing norms for tests in a wide range of different populations (especially norms for age, education and individual ethnic groups).

Modification of existing tests

In response to the need for cross-cultural neuropsychology, there has been a recent explosion of translations, modification and adaptations of existing instruments for a range of language and ethnic groups, many of these in rural settings. These include Cree (Cree-speaking natives on reserves in Manitoba), Czech, Chamorro (Guam), Chinese (Shanghaiese, Cantonese, Mandarin, Kinmen- a Chinese Islet), Croatian, Danish, Dutch, Finnish, French, German, Spanish, Hindi (India, Pakistan, Bangladesh), Icelandic, Italian, Japanese, Malay in Singapore, South African, Vietnamese and Yoruba (Yoruba-speaking population of Ibadan, Nigeria).

Increasingly, however, emphasis in cross-cultural neuropsychology has been shifting away from emphasis on translation and adaptation (Brislin et al., 1973; Karno et al., 1993), toward test development *de novo*, that is, construction of totally new tests specifically designed for cross-cultural use (Wolfe, 1993).

Three Newer Cross-Cultural Dementia Screening Instruments:

In an attempt to assess elderly and demented subjects with reduced cultural bias, there have been several excellent instruments developed over the past few years. Three of these are briefly described below.

Cognitive Abilities Screening Instrument (CASI) (Teng et al., 1994)

An excellent example of an instrument specifically designed for cross-cultural neuropsychology of the elderly is the CASI (Teng, 1996). Evolved over years of research by Evelyn Teng and colleagues in the area of epidemiology of dementia, the CASI offers tremendous advances in the field. The CASI has increasingly gained attention as a neuropsychological screening instrument for dementia that was designed for cross-cultural use. This instrument offers several advantages and has been applied especially in the international collaborative epidemiological research of dementia between Japan and the U.S. and in China. White et al (1996) used the CASI as the screening assessment instrument in a large-scale epidemiology study of dementia: Honolulu-Asia Aging Study. Briefly described: "The CASI ... provides quantitative assessment on attention, concentration, orientation, short-term memory, long-term memory, language abilities, visual construction, list-generating fluency, abstraction and judgement." Scores of the Mini-Mental State Examination, the Modified Mini-Mental State Test, and the Hasegawa Dementia Screening Scale can also be estimated from subsets of the CASI items. Pilot testing conducted in Japan and in the U.S. has demonstrated its cross-cultural applicability and its usefulness in screening from dementia, in monitoring disease progression and in providing profiles of cognitive impairment. Typical administration time is 15 to 20 minutes. The CASI has a Short Form (4 item) which has been reported to perform comparably to the Mini-Mental State Examination (MMSE) and the 3MS and the Hasegawa Dementia Scale in sensitivity and specificity for detecting dementia in individuals age 51-93 in U.S. vs Japan (Teng et al., 1994). The CASI requires literacy, however, and thus may be less appropriate for populations with little or no formal education.

The Cross-Cultural Cognitive Examination (CCCE) (Glosser et al., 1993)

Filling a niche for use in non-literate populations and particularly useful in rural settings, the CCCE is an instrument similar to the CASI, designed for cross-cultural neuropsychological screening for dementia. The CCCE was also designed for epidemiological applications but specifically evolved out of demand for screening in non-literate populations. Originally constructed for an NIH neuroepidemiologic study of Guam-Parkinsonism-Dementia-Complex, the CCCE offers several unique advantages (Glosser et al., 1993). The CCCE was designed to assess a range of basic cognitive functions over eight domains: attention, language, visuo-spatial, verbal memory, visual memory, recent memory, abstraction, and psychomotor speed. Incorporated in the CCCE is the two-stage method of case identification used in population surveys. Thus, the test includes a five-minute brief screening procedure (designed to be highly *sensitive*), followed by a more extended 20-minute mental status examination (designed to be more *specific* for identifying dementia) intended for individuals who fail the screening portion. In several validation studies in mainland U.S. populations, Chamorro villagers on Guam, and in Japan, language, education and social factors did not significantly compromise the high sensitivity and specificity of the CCCE for identifying cases of dementia (Wolfe et al., 1992; Tanaka et al., 1992; Glosser et al., 1993). Criterion validity of the CCCE with respect to other accepted dementia screening measures was also demonstrated (Glosser et al., 1993). These findings support usefulness of the CCCE in cross-cultural neuroepidemiological research.

Community Screening Instrument for Dementia (CSID) (Hall et al., 1996)

The purpose of the CSID is, like the CCCE, to screen for dementia particularly in epidemiological studies. The CSID has a unique two-part design. One part includes cognitive and risk factors, and the other an interview with a relative about daily functioning and general health of the subject. The inclusion of information on daily functioning has been recommended, for example, by Jorm and Jacomb (1989) as a way to avoid the educational bias in cognitive testing. This approach is particularly useful in adapting a screening instrument to rural settings. The CSID was developed and validated in a study comparing Cree Indians in Manitoba and Manitobans of European extraction (Hall et al. 1993). It has been further applied to study incidence and prevalence of dementia in a cross-cultural study of elderly community-dwelling African-Americans in Indianapolis and Yoruba in Ibadan, Nigeria. In each application, the instrument was adapted for the particular language and cultural setting. Although both the Cree language and Yoruba have written forms, they are predominantly spoken languages, and the subjects tested were largely unable to read or write.

In an interview of approximately 20 minutes, the cognitive items are designed to measure: memory, abstract thinking, judgement, other disturbances of higher cortical function, personality changes and functioning at work and in social relationships. Hall's careful development of the included item selection, adaptation, two independent translations, consensus translations, back-translation, two pilot tests and subsequent revisions, and determination of cut off scores for screening. (Hall et al., 1996, p. 131).

In their study of the CSID (Hall et al., 1996) the screening stage was followed by a detailed diagnosis. Individuals identified as possibly demented based on performance on the CSID then completed a range of other evaluations (CERAD-NB, CAMCOG, CT scans, relative interview, neurological assessment and laboratory tests). Results suggest the sensitivity and specificity of the instrument in both sites combined was 87.0% and 83.1% respectively (Hall et al., 1996).

The three instruments above are among the best brief screening instruments for detecting possible dementia. They are all well applied in the rural setting. But this list is not comprehensive. Tests of specific domains include "The Taussig Cross-Cultural Memory Test" (Taussig et al., 1993) And, instruments relying on particularly on informant sources have also been developed for cross-cultural neuropsychological screening. One recent example of these is the Informant Questionnaire on Cognitive Decline in the Elderly (IQCODE) (Fuh et al., 1995). Valle (1994) has presented a so-called "culture-fair behavioral assessment and intervention model" for *non-cognitive* behaviors. It permits access to cultural data and differentiates influence of socioeconomic status. (Valle, 1994) For more in-depth clinical neuropsychological assessment there is the Spanish and English Neuropsychology Assessment Scale (SENAS) (Mungas, 1996; Mungas et al., 2000). The SENAS has been designed with 12 tests, six verbal and six non-verbal assessments of a range of cognitive domains. Ideally suited for assessment of elderly and demented subjects, it could have broader applications as well (Mungas et al., 2000). This instrument should represent a substantial advance over available methods, as it is specifically designed *de novo* with the cross-cultural application in mind using rigorous item response theory methods.

Some Methods for Constructing New Cross-Cultural Instruments *(de novo)*

Some of the psychometric methods recommended by Mungas to reduce cultural bias are outlined an excellent chapter in "Ethnicity and the dementias", (Mungas in Yeo & Gallagher-Thompson, 1996). Cultural sensitivity of the test developer may not be sufficient. Mungas suggested that one cannot always anticipate bias. Instead he recommended specifically testing for bias. He emphasized the importance of combining knowledge and experience with rigorous empirical methods (Mungas, 1996).

III. Recommendations

Defining "Culturally Equivalent"

Ideally a neuropsychological instrument or item used in cross-cultural application would be "culture fair" or "culturally equivalent". Cultural equivalence might be defined as equivalence of scores across national, cultural boundaries or ethnically non-discriminatory use within a society. Early attempts based on non-verbal test and performance tests (Anastasi, 1988; Cattell, 1940) did not prove to be as "culture fair" as hoped (Anastasi, 1988; Vernon, 1969). Unfortunately, non-verbal testing does not necessarily reduce cultural bias, and many non-verbal abilities (such as the ability to draw in three dimensions) are highly education dependent (Cattell, 1979). Thus, it is probably more realistic to aim for "culturally-reduced tasks" rather than "culturally-loaded tasks".

Documenting population demographics

In cross-cultural applications of neuropsychology it can be particularly helpful to start with a thorough delineation of population demographics. These include the more routinely obtained age, sex, and education information. In addition, to fully describe the socio-cultural context many other variables are relevant. These include size of community (urban versus rural), race, socioeconomic status, occupation, religion and language preference. Demographic information is especially important when attempting to match samples and to compare two cultural groups (Wolfe et al., 1992). Ardila has emphasized the importance of clearly distinguishing education and cultural variables. Differences resulting from education are sometimes attributed to cultural and even ethnic differences (Ardila 1995). Ardila (1995) noted that less educated individuals sometimes perform on neuropsychological tests like some brain-injured subjects. This is called the "Ardila effect". Thus, education should be coded and analyzed rigorously, including years of education, and country of origin which might contribute to a cohort effect (Taussig and Ponton, 1996).

Ethnicity can be difficult to define. Self-report is often relied upon; however, in ethnic minorities variables such as the degree of acculturation and assimilation are difficult to quantify (Sue, 1996). In many cross-cultural applications (for example with immigrant populations) it helps to assess an individual's degree of acculturation and bilingualism. This can be accomplished with the aid of acculturation scales, and by allowing for multiple responses in regional dialects. Multi-site studies help as well (Taussig & Ponton,1996). Measures of acculturation generally include items such as age at immigration, educational history, social class, health care preferences and beliefs.

Translation and back-translation

Several useful translation methods outlined by Brislin (1980) include:
1. Back-translation – a bilingual translator performs independent translation into the original language to ensure original meaning is preserved.
2. Bilingual technique – two groups of bilinguals (one in each language); items which yield discrepant responses can be identified.
3. Committee approach – translation by a committee of bilinguals.
4. Pre-test procedures – field testing to ensure items are well understood (Brislin, 1980).

Careful translation still does not necessarily solve all problems. Standard screening instruments such as the Mini-Mental State Exam (Folstein et al., 1975) have been translated but still require attention to individual items. For example, Katzman et al. (1988) noted that the item which asks individuals to read "CLOSE YOUR EYES" had a death connotation in Shanghai, and was changed to the less offensive "RAISE YOUR ARMS". Adaptation of individual test items must also preserve the same difficulty level. For example, for Digit Span tests, repetition may be easier in languages where each digit is a spoken in single syllable, reducing the time and complexity of the task. Similarly the task of naming the months of the year may be easier in Japan vs the U.S. since names of the months are simply in numerical order (month one, month two etc).

Selection and adaptation of individual test items

Jensen (1980) recommended several general methods in test construction that can help to reduce cultural loading. These include choosing the following: Performance tests, oral instructions, pictorial responses, power tests (instead of speed tests), non-verbal content, abstract reasoning (instead of specific factual knowledge), non-scholastic tasks, and solving novel problems (instead of recall of past-learned information) (Jensen, 1980).

Several general principles for selecting items are suggested below. Items should be understandable and meaningful to all subjects. That is, items should have maximum *ecological validity*. For example, items used in a rural setting should not be based on experiences of city life. Items should be interpretable by other neuropsychologists. Previously normed tests should be used where possible. Items should be able to be scored in an objective fashion. Items should be readily translatable. Items should not be obviously biased in one culture. Items should not require special training that some subjects do not have (for example literacy or mathematical ability). Items should be practical for administration. Items should be as non-threatening as possible. Mungas (1996) suggested making more items than needed in order to have room to eliminate biased items during test development; and including a range of difficulties such that demented subject are able to pass some items and healthy individuals could fail some items.

A key methodological consideration in new test construction is that two versions of an instrument must be match for overall difficulty level. Chapman and Chapman (1973, 1988) note that instruments must be matched according to their psychometric characteristics to reach valid conclusions about the presence of differential deficits in one ability.

Defining item bias

An item can be defined as biased if: "individuals with the same amount of an underlying trait, from different sub-populations, have different probabilities of responding to an item correctly." (Hulin, Drasgow, & Parsons, 1983). The use of item-response theory is described well by Mungas (1996) in his development of the Spanish English Neuropsychological Assessment Scale (SENAS). The item-response approach is well suited to this cross-cultural application because it uses non-linear regression of the probability of passing each item. An item is non-biased if the item curves are equal in two groups. That is, if two individuals of equal ability from different groups have the same expected outcome. The difficulty with using item-response theory in the development of cross-cultural tests is the reliance on large normative sample sizes. While this has been somewhat easier to obtain with multiple-choice tests used in educational assessment, the longer, more complex administration of the neuropsychological batteries makes large samples more difficult to obtain.

Specific adaptations to "control" for education differences

Education clearly affects performance on neuropsychological tests, and differs tremendously between socio-cultural, racial and ethnic groups. Two major methods for management of education effects have been proposed. A neuropsychological instrument could be statistically adjusted for education (Kittner et al., 1986)(using a stratified regression or non-parametric method), or it could be designed to be less sensitive to education effects (Berkman, 1986). These two approaches, however, are not mutually exclusive. The best methods may be those which design instruments to be less sensitive to education effects and also adjust for education level. Investigators differ in opinion, however, on whether to develop items which are not education-biased. Some explain that since underlying abilities (cognitive processes) are education-biased it is not appropriate to eliminate educational effects from instruments.

In order to reduce the cultural bias that is due to more than just educational differences, Mungas (1996) described psychometric methods (for example, the use of ANCOVA) which examine the relationship between scales, or items and variables such as age, education, and language.

Validity and reliability

The principles of test construction, including establishing validity and reliability are particularly important in cross-cultural neuropsychology. New instruments require structured clinical validation protocols (LaRue and Markee, 1995). Studies of criterion validity, comparing the new instrument to some existing "gold standard", are especially important to ensure interpretability of the new instrument in each culture. An example of the design of such a study can be found in Wolfe et al. (1992). Excellent examples of test-retest and inter-rater reliability studies are also available (Hall et al., 1996).

Test administration / training goals

How does one adapt to "culture" that is not static? Training individuals for cross-cultural neuropsychology includes increasing awareness and knowledge of test items' relevance to different cultures, keeping abreast of research related to culturally diverse groups, and achieving some cultural competency greater than only written and spoken language (Hinkle, 1994). Researchers can familiarize themselves with those dimensions of culture most relevant to neuropsychological assessment such as language (dialects and idioms), religions, family structures, recent history, attitudes toward disclosure, non-verbal conventions (such as eye contact and interpersonal distance), and attitudes toward health and disability.

Some suggestions for the administration of cross-cultural instruments (Ardila, 1995)

Testers should speak the same language or dialect as the examinee. They should be familiar with principles of neuropsychological assessment such as: maintaining a non-judgmental attitude, offering encouragement, confidentiality, and explaining the goals of the evaluation. Furthermore, test instructions should not be in a formal language that people do not use themselves and could be misunderstood (Ardila 1995). Testers should be well trained in the instruments to be administered. An example of a sample tester training program is outlined below:

- Select testers (bilingual, educated, motivated),
- Review goals of neuropsychological testing,
- Provide detailed training with a written manual, video and verbatim instructions,
- Encourage testers to practice, provide detailed feedback,
- Evaluate tester competency (e.g. quiz) to qualify the tester, and
- Adapt the instrument and testing methods based on pilot results.

Implementation of some of the recommendations outlined above could help to reduce cultural bias, making neuropsychological assessment more cross-cultural.

Future Directions in Cross-Cultural Neuropsychology

In some regions of the United States, ethnic minorities will soon be the majority of those over 65 years old. Thus, the demand for cross-cultural neuropsychology of aging is urgent. In response to immediate needs, investigators have been working to establish norms and to construct new cross-cultural neuropsychological instruments. The progress described in this chapter represents the first advances in this rapidly emerging field.

References

Ardila, A. (1995). Directions of research in cross-cultural neuropsychology. *Journal of Clinical and Experimental Neuropsychology. 17*, 143-150.

Anastasi, A. (1988). *Psychological testing.* New York: Macmillan.

Anthony, J.S., Le Resche, L., Niaz, U., Vo-Korff, M.R., & Folstein, M.R. (1982). Limits of the "Mini-Mental State" as a screening test for dementia and delirium among hospital patients. *Psychological Medicine, 12*, 397-408.

Berkman, L.F. (1986). The association between educational attainment and mental status examinations, of etiologic significance for senile dementia or not? *Journal of Chronic Disease, 39,* 171-173.

Blessed, G., Tomlinson, B.E., & Roth, M. (1968). The association between qualitative measures of dementia and senile change with cerebral matter of elderly subjects. *British Journal of Psychiatry, 114,* 792-811.

Brislin, R.W. (1980). Translation and content analysis of oral and written materials. In H.C. Triandis, J.W. Berry (Eds.). *Handbook of cross-cultural psychology. Methodology.* Vol. 2. (pp. 389-444). Boston: Allyn and Bacon, Inc.

Brislin, R.W., Lanner, W.J. & Thorndike R.M. (1973). *Cross-cultural research methods.* New York: John Wiley.

Cattell, R.B. (1940). A culture free intelligence test. Part 1. *Journal of Educational Psychology, 31,* 161-179.

Cattell, R.B. (1979). Are culture fair intelligence tests possible and necessary? *Journal of Research and Development in Education, 12,* 3-13.

Chapman, L.S., & Chapman, J.D. (1973). *Disordered thought in schizophrenia.* New York: Appleton-Century-Crofts.

Chapman, L.C., & Chapman, J.C. (1988). Artifactual and genuine relationships of lateral difference scores to overall accuracy in studies of laterality. *Psychological Bulletin, 104,* 127-136.

Escobar, J.I., Burnam, A., Karno, M., Forsythe, A., Landsverk, J., & Golding, J.M. (1986). Use of the Mini-Mental State Examination (MMSE) in a community population of mixed ethnicity. Cultural and linguistic artifacts. *Journal of Nervous and Mental Disease, 174*(10), 607-614.

Folstein, M.F., Folstein, S.E., & McHugh, P.R. (1975). The Mini-Mental State. A practical method of grading the cognitive state of patients for the clinician. *Journal of Psychiatric Research, 12,* 189-198.

Friedland, R.P., & Kalaria R.N.T. (1998). The East African Dementia Project. Establishment of the Nyeri dementia study and training workshops in the clinical neurosciences. *IBRO News, 1,* 3.

Fuh, J.L., Teng, E.L., Lin, K.N., Larson, E.B., Wang S.J., Lui, C. Y., Chou, P., Kuo, B.I., & Lui, H.C.(1995). The Informant Questionnaire on Cognitive Decline in the Elderly (IQCODE) as a screening tool for dementia for a predominantly illiterate Chinese population. *Neurology, 45,* 92-96.

Glosser, G., Wolfe, N., Albert, M.L., Lavine, L., Steele, J.C., Calne, D.B., & Schoenberg, B.S. (1993). Cross-cultural cognitive examination: Validation of a dementia screening instrument for neuroepidemiological research. *Journal of the American Geriatric Society, 41,* 931-939.

Golden, R.R., Teresi, J.A., & Gurland, B.J. (1983). Detection of dementia and depression cases with the Comprehensive Assessment and Referral Evaluation interview schedule. *International Journal of Aging and Human Development, 16,* 242-254.

Gurland, B.J., Wilder, D.E., Cross, T., Teresi, J., & Barrett, V.W. (1992). Screening scales for dementia: Toward reconciliation of conflicting cross-cultural findings. *International Journal of Geriatric Psychiatry, 7,* 105-113.

Graves, A.B., Larsen, E.B., White, L.R., Teng, E.L., & Homma, A. (1994). Opportunities and challenges in international collaborative epidemiologic research of dementia and subtypes. Studies between Japan and the United States. *International Psychogeriatrics, 6*(2), 209-223.

Hall, K.S., Hendrie, H.C., Rodgers, D.D., et al. (1993). The development of a dementia screening interview in two distinct languages. *International Journal of Methods in Psychiatric Research, 3,* 1-28.

Hall, K.S., Ogunniyi, A.O., Hendrie, H.C., Osuntokun, B.O., Hui, S.L., Musick B.S., Rodenberg C.A., Unverzagt F.W., Guerje, O., & Baiyewu, O. (1996). A cross-cultural community based study of dementias: methods and performance of the survey instrument in Indianapolis, U.S.A. and Ibadan, Nigeria. *International Journal of Methods in Psychiatric Research*, 6, 129-142.

Hinkle, J.S. (1994). Practitioners of cross-cultural assessment: A practical guide to information and training. Special Issue: Multicultural assessment. *Measurement and Evaluation in Counseling and Development*, 27, 103-115.

Hulin, C.L., Drasgow, F., & Parsons, C.K. (1983). *Item response theory: Application to psychological measurement*. Homewood: Dow Jones-Irwin.

Jensen, A.R. (1980). *Bias in mental testing*. New York: Free Press.

Jorm, A.F., & Jacomb, P.A. (1989). The informant questionnaire on cognitive decline in the elderly (IQCODE): socio-demographic correlates, reliability, validity and some norms. *Psychological Medicine, 19*, 1015-1022.

Kahn, R. L., Goldfarb, A.I., Pollack M., & Peck, A. (1960.) Brief objective measure for the determination of mental status in the aged. *American Journal of Psychiatry, 117*, 326-328.

Karno, M., Burman, M.A., Escobar, J.I., & Eaton, W.W. (1993). Development of the Spanish-language version of the National Institute of Mental Health diagnostic interview. *Archives of General Psychiatry*, 40, 1183-1188.

Katzman R., Zhang, M., Orang-Ya-Qu, Wang, S., Liu, W.R., Wong, S., Salmon, D.P., & Grant, I. (1988). A Chinese version of the Mini-Mental State Examination: Impact of illiteracy in a Shanghai dementia survey. *Journal of Clinical Epidemiology, 41*, 971-978.

Kittner, S.J., White, L. R., Farmer, M. E., Wolz, M., Kaplan, E., Moes, E., Brody, J.A., & Feinlieb, M. (1986). Methodologic issues in screening for dementia: the problem of education adjustment. *Journal of Chronic Disease, 39*, 163-170.

LaRue, A. (1987). Methodological concerns: Longitudinal studies of dementia. *Alzheimer's Disease and Associated Disorders, 1*, 180-192.

Loewenstein, D.A., Arguelles, T., Arguelles, S., & Linn-Fuentes, P. (1994). Potential cultural bias in the neuropsychological assessment of the older adult. *Journal of Clinical and Experimental Neuropsychology, 16*(4), 623-629.

Matthews, C.G. (1992). Truth in labeling: Are we really an international society? *Journal of Clinical and Experimental Neuropsychology, 14*, 418-426.

Mungas, D. (1996). The process of development of valid and reliable neuropsychological assessment measures for English- and Spanish-speaking elderly persons. In G. Yeo & D. Gallagher-Thompson (Eds.), *Ethnicity and the dementias* (pp. 33-46). Washington, D.C.: Taylor and Francis.

Mungas, D., Reed, B.R., Marshall, S.C., & Gonzalez, H.M. (2000). Development of psychometrically matched English and Spanish language neuropsychological tests for older persons. *Neuropsychology, 14*(2), 209-23

Pfeiffer, E. (1975). A short portable mental status questionnaire for the assessment of organic brain deficit in elderly patients. *Journal of the American Geriatric Society, 22*(10), 433-444.

Rosselli, M., & Ardila, A. (1993). Effects of age, gender and socioeconomic level on the Wisconsin Card Sorting Test. *The Clinical Neuropsychologist, 7*, 145-154.

Sue, S. (1996). Measurement, testing and ethnic bias: Can solutions be found? In G.R. Sodowsky & J.C. Impara (Eds.), *Multicultural Assessment in Counseling and Clinical Psychology* (pp. 7-36). Lincoln: Buros Institute of Mental Measurements.

Tanaka, Y., Miyazaki, M., Sugimoto, K., Yamaguchi, T., & Wolfe, N. (1992). Preliminary validation study of the Mental Status Examination (MSE). *Neurological Medicine* (in Japanese with English Abstract) 36, 1.

Taussig, I.M., Dick, M., Teng, E., & Kempler, D. (1993). *The Taussig Cross-Cultural Memory Test*. (Available from Andrus Gerontology Center, University of Southern California, Los Angeles, CA 90089-0191).

Taussig, I.M., & Ponton, M. (1996). Issues in neuropsychological assessment for Hispanic older adults: Cultural and linguistic factors. In G. Yeo & D. Gallagher-Thompson (Eds.), *Ethnicity and the dementias* (pp.47-58). Washington, D.C.: Taylor and Francis.

Teng, E.L. Hasegawa, K., Homma, A., Imai, Y., Larson, E., Graves, A., Sugimoto, K., Yamaguchi, T., Sasaki, H., Shui E., & White, L.R. (1994). The Cognitive Abilities Screening Instrument (CASI): A practical test for cross-cultural epidemiological studies of dementia. *International Psychogeriatrics*, 6, 45-58.

Teng, E.L. (1996). Cross-cultural testing and the Cognitive Abilities Screening Instrument. In G. Yeo & D. Gallagher-Thompson (Eds.), *Ethnicity and the dementias* (pp. 77-85). Washington, D.C.: Taylor and Francis.

Valle, R. (1994). Culture fair behavioral symptom differential assessment and intervention in dementing illness. *Alzheimer's Disease and Associated Disorders*, 8, Suppl. 3: 21-45.

Vernon, P.E. (1969). *Intelligence and cultural environment*. London: Methuen.

White, L., Petrovitch, H., Ross, G.W., Masaki, K.H., Abbott, R.D., Wergowske, G., Chiu, D., Foley, D.J., Murdaugh, D., & Curb, J.D. (1996). Prevalence of dementia in older Japanese-American men in Hawaii: the Honolulu-Asia Aging Study. *Journal of the American Medical Association*, 276(12), 993-995.

Wolfe, N., Imai, Y., Otani, C., Nagatani, H., Hasegawa, K., Sugimoto, K., Tanaka, Y., Kuroda, Y., Glosser, G., & Albert, M.L. (1992). Criterion validity of the Cross-Cultural Cognitive Examination (CCCE) in Japan. *Journal of Gerontology*, 47(4), 289-291.

Wolfe, N. (1993). Psychometric issues in cross-cultural neuropsychology. *Cross-cultural issues in neuropsychological assessment*. A Symposium held during the Twenty First Annual Meeting of the International Neuropsychological Society, Galveston (Texas, USA) February, 1993.

Yeo, G., & Gallagher-Thompson, D. (Eds.). (1996). *Ethnicity and the dementias*. Washington, D.C.: Taylor and Francis.

Chapter 16

CROSS-CULTURAL NEUROPSYCHOLOGY IN SAUDI ARABIA

Vincent A. Escandell, Ph.D.
King Faisal Specialist Hospital and Research Center, Riyadh, Saudi Arabia

Abstract

Neuropsychology is a method of studying brain functioning by making inferences about brain-related behavior. This chapter will review the culture of Saudi Arabia and its influence on the validity of these inferences. Saudi Arabia is the epitome of the Arabic Culture, due to the Saudi origin of the Arabic language and the Muslim religion. The culture's influence on neuropsychology as a science of deficit measurement will be highlighted through the different meaning of it's demographics and other changes needed to the neuropsychologist's use of a premorbid baseline. Questions about the need for both culture-fair and culture-specific methodology are presented. The emphasis on cross-validation studies is displayed by the actual adaptive methods for language and non-language items being used in Saudi Arabia and other Arabic countries. The problems with translation and other methodologies short of cross validation are addressed in response to the Saudi-Arabic culture and other Arabic cultures. The summeray of these facets of cross-cultural neuropsychology in Saudi Arabia will be the vignettes of actual cases that would be misrepresented by the simple presentation of scores.

Introduction

Neuropsychology makes inferences about the brain and its behavior by studies of their relationship. Suzuki et al. (1996) question the use of cognitive and personality instruments with diverse racial and ethnic populations. They state these tests discriminate by underestimating the potential or overpathologizing the unsampled groups. These studies and their inferences are often specific only to the sampled groups. The samples of behavior and subjects are sterilized by the standardization of the instructions and the apparatus used. The standardization allows statistically reliable inferences but not always ecologically or culturally valid inferences. In Saudi Arabia, the patient may be able to score within the normal range on social judgment tests. However, the Saudi culture requires the patient to conform with the decision of the family's oldest male. The elder's views for treatment may be in conflict with the views of the patient. This chapter will review the culture of Saudi Arabia and its influence on the validity of these inferences.

Saudi Arabia is the epitome of the Arabic culture because it is the birthplace of both the Arabic language and the Muslim religion. The Saudi-Arabian culture's influence on neuropsychology as a science of deficit measurement will be highlighted. Culture influences the different meaning of demographics. The chapter presents adaptations for the data normally used in acquiring a premorbid baseline. Several questions about the need for both culturally fair and culturally specific methodology are answered. The emphasis in adaptation is on cross-validation studies. The actual adaptive methods for language and non-language items being used in Saudi Arabia and other Arabic countries will be displayed. The problems with translation and other methods short of cross-validation, are addressed in response to the Saudi-Arabian culture. The summary of these facets of cross- cultural neuropsychology in Saudi Arabia will be vignettes of actual cases that would be misrepresented by the simple presentation of scores.

In some western cultures, there are personal beliefs that separate an individual from complete conformity with his native culture. In Saudi Arabia, individualism is not accepted. Therefore, the interpretation of Saudi behavior must include an awareness of this culture to which he or she is attempting to conform.

The task of cross-cultural neuropsychology is to identify and differentiate between what is universal, what is culturally variable, and what is unique to the individual (Perez-Arce, 1999). The concept of cross-cultural deficit measurement is the central element of our neuropsychological evaluation. Customary or universal standards, standards that vary by culture, and standards unique to the individual in Saudi Arabia will be the basic format. This concept of deficit measurement will be the axis around which we order the presentation.

Saudi Arabia and the Arab

This paper focuses on Arabic groups or, more specifically, Muslim Saudi-Arabian groups. Hourani (1970) gives a definition that appears to be the consensus of most Arabs. The use of the term Arab may include all people who speak the Arabic language and claim a link with the nomadic tribes of Arabia, whether by descent, affiliation or by appropriating the traditional ideals of human excellence and standards of beauty (Hourani, 1970). Saudi Arabia is the center and origin of the Arabic language, Muslim religion and Islamic values.

Saudi Arabia and the Arabic Language

Arabic is spoken by 130 million people and is the sixth official language of the United Nations. It is ranked as the fourth most widely spoken language in the world (tied with Bengali). Classical Arabic and written Arabic are the same in all Arab countries and used for formal speech, broadcasting, and writing. Because the term Arab is based on the person's language and culture and is not an ethnic origin, there is a great deal of diversity among Arabs (Abudabbeh, 1996). The only country considered Arabic but not dominated by the Arabic language is Iran. Iran's spoken language is Persian (Farsi) and Arabic is integrated into their writings. All other Arabic groups use Arabic as their spoken and written language (Jalali, 1996). An interesting note is the interpretation beyond the simple meaning of a sentence's words or grammar. It is important for the psychologist to realize that it is the grace of the word and the fluency of the expression rather than the logic of the argument and veracity of the statement that count (Khalid, 1976). The Saudi-Arabian language is Arabic. Despite more than 4.6 million residents who are not citizens, the population of over 12 million Saudi-Arabian citizens maintain Arabic as the vibrant dominant language. Literacy is estimated at 62%; with 73% of the men and 48% of the women considered able to read and write (Central Intelligence Agency, 1994).

Saudi Arabia and the Muslim Religion

Although approximately 14 million Arabs follow the Christian faith, or 10% of overall Arab population, and 50% of Lebanon is Christian (Simon, 1996), Christianity remains a minority in all other Arab countries. Muslim is the religion of the vast majority. (Abudabbeh, 1996). Saudi Arabia does not tolerate the practice of any religion except Islam. Saudi Arabs can not belong to another religion without severe adverse cultural effects.

Islam is divided into two major sects, Shiism and Sunnis. This differentiates Shiite Iranians from most of the Muslim world who are Sunnis. Currently, 98% of the Iran's population is Moslem and 93% of these are Shiites. Shiism is an emotional, mystical form of Islam which focuses on a series of martyrs; the twelve divinely designated martyred descendants of the prophet or the Imams (Jalali,1996). The Saudi-Arabian population is mostly Sunni.

Religion and culture enmesh in Saudi Arabia. Sunni is the predominant sect. Islam means absolute submission to God's will in everything. Islamic belief states that Gabriel gave the Prophet Mohamed the Qu'ran in 610 A.D. near Makkah. Islam has five pillars or obligations. The five pillars are a profession of faith, prayer five times a day facing Makkah, almsgiving, fasting, and a pilgrimage to Makkah. The spiritual center of the Islamic world, the Ka'abah, lies in Makkah. Saudi Arabia is a leader in the pursuit of worldwide Islamic solidarity. The Muslim World League and the Organization of Islamic Conference are both headquartered in the Kingdom of Saudi Arabia (Royal Embassy of Saudi Arabia, 2000). Islam is without ordained clergy but an ever-present "mutawah" (religious police) maintains public adherence to Islamic principles. The Sharia is the law of the country. Sharia law is not based on common law or secular principles but is based on ethical Islamic beliefs. The Sharia system of law is the result of a belief that the community is the highest order and individuality has little value. The courts follow the Hanbali sect from the Shaikh Muhammad Bin Abd Al-Wahhab and are considered conservative. This minimizing of individual value must be recognized in establishing consent for treatment, assessment and support for the family that follows the recommendations.

Saudi Arabia and the Arabic Culture

This article will review that which is culturally variable and culturally specific to the Muslim Arabic culture as defined in Saudi Arabia. Saudi Arabia is the Muslim Arabic culture. It is the birthplace of the Arabic language and the birthplace of the Muslim religion that the majority of Arabs use to define their culture.

Saudi-Arabian culture has survived the millennia by its isolation and its rigid view of itself as different from others. Its location, its people and their language define Saudi Arabia. The kingdom presents a range of landscapes dominated by a rocky surface devoid of water and absent of topsoil. The Empty Quarter is the large southeastern region. This is no misnomer. Water, animals, nor people prevail there. A short five- to ten-minute car ride from Riyadh brings you to a rocky arid land more similar to the barren waste of the moon than to land immediately adjacent to a metropolis of 4 million people. The Saudis have found a way to farm, even to export wheat, but all by optimal use of minimal water. The abundance of oil allows a society subsidized for jobs, agriculture, education, power and water. The focus of this culture through religion and customs is the preservation of the family or tribe over any individual aspirations. The history of the extended family and the genogram become increasingly important in order to understand the individual in the Saudi culture. This becomes more relevant as we discuss women later in the chapter. Despite new laws, deeply rooted social customs assert and preserve the domination of the male. That girls should marry early, marriages should be arranged by the family and wives could easily be repudiated are firmly rooted ideas, preserved by women themselves; the mother and the mother-in-law are often pillars of the system (Hourani, 1991). The chief employer, the government, entitles the indigenous people to free services, including health care. This chief employer produces a culture dependent on the larger extended family. This extension of the family culture encompasses the Royal Family and the father of this extended family is the king. In the newspapers, the King of Saudi Arabia is always identified as Custodian of the Two Holy Mosques King Fahad.This is a macrocosm of the immediate family.

Neuropsychology

Neuropsychology focuses on brain-behavior relationships. Lezak (1995) posited American neuropsychology evolved mainly from psychology with its rich operational/statistical techniques for defining constructs and assigning diagnosis based on actuarial bases. Conclusions are from scores obtained from highly standardized testing procedures. She conceptualized behavior as cognitive, emotional, and executive. We will attempt to review all these constructs of the brain-behavior relationship.

The concept of deficit measurement is the central element of neuropsychological evaluation. Customary or universal standards, standards that vary by culture, and standards unique to the individual in Saudi Arabia will be the basic format. Examples of the culture's influence on neuropsychological assessment will allow new methods for measurement. In agreement with Friedman and Clayton (1996), it is necessary to validate measurements with diverse populations. The use of specific normative data to fit the client will enhance the inferences we use as our special identity. In the meantime it will be necessary to use a wide spectrum of cognitive, emotional, and executive measures to ensure a consistency in the pattern we use as the base to make these inferences. These measures are either specific to a culture or culture-free. The latter part of the chapter will place these circumstances within the context of actual patients in Saudi Arabia.

Saudi Arabian Demographics

For success in diagnostic normative testing, the subject examined must be the "best fit" between the subject's demographic profile and the demographic profile of the sample to which he is compared. If the patient is not truly representative of the sample, normative comparison is not advised. To make optimal use of the normative test data, the diagnostician must have an understanding of normal performance on the tests before an opinion regarding the strengths or weaknesses of various neurobehavioral capacities can be offered (Mitrushina, Boone, & D'Elia, 1999).

In a review of clinical and forensic instruments, Gray-Little and Kaplan (1995) state that the use of psychometric instruments reflects the need for sensitivity towards attributes of ethnicity and socioeconomic status. Usually this reflects the need for covariance of race and education or occupation. In Saudi Arabia, these qualities do not differentiate test performance scores. The division of the country by race does not exist in any formal acknowledgement by public or government documents. We are unable to identify the racial divisions for comparative assessment. The Saudis do not claim racial discernment. There is no obvious discernment by color or race. Most divisions are by tribal characteristics. This division is reflected in the surname. Many use their tribal name to represent their political organization or structure. This name can apply to a region but often can describe someone within their family structure. This could be someone who lives between the areas of Egypt and Iraq or farther. The closer the name or ethnic grouping, the closer the suggestion of an ancestor or lineage that goes back to a central family on the Arabian peninsula. The name identifies a marriage candidate or an ally. The preferred marriage is to a first cousin. The father is the undisputed head of a family and the eldest male is the authority of his extended family. No family member publicly questions the male head of the family. The father's role is to keep the family cohesive, to resolve conflicts, provide material support and social support for the members of his family, extended family, and tribe. This line of authority gives power to the tribal names and their influence. The family members use each other in relation to their status to communicate problems with outsiders. This leads to indirect communication but allows a reduction of conflict. Many westerners expect their Arabic counterparts to express concerns openly and are alarmed when other third parties are introduced into the fray. A westerner identifies himself and his private or public boundaries as separate from his enemy or his friend. An Arab will see his friend as identified and intimately connected with himself. There are few boundaries between family and friends and the patient. The patient polarizes any contact as friend or enemy. Friends are an integral part of the Arabic patient's resources, inasmuch as a westerner will see his immediate family. No patient is ever seen in outpatient or inpatient setting without the physical presence of one or more family members. Saudi-Arabian hospitals give family members beds, meals, airline tickets and other amenities while they stay with the identified patient. These additional extended relationships make the socioeconomic lines more specific to the name and family. This requires an assessment of the family and allied resources, not just the individual patient. This is most important when recommendations are being assessed as to their feasibility within this patient's context.

Premorbid Functioning

A neuropsychologist identifies and monitors deficits in order to describe the behavioral relationships to impaired brain behavior. This deficit measurement is done by assessing the patient's previous scores on that same or a similar measure, against the patient's own behavior and against the normative data from a selected sample.

The use of previous scores for comparison to current performance is near impossible in Saudi Arabia. There are no formal academic achievement or aptitude measures accomplished in the school or other large groups such as done by the school system or the military in the United States. There is a literacy program for the Saudi National Guard but these scores are not available to any practitioner. Except for serial assessment in the clinic or hospital setting, any form of direct comparison of two scores is not available.

Neuropsychologists in the United States use premorbid measures based on demographic data in order to make comparisons for diagnosis within the deficit measurement formula. Demographic formulae give an IQ score. This IQ score provides a benchmark to compare the current cognitive performance. Any difference is the deficit measurement. The most commonly used demographic characteristics are age, sex, race, and education (Wilson, Rosenbaum, Brown, Rourke, & Whitman, 1978; Barona, Reynolds, & Chastain, 1984). The variables for geographic region (urban/rural) and occupation are used in creating an index of premorbid intelligence. These characteristics are compromised in this area of the world.

The use of age, a subject-specific variable, is known to influence neuropsychological results (Cimino, 2000; Heaton, Grant, & Matthews, 1986). Most neuropsychological measures have specific normative data for different age groups (Heaton et al., 1991). In Saudi Arabia, age and birthdays are not recognized or kept within the family history. The family can give an approximation of the patient's age. This age approximation was inconsistent for greater than one half of all the elderly, those more than 55 years of age. When the family gave the patient's age they differed by as much as twenty years. The patient and the family rarely agree as to the patient's age. Often neither the patient nor his family's report of his age is the same as the age stated in the hospital chart. This is more of a problem when working with children. The family usually states the child's age with some confidence within a two-year range. All cognitive tests of development use specific age norms to produce a score for inference. Sometimes the age norms are specific to years, months or even days in determining the age of the child. The Wechsler is the most translated and widely given test in this region and yet this approximate age of the patient is the basis for all scoring. Developmental ages on the Visual Motor Integration test, the Raven's Progressive Matrices and other language age scores and cognitive index scores are influenced by these data. When inferences or results are dictated, qualifiers must be stated.Therefore a higher standard of error and greater disclaimers are necessary in the body of the report. A review of the chart for children often will give a beginning service date. This approximation of age by the initial attending doctor is a good starting point to estabish a premorbid index. In the premorbid formula more than one estimation may be necessary. A use of the extremes of the age ranges presented by the chart or family is helpful as input into the premorbid formula.

Education and occupation are not highly correlated with intellectual assessment as they are in the West. Therefore, their use as an indicator of premorbid level of functioning needs qualification. The formulation of pre-morbid scores based on years of education is minimally effective as Saudi students may complete primary school grades and high school grades many times. The grades completed do not always reflect the ability of the student or his academic achievement. A large percentage of patients who are seventeen to twenty one are still in high school. An even larger group is not allowed to stay in school due to seizures or other physical disorders. Consequently, this group does not complete grammar school despite average intellectual performance on aptitude tests. Therefore, intellectual abilities do not have the same correlation to education or the number of academic years completed as they would in the United States or western Europe.

Occupation is highly correlated to the status of the patient's family or the trade of the patient's father. The son will often follow into the business of the father. Most of the nomads and rural people are in the same trade as their father. The mother and daughter are predominantly homemakers. There is a growing number of women working, especially in the professional domain. These data are skewed and suggest a higher premorbid point value for those who work outside the home than the point value used in the West.

A better correlation is present between IQ and a literacy test. Axelrod, Vanderploeg, and Schinka (1999) review the use of ability tests and demo-graphic data for a more complete estimation of the patient's prior ability. Reading tests, simple written story of the patient's choosing, or the patient's success in reading the local paper provide literacy normative data for comparison. An inherent problem is that adding psychometric tasks to formulate premorbid skills is counter to the idea of establishing premorbid skill level from demographic data alone. If psychometric achievement tests are used then there is a direct measure of the current skill level. This removes the need to predict intellectual functioning by demographic data or any other indirect data. However, if the patient is currently unconscious or unable to complete the cognitive assessment then the indirect valid premorbid measurement with demographic data may be helpful.

Culture-Fair and Culture-Specific Instruments

Culture-fair instruments are preferred when demographics are dissimilar to the normative database used to assess the patient. Culture-specific instruments are appropriate when the demographics are similar to the normative database used to assess the patient. Culture-fair instruments are often non-verbal, devoid of cultural context cues and emphasize problem-solving flexibility in thought and response. Culture-specific instruments are both verbal or non-verbal, are with context cues throughout, and emphasize repetitive episodic or rote learning.

The use of simple words does not always result in a shorter test. Arabic colors and numbers are at least two syllables. This initially changed the use of these tests on the color naming test and the digit span test. The tasks give the same normative data. These tasks are so familiar they are essentially automatic statements. The length of the utterance and simplified language did not change any scores from the traditional scores on simple activities of daily living scales. For discourse competence and strategic competence, measures requiring activities of daily living scales were effective.

Adjustment Scores

Cross-validation studies show mixed results for use of adjustment scores. Some previous psychological systems attempt to adjust scores on a non-linguistic basis. With much publicity and with many national workshops, Mercer (1979) and the Psychological Corporation introduced The System of Multicultural Pluralistic Assessment. In this system, a child's score on the Wechsler Intelligence Scale for Children is converted to Estimated Learning Potential on the basis of acculturation and other sociocultural variables. This adjusted score does not demonstrate a statistically better measure of intelligence in children whose language is in the minority (Figueroa & Sassenrath, 1989).

In a review of dementia-screening measures, the Mini-Mental Status Exam (MMSE) was often translated or adapted with arbitrary methods. More explicitly stated, the test was used with changes in words and procedures without a new normative database. As with previous attempts, simple translation does not account for cultural factors in the test questions or the subjects responses in Saudi Arabia. The western MMSE scores are inadequate due to the high illiteracy rates in Saudi Arabia. To increase the test's sensitivity to dementia, the author added two tests. One was culturally specific and one was culture-fair. The Clock test and the Kings Test increased the sensitivity with illiterate patients.

The Kings Test is culture-specific and able to differentiate memory disorders for dementia without respect to education and age for only Saudi-Arabian groups. The Kings Test is similar to the Presidents Test by Roberts, Hamsher, Bayless, and Lee (1990). The Kings Test requires the subject to freely recall, verbally name and verbally sequence the names of the kings of Saudi Arabia. After naming them verbally the subject visually identifies and visually orders the sequence of the pictures of the kings of Saudi Arabia.

The five kings of Saudi Arabia are prominently displayed throughout the kingdom. Saudi children must learn these facts in school. Anyone who lives in this country also learns these facts. The score on this test identifies quite clearly if the subject is from Saudi Arabia or has lived in Saudi Arabia for greater than six years and has become familiar with the cultural norms. This appeared irrespective of language or dialect.

The Clock Test is culture-fair and helps identify global or right-hemisphere disorders independent of literacy, language use and education. This test has six places to draw clocks. Within the first two panels, a circular clock face with appropriate numbers is available. The patient is asked to draw in the clock's hands in the upper visual fields. In each of the bottom four panels the subject is asked to draw in the circles for the clocks, numbers, and the hands for the requested time. The hands requested require adequate visual ability in each of the four visual fields. The Clock Test score with the Kings Test score has differentiated the means ($p > .05$) between 20 patients and 20 controls matched for age with reference to disorders found on imaging studies and decline in adaptive living skills.

In an attempt to find measures that cross cultural boundaries, a cross validation of a dementia screening test in a heterogeneous population was accomplished. Jewish, Russian, Romanian, Moroccan, Polish, Argentinean, and Iraqi elderly illiterates were assessed. The investigator used the Temporal Orientation test, the Controlled Word Association test, and the Benton visual retention test. Ritchie and Hallerman (1989) found 85% sensitivity with the three illiterate groups (Russian, Jewish, and Romanian) when compared to changes in activity of daily living scales or neurological exam using Riesberg Criteria for classification of dementia. This would be a use of a culture-specific measure, the Controlled Word Association test, and culture-fair measure, the visual retention test.

Salmon completed a multicenter cross-cultural study of dementia. He adapted the Mini-Mental State Examination. He and his colleagues assessed elderly patients in Finland and China. They found that the difference between persons with greater or lesser education was greater than the differences between countries for persons within a similar educational level (Salmon et al, 1989).

Cultural Identification

The Diagnostic and Statistical Manual of Mental Disorders, Fourth Edition (DSM-IV) of the American Psychiatric Association declares the need to identify all patients with information to establish the cultural identity of the individual. They suggest a note to establish the individual ethnic or cultural reference groups. For immigrant and ethnic minorities, they include a separate note regarding the degree of involvement in both the culture of origin and the host culture. It is further recommended to document the patient's language abilities, use and preference (including multilingualism). Terms used in DSM-IV that apply to the local culture include a set of cultural interpretations that ascribe illness to hexing, evil eye, and gin. They will be partially described here and then used in the case studies at the end of the chapter.

1) Hexing, witchcraft, sorcery or the evil influence of another person. Symptoms may include generalized anxiety and gastrointestinal complaints (i.e. nausea, vomiting, diarrhea) weakness, dizziness, the fear of being poisoned and sometimes the fear of being killed.

2) Evil eye. A concept widely found in Mediterranean cultures and elsewhere in the world. Children are especially at risk. Symptoms include fitful sleep, dying without apparent cause, diarrhea, vomiting and fever in a child or infant. Sometimes adults, especially, women have the condition.

3) Zar or Gin. A general term applied in Ethiopia, Somalia, Egypt, Sudan, Iran, and other North African and Middle Eastern societies to the experience of spirits possessing an individual. Persons possessed by a spirit may experience dissociative episodes that may include shouting, laughing, hitting the head against a wall, singing, or weeping. Individuals may show apathy and withdrawal, refuse to eat or carry out daily tasks, or may develop a long-term relationship with the possessing spirit.

4) Locally, such behavior is not considered to be pathological.

Translation

Despite being the most common attempt at cultural intervention, the use of translation may not be effective. Loewenstein, Rupert, Arguelles, and Duara (1995) produced identical English and Spanish versions of the Direct Assessment of Functional Status, a test battery designed to assess the functional capabilities of patients with neurological damage through an extensive process of back translation and translation by committee. When scores on both versions of the battery were correlated with a standard battery of neuropsycholgical tests, different neuropsychological tests predicted different patterns of functional abilities in English- and Spanish-speaking patients. This finding is particularly striking in light of the fact that the Direct Assessment of Functional Status Test has been widely used in the assessment of both English- and Spanish-speaking patients (Loewenstein et al., 1995). Gray-Little and Kaplan (1998) reflect "It is clear that even when great care has been taken to develop linguistically appropriate assessment instruments the ability to base conclusions or make predictions about the performance of a ...group... using other culture norms is not guaranteed."

Escobar et al. (1986) examined the higher prevalence of cognitive impairment using the Mini-Mental Status Exam. They revealed items on orientation, attention and calculation, and speech were affected by language and ethnicity. When these items were removed the scores on registration, recall, following a three-step command, reading, writing and construction between Hispanic and non Hispanic groups did not differ.

As a caveat, Sandoval and Duran (1998) cite Figueroa (1990). These comments are worth repeating as translation is the number one method used to adapt materials in Saudi Arabia,

> "During testing, an interpreter should never have to translate any part of the test being administered. Interpreters should only be used when there is a valid, normed translation of the test or when there are age-appropriate written instructions for a nonverbal test. There should be no problem in administering a test. The interpreter should know how to administer the test. The seating arrangements should be predetermined. And the pattern of communication(s) (who can talk to whom when) should be set up before testing" (p.102).

Timed Tests

Timed tests are observed to be culture-laden as the burden of quick responses is more difficult for patients where the language of the test is different from the language of the subject. Therefore, a lower score may differentiate the difference in speed of language processing rather than the true measure of the task being assessed. In a comparison of the digit symbol task with 30 pre- and post-epilepsy surgery patients, the task in English required significantly more time than the task with the numbers translated into Arabic numbers to Saudi patients with intractable epilepsy ($p < .01$) or tumor.

Culture-fair instruments are the appropriate choice when demographics are dissimilar to the normative data base being used to assess the patient. Culture-specific instruments are appropriate when the demographics are similar to the normative database being used to assess the patient. Culture-fair instruments are often non-verbal, devoid of cultural context cues and emphasize problem-solving flexibility in thought and response. Culture-specific instruments are verbal or non-verbal, with context cues throughout, and emphasize repetitive episodic or rote learning.

The neuropsychologist can make individual comparison standards whenever a psychological trait or function that is normally distributed in the intact adult population is evaluated for change. Species-wide, population or customary norms are the names for these normative studies. This type of comparison is most often used when child development is measured. Also this is a beneficial method for comparison when certain customary norms for all intact adults such as motor speed and other cognitive skills are expected and other group performances for a selected sample are discovered. The assessment of an expected skill level of development helps in the comparison of various genetic diseases that were assumed specific to a single geographic region. An example includes progressive myoclonus epilepsy of the Mediterranean. This genetic disorder has the same characteristics as the Baltic and other regional myoclonus disorders. When the genetic factor is established it can be shown to manifest itself in similar cognitive, motor, and emotional patterns which help reflect the disease as a single entity. They are all subsumed under the Unverricht-Lundborg type. Disease-laden group assessments can reflect genetic disorders that cross beyond the cultural barriers of language or geographic region. Jensen's table (as cited in Sandoval and Duran, 1998) lists culture-reduced or culture-fair measures, including tests which are performance-oriented, pantomime instructions, preliminary practice items, purely pictorial, abstract figural, oral response, answers written on the test, non-language tests, power tests, non-verbal content tests, non-scholastic skills, solving of novel problems, difficulty based on complexity of relation education.

These culture-fair measures may include non-verbal and motor scales where standards of customary development are expected for the species. Ten Saudi patients with progressive myoclonus epilepsy of the Mediterranean variety were similar to other progressive myoclonus disordered patients from the Baltic region, Southern Europe, North Africa, French Canada, the United States, Japan and Iran on measures from the Tinetti scale of balance and gait and the Aims scale for Involuntary movement (Escandell et al., 2000). Therefore, this group of patients who were identified by movement disorder scales appear to be like others (Unverricht- Lundborg) with cystatin B on chromosome 21 deficiency (Engel & Pedley, 1997).

Assessment of Language

There is a growing trend toward a more complex characterization of the construction of language especially as it is manifest in everyday situations. These characterizations build on notions such as communicative competence, communicative language ability and communicative proficiency. Communicative competence is knowledge about the appropriateness of language form. This content and usage reflects an understanding of other immediate purposes of communication. This may include the social and structural characteristics of communicative settings. Traditional language proficiency tests have emphasized the accuracy of language form as the main issue for language assessment. Communicative competence theory raises the importance of assessing the appropriateness of the functional uses of language in sociocultural contexts. Language assessment researchers have proposed that communicative competence encompass four major capacities: grammatical competence, discourse competence, sociolinguistic competence, and strategic competence (Canale and Swain, 1980). In the creation of a normative base for the Arabic-language measures to be used in our intractable epilepsy program, we had to take all of the above into account. A presentation of the changes as applied to neuropsychological language tests follows.

Repetition

The creation of the Arabic Sentence Repetition test revealed a grammar emphasis for success in differentiating impaired patients. This test is based on the methodology of the Multilingual Aphasia Exam (Benton, Hamsher, & Sivan, 1994) and requires examples of the grammatical structure of positive declarative, positive interrogative, imperative, negative declarative, negative interrogative, compound and complex sentences. In the Multilingual Aphasia Exam Sentence Repetition test, the degree of difficulty progresses by increasing the length of the sentence. The simple use of translation did not work as the Arabic grammar reduced the length of some translated sentences and increased the length of others. A local normative base was established. Attached is a copy of the form.

Another sociolinguistic problem requires a culture-specific response. The prefix and suffix and other grammatical changes in the expressions translated increases or decreases the length of the translated expression. This change in length can occur if the speaker is someone of lesser or greater rank, is different in age, or different in gender, or from a different region. This requires the interpreter to become familiar with the test form and the patient's demographics prior to administration. In the instructions, for the repetition of words and sentences, the examiner must inform the subject that the grammar of the test must be repeated even if not correct in that examiner/subject testing context/situation.

Fluency

The use of fluency or word generation tests as exemplified by the Multilingual Aphasia Exam (Benton et al., 1994) is based on the frequency of letters in the language to be measured. In Arabic, this is not possible because male and female verbs are formed by addition of the prefix "aliph "or "teh" . This means every verb can use these letters as a prefix to identify male or female forms. Aliph is also used as a prefix to create collective proper names. For instance, "Al arnab" means all the rabbits. This changes the frequency rates of the letters and changes the rules of the task. The author therefore produced normative data for six letters instead of three. A dictionary frequency established the base rate of expected scores in order to run the pilot. Six letters resulted in an adequate normative base for normal and neurologically impaired patients. In the instructions to the task, subjects cannot use the initial letters "alif" and "teh" for verbs nor alif as a prefix such as in collective nouns. The traditional instructions do not use the proper names for people or places. Normative data for the verbs are also available. This test form is given as an appendix to this article. The resultant letters and their frequency in Arabic are meem (215), alif (199), teh (139), ha (55), ain (50), and waw (17). The frequency is the fraction produced from a total possibility of 1204 units for the language as recorded in the Al-Mawrid Dictionary (Baalbaki & Baalbaki, 1998). This appears to be a very robust task and is highly significant for Arabic left frontal lobe and anterior cerebral disorders.

A fluency problem may demonstrate a deficit in speech, reading and writing. Generally fluency deficits will affect all three activities (Perret's and Taylor's studies as cited in Lezak,1995). Fluency deficits are found in both free and responsive speech (Feyereisen, Verbede-Dewitte, C., and Serron's study as cited in Lezak, 1995). However, with aging writing fluency tends to slow down much earlier than speech fluency, which healthy persons maintain well into the 70s (Benton, 1984). Problems in word generation are prominent among the verbal dysfunctions of dementia. This is a common test administered by neuropsychologists in Saudi Arabia. This measure was found to be sensitive in global and left frontal lobe measures with epilepsy and frontal lobe tumor patients as well as dementia.

Naming

The development of a visual naming test was problematic. In the formation of our test battery, several different items from western tests and their names were found to be unfamiliar to the people of Saudi Arabia regardless of their geographic home or original dialect. Many western tests such as the Boston Naming Test (Kaplan, Goodglass, & Weintraub, 1983) achieved zero correct identifications from the subjects tested ($n = 160$) regardless of education. These items have cultural bias within the Saudi-Arabian sample. The words: pretzel, snail, canoe, beaver, harmonica, stilts, igloo, hammock, pelican, unicorn, accordion, asparagus and tripod were at a zero recognition. A possible acceptance to increase the frequency was "karob " or small boat for canoe and "bet thalj" (icehouse) for igloo. Although on further investigation subjects named the icehouse as a bear (dub) house and therefore, an incorrect response. The small boat is a much larger classification, supraordinate, not unique to a canoe. It would be like accepting ship for a canoe. This remained equivocal. More words were known to urban rather than rural subjects. In other tests such as the Multilingual Aphasia Examination for Visual Naming (Benton, Hamsher, & Sivan,1994), many words were also unfamiliar or difficult to perceive. The piano is not a common musical instrument in Saudi Arabia. The letter, stamp, and postmark are unknown to children as the postal system does not use stamps in the same manner. Postal service does not go to the homes but to the workplace or other central depositories. Therefore, women and children are not actively engaged in this service. Simple words for bed, the initial item of the Boston Naming Test, have different names within Bedu (nomadic) or urban groups. This picture naming list had to be renormed for various internal groups. The author kept the subjects' responses in a bank for different words. We recorded the word's frequency and the subject's home geographic region in order to see if the word was peculiar to a specific geographic region. We are using a shortened form with some success. Morris, Heyman et al., 1989 (as cited in Lezak, 1995) reported the CERAD (the Consortium to Establish a Registry for Alzheimer's Disease) uses only 15 words and is sensitive to the presence and severity of dementia.

Similarities

The similarities subtest of the Wechsler Adult Intelligence Scale – III required minimal changes. The piano was replaced by a guitar-like instrument (orud) and the scores resembled American normative patterns for the items by level of difficulty and posterior cerebral or language sensitivity for deficits. The patient's problems with the poem-statue item revealed the infrequency of statues in their culture. Their religion does not permit the display of statues due to Islamic fears of idol worship. Therefore, we substituted a painting and music item, also used in the Cognistat test (Kiernam, Mueller, Langston, & Van Dyke, 1983). The scores then returned to a familiar pattern for interpretation. The Information and Comprehension subtests of the WAIS-III are culturally biased as expected. Many of the questions have to be adapted and renormed (i.e. the question related to taxes is inappropriate in this culture as there are no taxes in Saudi Arabia). These measures appear to be reliable scores for convergent language. However, the comprehension, picture arrangement, and information subtests are invalid due to cultural influences such as being unfamiliar with the items. Epilepsy patients in Saudi Arabia display problems with the picture arrangement subtest regardless of the site of their lesion. Our answer at this time is to use other types of questions for social judgement. The social judgement test scores of the Cognistat allow greater interpretation.

Vocabulary

A patient's vocabulary performance is the most significant correlate of his general intellectual functioning if there is integrity in the patient's dominant hemisphere. If deficits are found on vocabulary tests the deficits may reflect problems with the patient's brain functioning or the patient's integration into his culture. Education affects vocabulary scores to a greater extent than age and the problems with education-level correlates have been noted previously. Therefore, the adaptation of a vocabulary test is still being developed. We are trying to find words of graded difficulty that are similar to the WAIS-III items. We are having greater success with the multiple-choice items selected by Kaplan, Fein, Morris and Dellis (1991) in the WAIS-R as a neuropsychological instrument.

Early socialization experiences tend to influence vocabulary development even more than educational experiences. Therefore, the vocabulary score is more likely than information or arithmetic to reflect the patient's socioeconomic and cultural origins and less likely to have been affected by academic motivation or achievement (Anastasi, 1988). Vocabulary scores represent the skill level for language usage.

Many words in the vocabulary subtest on the WAIS-III had a partial relationship to Arabic words. The English cognates for "regret" have similar but not identical word meanings to Arabic words such as mercy. The word for epic has two meanings that became confusing to the patient. One meaning referred to a butcher shop while the other was consistent with a heroic story. The problem was to find a word that had a one-to-one correspondence with the target word. As earlier discussed, simple translation is a poor method for cultural adaptation of an item used to interpret brain deficits in a neurosurgical candidate.

Memory Span

While the numbers are simple one-,syllable structures in English they can represent two (whahid, ithnain, arba, hamsa, sita and saba, tisa) and three syllables (tellata, thumana, ashera) in Arabic. We found normative data based on syllables as well. However word length was not statistically different on memory testing from letter or digit span length (n= 30) (Escandell, Al-Semari, Sandridge, & Escandell, 2000).

When creating a memory word list, some of the words in the western tests such as the Wechsler Memory Scale , Rey Complex Figure, and Buschke word lists are not known in the Arabic language/culture. Raccoon, a word unknown in Arabic, was changed to rabbit (arnab) with no apparent harm to the epilepsy patients' pilot study for differentiating memory disorders (n=30). Cultural aspects required changes in the stories for logical memory. The story of Sarah Thompson had to change. Women rarely work outside the home. Any reports to a police station would be done by the highest ranking male in the family, etc. The stories in the Wechsler Memory Scale – III were easier to change and use. Translations and adaptations of the truck driver story and the weather story are being validated by local normative data. The initial results of the pilot study provided similar deficit patterns to those noted on western exams.

Non-Verbal Tests

On non-verbal measures, many tests that do not use language or timed tasks are able to be adapted to the culture. An excellent example is the Continuous Visual Memory Test (CVMT) by Trahan and Larrabee (1988). This measures ability to correctly differentiate non-dominant from dominant memory disorders in 30 patients with intractable epilepsy better than the Faces or Family tests of the Wechsler Memory Scale –III (Escandell et al., 2000). The Faces test and the Family test both have unfamiliar content to the normally face-covered Saudi. The male wears a traditional covering called a gutra and the female has her face covered in public. Adding to the benefit of the task, the CVMT has visual recognition items, delayed visual memory items, and visual items difficult to verbalize. The same applies to the clock test. It is culture-fair, as long as an analog clock is familiar in the culture. Freedman, Leach, Kaplan, Winocur, Schulman, & Dellis (1994) present an encyclopedic review of the clock test. They present comparison tables to the percentage of people with norms for the construction of items as well as norms for various disorders and focal lesion examples.

The Rey Complex Figure task is well received by the patients and the scores are reliable. The scores are consistent in representing right-hemisphere disorders in memory and construction (Escandell et al., 2000). Constructional tasks have done well in correlation with imaging studies. The use of visuo-perceptual tests and perceptual motor tests are consistent in correlation with disease. The belief that desert nomads would do better on these tasks or have a higher base rate on scores in this area did not hold up on initial inspection of a small sample ($n = 8$). Tasks that do not require language have been easily modified and show reliable normative data consistent with anatomical correlates (Escandell et al., 2000). The problems of deficit measurement reflect the need for further validation with normal subjects. The data currently available are with neurologically impaired patients.

Adaptation of Tests from Other Cultures

The acquisition of local normative data stratified by age, sex, education, occupation, and geographic region is the preferred method when hoping to use new instruments that show great sensitivity or selectivity but are from another culture. They must first become effective tests in the new locale. This is similar to new drugs that have great promise but must be tested before use. Local norms give purpose to the measure. Its use for interpretation requires validation on the group that will be interpreted. Many attempts to find significant tests that could short-circuit these methods are problematic as base rates for disease and functional disorders are unknown here. The use of many single-item tests like those presented by Fischer, Luria, Mensulam, Reitan and others (i.e., Aphasia Screening Tests), are at best heuristic devices. However, collecting local normative data takes time, money, and long-range planning. Assistance from the Royal Minister of Health will produce these elements through a national study. Currently simple clinical outpatient and inpatient visits allow the accumulation of this data.

The demographics of the country would suggest a need to have a census in order to apply a sensible stratification of the demographic measures and cognitive measures.

Case Studies

Religion has an impact on many issues including medication use, resuscitation directives, competency criteria, consent for treatment, and the use of images in drawing tests. In consults on the neurosurgical units and the palliative-care unit these issues are more evident. A consult that requests a competency evaluation reflects more about the issues surrounding the patient's cognitive integrity and the family's resources for rehabilitation than the narrow assessment of the patient alone. Women and children do not give consent. The husband, father or oldest brother may give consent or deny interventions by neurosurgery, oncology or any service provider. The western concept of a patient's bill of rights does not exist yet in Saudi Arabia. The hospital that attempts to pass an international accreditation will have to work through the controversy of authority over treatment and how much information the patient should have about the services he or she is to receive. A proposed Bill of Rights similar to western standards has been in committee for over a year, however cultural issues abound. For the neuropsychologist the major concern is the use of tests that may conflict with traditional restrictions on behavior. This includes drawing the human form, removing the abaya (or protective veils) in order to display the female movement and to display facial affect.

Cases exemplifying the cultural issues in Saudi Arabia

A 65-year old male Sharia judge was referred for cognitive evaluation due to memory problems. A female technician was unable to examine a him as he refused to draw figures or follow gestures preceded by pantomine. He was a highly religious man, he felt corrupted by looking at the female technician.

A mutawah was referred because of continued cognitive problems at work after a gamma knife surgery for removal of an aneurysm. He continued to berate a female technician working with him because she did not have her face veiled. As the conversations are in Arabic, the neuropsychologist must pay close attention regarding the differences in the demographics between the examiner (including the technician) and the subject.

When the woman is veiled, making her essentially unobservable, a male family member is required to give the permission for the female to expose her face to the examiner.

The tests of Faces in the Wechsler Memory Scale – III and Facial Recognition in Benton, Hamsher,Varney and Spreen (1983) text procedures and other measures of the human form must be approved by a male family member before being presented to a child or female patient. Almost always the patient and male family member have agreed. They have always noted an appreciation of the courtesy. Any drawing of the human form, such as the drawing of a person on the Draw a House-Tree-Person Test must be cautiously approached with respect for the Islamic religion. Many people initially refuse do the test on religious grounds. All but one have complied when I allow them to draw a line through the item or produce some disfigurement of the drawing that is obvious and does not impair scoring. This allows them to indicate to their god that they are not participating in idol worship. The reliability of projectives, scales of depression and scales of anxiety are about the same as in the West. The Graph Projective Test uses graph paper wherein the patient places a wooden form on an x axis to display the subjective level of physical distress. The patient then moves the wooden form over on a y axis to indicate his or her subjective level of psychological distress. From this resulting placement, additional wooden figures representing other family members are placed on the graph paper. The distance of the family members from the subject is then calculated by counting the squares. This has been effective at seeing support systems and is highly correlated to family adjustment on the Quality of Life in Epilepsy (QOLIE). On this graphic projective technique a similar finding to Schwartz's (2000) presentation of values emerged. During the assessment of controls and in comparing the results of western assessments it was frequently noted that a Saudi's representation of the distance between himself and a friend were much closer than the western location of self to a friend. The actual scores represented the western self-location of his friend as closer to the enemy than to himself.

For patients in a coma or with multisystem failure, the male family member usually demands all heroic efforts including drugs and resuscitation be used regardless of the condition of the patient. They report that to do all that is humanly possible is a religious mandate. The use of the neuropsychologist to assess and measure the impaired level of consciousness or in counseling the family is more appropriate if done as a member of a multidisciplinary team. This will allow information to be presented from many sources and in many methods which improves communication with the family members. When information be given in both Arabic and in English there is an increase in the patient's trust and knowledge so that he can participate in his care.

Quality of Life Assessments

In reviewing Quality of Life scores for 45 male and female epilepsy surgery patients, it was noted that there is a general fatalistic view of their mood state with denial. Enshallah ("with God's will") is the most common expression. The role of mother and wife are the most important roles to the female. The idea of marriage is consuming to female patients. The males presented employment and driving a vehicle as most important functions. Despite this being the high score on scales in personal interviews, marriage was as important. Most patients had adequate insight about their disease and its debilitating role for them. One particular male patient reflected he wanted someone who would love him as he was, and he was willing to give the same in return. This represented a most modern thinking style as most marriages are arranged.

Almost all the patients on our Epilepsy Monitoring Unit have attempted traditional cures. Unfortunately, it is commonly believed that a spirit has possessed the epileptic patient. The term Zar is used in DSM-IV Glossary of Culture-Bound Syndromes. The local name given to the spirits is the gin. Westerners have heard of the word "genie" which is taken from this term. One culturally acceptable intervention is the use of a traditional medicine healer. The healer may burn the patient's body with heated iron brands. He may also strangle or make the patient vomit in order to make the host uncomfortable and thereby forcing the genie to leave the body. We have a skewed sample, but these traditional interventions are not successful with our patients. After undergoing physical pain and mental anguish with no decline in symptoms, the patient is not always happy to meet a new healer. Their trust is usually won by presenting a no-harm policy. Compliance is based on the patients' participation in devising a treatment plan. This means a great deal of patient education with regard to stopping medicine in order to have an increasing number of ward-bound seizures. This is necessary so the patient's seizures may be observed by video and measured by EEG. This allows the staff to observe and measure actual ictal events. Patient information books are written in Arabic and in English so the patient knows in advance what will happen. Further trauma to the patient is avoided.

On the neurosurgical floor, local traditional beliefs sometimes interfere with consultations for pain control or non-compliance. A patient with such a consult presented a history that accounted for his deficits. This young man who denied his family's desire for the marriage to a first cousin "felt" the wrath of the scorned cousin. The cousin told him he would lose the ability to walk if he left her to marry outside the family. He did not heed her warning and planned marrying another woman. The cousin responded by telling him she had cast the "evil eye" on him. As she stated, he began to lose the use of his legs. The neurosurgeons found and removed a tumor from his spinal column. Despite the decompression surgery, he lost the use of his lower extremities. Under relaxation strategies and suggestion, he was able to exhibit leg movement. He believed he was hexed by the evil eye and would not/could not walk since he had refused to marry his cousin. There were no signs of depression or anxiety (sympathetic arousal) on his personality and state measures. The patient was advised to seek traditional healers. This did not bring relief as he still did not marry his cousin.

A wife's fear of divorce is a common complaint. A woman in her late 30s began to have seizures with her pregnancies. She had persevered many assaults from her husband and traditional medicine interventions. Her husband presented her to the Epilepsy Monitoring Unit for intractable epilepsy surgery. She complied because her husband declared he would marry a new wife if she continued to have seizures. The law allows divorce by simple announcement of the husband "I divorce you" three times. The wife must return to her father or brother and receives no compensation beyond her initial dowry. This woman did well on the cognitive power performances. Her anxiety as noted by the QOLIE and her lack of education produced problems to her information-processing speed. Seizures had already compromised her memory performance.

A seizure disorder poses a particular dilemma for women. Women with seizure disorders are destined to remain single. Women marry to escape an eternal childlike dependency on male family members. Once married, the dependence is shifted to her husband. In Saudi Arabia courtship does not exist. By religious law and custom, single men and women do not mix socially. The mutawah regularly patrol public places looking for crowds of mixed company hoping to flesh out couples seen together in public who are not married. Unmarried couples are placed in jail. Families arrange the marriage; therefore, blind love does not cover obstacles like epilepsy. The young girls with epilepsy seen on neurology and neurosurgery wards consider the epilepsy surgery as a means to gain the capacity to marry. Marriage brings with it the status of adulthood. An even greater role for the female is the ability to bear children, particularly male children. Marriage and motherhood bring her great honor and prestige. The questions on quality of life surveys do not relate the intensity of this question to the female.

Arranged marriages are most often between first cousins. An old Arab expression says, "Marrying a strange woman is like drinking water from an earthenware bottle; marriage with a cousin is like a drink from a dish – you are aware of what you drink" (Cuddihy, 1997).

These first-cousin marriages produce a large number of genetic disorders. Within two years we have assessed ten young adults with progressive myoclonus epilepsy, Mediterranean variety. This is a movement disorder with a slow but inexhortable decline in cognitive skills and severe spontaneous or action myoclonus of the extremeties and trunk. This extreme movement disorder makes even the beginning designs of the Block Design subtest of the WAIS-III a very sensitive measure. Other tests, such as Grooved Pegboard, have shown to be too punishing as they produce frustration and despair before completion. On the Block Design subtest, the patient will often drop blocks and attempt compensatory strategies of moving all the blocks with their arm or whole hand like a palmar method of writing. This provides some success. We also use the Tinneti scale wherein the subject is asked to stand up, walk, turn, and tandem walk. This provides a measurement for balance and gait.

The most memorable case involved a mother, daughter-patient and myself. The family was nomadic and presented with henna-painted hands, a strong guttural dialect, and an unsettling distrust. The ritualized greeting gave us leeway to formally assess the daughter. We asked permission to videotape the young woman during the cognitive and motor measures. The patient wore an abaya, a required black robe, a black scarf covering her hair, a black veil covering her face, black gloves and black socks. She resembled an amorphic, black, opaque moving object. We asked for and received permission from the father to allow his daughter to remove her scarf, veil, gloves and socks. The mother shifted the patient's abaya to allow only partial observation of her movement disorder. The Tinneti test is a series of requests for various movements. The patient was asked to move her arms, stand still, walk forward, and produce alternating hand gestures. The mother moved nervously to and from her daughter in order to pull the abaya down for standing and sitting balance tasks. She would adjust the abaya up only so much for observing the feet during tandem walking or heel-shin movements. The face remained covered till we reviewed the extension of the tongue, and movement of oral facial muscles, and alternation of the articulator mechanisms of teeth and lips. This afforded the mother time to keep the patient's face partially covered at all times, unveiling minimally that which was requested to view the facial area being tested and observed. The mother moved in and out inspecting the objects and the neuropsychologist during confrontational naming and other parts of the exam. At the end of the examination the mother and the examiner were fatigued in our attempts to complete the assessment and maintain proper respect for the modesty of this mother's daughter.

In the serial assessment of another young seventeen-year old man with a progressive movement disorder, the accompanying younger brother appeared to be uninterested in the assessment of his older brother. He allowed us to observe and touch and move this patient, as he was a male. No restrictions were given on this patient. The patient demonstrated profound myoclonus. His attempts at walking and even sitting resulted in severe jerks that ended with him falling to the floor despite every caution. To further emphasize the severity of the disorder, while sitting at a desk he displayed an extreme jerking movement that resulted in his head striking the desk with great force. The honorable procedure for the younger brother was to ignore the problems of his older sibling in this public setting.

Children with handicapping conditions are kept out of the school and do not develop social skills nor do they have access to cognitive enrichment afforded more normal appearing children who attend school. Children with hemiplegia, epilepsy or other physically evident disorders were often unable to produce results on naming tasks expected for children their age despite absence of lesions in language areas. They display patterns of social and cultural deprivation.

A young woman of 20 years of age was unable to name animals and common objects reported by children two-thirds her age. This lack of cultural information made her a culturally deprived subject despite the tests being a product of local norms for her region. She had never been presented with this information. She was unfamiliar with objects commonly known to children. Her performance is similar to ghetto children, those who are deprived of cultural enrichment. The children are regularly told not to return to school if they have a seizure in the school setting. As a result, children with seizures rarely finish grade school. Despite their intractability, children with frontal-lobe seizures are often allow to continued school placement as the seizures occur more often at night.

Patients with seizures often feel ashamed. One twenty-year old female with an intractable seizure disorder rarely left her room. She felt embarrassed around the large extended family that occupied their family compound. On several occasions the children had observed her seizures and forever called her names and shunned any intimacy or normal physical contact. Older family members told the children the condition was contagious. Extended families of grandparents, mother, father, their children and the children's husband or wives and their resulting grandchildren all live in the same compound. The compound is a series of houses and wings of the house behind a wall usually about ten feet tall. This omnipresent wall keeps the family private and safe from outside influence. It also apparently brings a high price if someone has a condition considered to cause family shame or embarrassment. This daughter never came down for meals, and remained alone for days. Her coping strategy was to isolate herself and develop a stubborn, passive aggressive stance. On the neuropsychological exam, she scored well in naming and semantics. She showed impaired social judgement and presented as severely depressed even on western scales such as the Zung and the CES depression scale. Her drawings on the House-Tree-Person were shadowed and presented closed with withdrawn postures.

Consults to palliative-care units and neurosurgical units request assessement for cognitive competency and emotional status, interventions for pain control and emotional help with the response to death.

The cultural issues are everpresent here. Conflicts among the physician, family and patient regarding the type of information to impart is stressful for all involved. The focus is to get some type of information passed and to maintain the integrity of the patient/caregiver and medical team relationship. The father, husband, son or brother report they wish to protect the wife or daughter. The dynamics reveal the unwillingness of the male to show distress in front of the female family members. The males find it difficult to acknowledge fear, anger and pain in their male kin. A female patient often finds it difficult to accept the invitation to make personal decisions. She has not made decisions in the past. She has not decided where she will live, with whom she will live, nor has she had control of the money with which she lives. She normally has little or no education and has no input into family matters and no say over herself or her family. The father or husband makes all decisions. Women do not make decisions. It is presumptuous of the medical team to request new behavior when she is fighting a disease and requires the support from all her resources. The consent of treatment is a complex issue. It will require new skills for both the patient and the health-care provider.

The female patient cannot determine or control basic mobility. She is dependent on taxis or male family members for transportation to accomplish her independence.

The physician's desire to disseminate information to the patient often causes a conflict between the patient and the family. The patient may ask for information but the family may veto that request. They report they are providing protection. In Saudi Arabia the family can give consent for treatment or to inhibit treatment including surgery and medication despite the patient's knowledge or agreement. The culture and traditions of Saudi Arabia have a profound influence on neuropsychological care in the Kingdom.

References

Abudabbeh N. (1996). Arab Families. In M. McGoldrick, J. Giordano, & J. Pearce (Eds.), *Ethnicity and family therapy* (pp. 333-346). New York: Guilford Press.

American Psychiatric Association (1994). *Diagnostic and statistical manual of mental disorders* (4th ed.). Washington, D.C.: American Psychiatric Association.

Anastasi, A. (1988). *Psychological testing* (6th ed.) New York: Wiley.

Axelrod, B.N., Vanderploeg, R.D., and Schinka, J.A. (1999). Comparing methods for estimating premorbid intellectual functioning. *Archives of Clinical Neuropsychology, 14*, 341-346.

Baalbaki, M., & Baalbaki, R. (1998). *Al-Mawrid Dictionary. English- Arabic, Arabic-English*. Dar El-Ilm Lilmalayn.

Barona, A., Reynolds C. R., & Chastain R., (1984). A demographically based index of premorbid intelligence for the WAIS-R. *Journal of Consulting and Clinical Psychology, 52,* 855-887..

Benton, A. (1984). Constructional apraxia; An update. *Seminars in Neurology, 4,* 220-222.

Benton, B.L., Hamsher, K. deS., Varney, N.R., & Spreen, O. (1983). *Contributions to neuropsychological assessment.* New York: Oxford University Press.

Benton A., Hamsher, K. deS., & Sivan A. (1994). *Multilingual aphasia examination manual of instructions* (3rd ed.). Iowa City: The University of Iowa, Department of Neurology and Psychology.

Canale, M., & Swain, M. (1980). Theoretical bases of communicative approaches to second-language teaching and testing. *Applied Linguistics, 1,* 1-47.

Central Intelligence Agency (1994). *The World Factbook.* Washington D.C.: The Office of Public and Agency Information.

Cimino, C. (2000). Principles of neuropsychological interpretation. In R. Vanderploeg (ed.), *Clinician's guide to neuropsychological assessment* (2nd ed.) London: Lawrence Erlbaum Associates.

Cuddihy, K. (1997). *Saudi customs and etiquette*. Riyadh: Published by the Author.

Engel, J., & Pedley, T. (Eds.) (1997). *Epilepsy: A comprehensive textbook*. New York: Lippincott Raven.

Escandell, V., Al-Semari, A., Sandridge, A., & Escandell, C. (2000). The amobarbital test, pre/post epilepsy surgery psychometrics and functional reserve/capacity [Abstract]. *International Journal of Psychology, 35,* 423.

Escandell,V., Al-Semari, A., Escandell, C., & Sandridge A. (2000). Neuropsychological measures of Mediterranean progressive myoclonus epilepsy [Abstract]. *International Journal of Psychology, 35,* p.375.

Escobar, J. I., Burnam, M.A., Karno, M., Forsythe, A., Landsverk, J., & Golding, J. A. (1986). Use of the Mini Mental State Examination (MMSE) in a community population of mixed ethnicity. *Journal of Nervous and Mental Disease, 174,* 607-614.

Figueroa, R., & Sassenrath, J.M. (1989). A longitudinal study of the predictive validity of SOMPA. *Psychology in the Schools, 26,* 5-19.

Figueroa, R.A. (1990) Best practices in the assessment of bilingual children. In A Thomas & J.Grimes (Eds.), *Best practices in school psychology*, Vol. 2 (pp. 93-106). Washington, D.C.: National Association of School Psychologists.

Freedman, M.,Leach, L., Kaplan, E., Winocur, G., Shulman, K., & Dellis, D.C., (1994). *Clock drawing: A neuropsychological analysis*. New York: Oxford University Press.

Friedman, C.A., & Clayton, R.J. (1996). Multiculturalism and neuropsychological Assessment. In L.S. Suzuki, P.J.Meller, & J.G. Ponterotto (Eds.), *Handbook of multicultural assessment: Clinical, psychological, and educational applications*. San Francisco: Jossey Bass.

Gray-Little, B., & Kaplan, D. A. (1995). Interpretation of psychological tests in clinical and forensic evaluations.

Heaton, R.K., Grant, I., & Mathews, C. G. (1986). Differences in neuropsychological test performance associated with age, education, and sex. In I. Gtant & K.M. Adams (Eds.), *Neuropsychological assessment of neuropsychiatric disorders* (pp. 100-120), New York: Oxford University Press.

Heaton, R. K., Grant, I., & Matthews, C. (1991). *Comprehensive norms for an expanded Halsead Reitan battery: Demographic corrections, research findings, and clinical applications*. Odessa, FL: Psychological Assessment Resources.

Hourani A. (1970). *Arabic thought in the liberal age 1778-1939*. London: Oxford University Press.

Hourani, A. (1991). *A history of the Arab peoples*. New York: Warner Books.

Jalali B. (1996). Iranian families. In M. McGoldrick, J. Giordano, & J. Pearce (Eds.), *Ethnicity and family therapy* (pp. 347-363). New York: Guilford Press.

Kaplan, E., Fein, D., Morris, R., & Dellis, D. (1991). *WAIS-R as a neuropsychological instrument*. San Antonio: The Psychological Corporation.

Kaplan, E.F., Goodglass, H., & Weintraub S. (1983). *The Boston Naming Test* (2nd ed.). Philadelphia: Lea and Febiger.

Khalid, M. (1976). The sociocultural determinants of Arab diplomacy. In G. N. Atiyeh (Ed.), *The conference on Arab and American cultures* (p. 130). Washington, D.C.: American Enterprise Institue for Public Policy Research.

Kiernam, R.J. , Mueller, J., Langston, J.W., & Van Dyke, C. (1983). The Neurobehavioral Cognitive Status Examination: a brief but differentiated approach to cognitive assessment. *Annals of Internal Medicine, 107*, 481-485, 1987.

Lezak, M. (1995). *Neuropsychological assessment*. New York: Oxford University Press.

Loewenstein, D.A., Rupert, M.P., Arguelles, T., & Duara, R. (1995). Neuropsychological test performance and prediction of functional capacities among Spanish-speaking and English-speaking patients with dementia. *Archives of Clinical Neuropsychology, 10*, 75-78.

Mercer, J.(1979). *The System of Multicultural Pluralistic Assessment: technical manual*. New York: Psychological Corporation.

Mitrushina, M., Boone, K., & D'Elia, L. (1999). *Handbook of normative data for neuropsychological assessment*. Oxford: Oxford University Press.

Perez-Arce P. (1999). The influence of culture on cognition. *Archives of Clinical Neuropsychology, 14*(7), 581-592.

Ritchie, K. & Hallerman, E. (1989). Cross validation of a dementia screening test in a heterogeneous population. *International Journal of Epidemiology, 18*, 717-719.

Roberts, R.J., Hamsher, K. deS., Bayless, J.D., & Lee, G.P. (1990). Presidents test performance in varieties of diffuse and unilateral cerebral disease. *Journal of Clinical and Experimental Neuropsychology, 12*, 195-208.

Royal Embassy of Saudi Arabia (2000). *Saudi Arabia, History and Islam*. Riyadh: Royal Embassy of Saudi Arabia.

Salmon, D.P., Riekkinen, P.J., Katzman, R., Zhang, M., Jin, H., & Yu, E.(1989). Cross-cultural studies of dementia. *Archives of Neurology, 46,* 769-772.

Sandoval, J.& Duran. R.P. (1998). Language. In J. Sandoval, C. Frisby, K. Geisinger, J. Seuneman, & J. Grenier (Eds.), *Test interpretation and diversity.* Washington, D.C.: American Psychological Association.

Schwartz, S. (2000). *Stop the confusion! Conceptual and empirical differences between cultural and individual dimensions of values.* XXVII International Congress of Psychology, Stockholm, Sweden.

Schwartz, S. (2000). National value cultures: Do they underpin democracy or undermine it? [Abstract.] *International Journal of Psychology, 35,* 95.

Simon, L. (1996). Lebanese families. In M. McGoldrick, J. Giordano, & J. Pearce (Eds.), *Ethnicity and family therapy* (pp. 347-363). New York: Guilford Press.

Suzuki, L.S., Meller, P.J., & Ponterotto, J.G. (1996). *Handbook of multicultural assessment: clincal, psychological, and educational applications.* San Francisco: Jossey Bass.

Trahan, D.E., & Larrabee, G.J. (1988). *Continuous Visual Memory Test.* Odessa: Psychological Assessment Resources.

Wilson, R.S., Rosenbaum, G., Brown, G, Rourke, D., & Whitman, D. (1978). An index of pre morbid intelligence. *Journal of Consulting and Clinical Psychology, 46,* 1554-1555.

PART VII

EPILOGUE / FUTURE DIRECTIONS

Chapter 17

NEUROPSYCHOLOGICAL AND PSYCHOLOGICAL ISSUES ASSOCIATED WITH CROSS-CULTURAL AND MINORITY ASSESSMENT

Amir Poreh
Dept. Psychology, Hebrew University, Jerusalem, Israel

Abstract

During the past 20 years, psychologists have become more aware of the importance of cross-cultural and minority variables in psychological assessment. In contrast, neuropsychologists have lagged behind and have only recently begun to examine these issues. The present chapter examines various factors that have contributed to this neglect from a review of the theoretical and research-based literature on these issues. In doing so, the number of psychological and neuropsychological studies addressing cross-cultural and minority issues that have been published in the past two decades are compared. The chapter then examines the various guidelines proposed by clinical psychologists to ramify the neglect of minority issues in assessment and addresses whether and in what manner neuropsychologists can apply such guidelines to their clinical practice. Additionally, suggestions for the integration of cross-cultural and minority issues in neuropsychological assessment brought forth by neuropsychologists themselves are examined. Finally, overall guidelines regarding the evaluation of culturally diverse patients are outlined with an emphasis on ethical issues.

Introduction

Early research on cross-cultural psychology originated from the field of cultural anthropology. Studies in this area emphasized differences in personality temperament and traits (i.e., Boas, 1911). However, most of the work during that era was ethnographic and lacked an empirical emphasis. Whenever personality and intellectual measures were applied they were literally translated into the local dialect or language. The end result is a collection of data that is difficult to interpret and of questionable validity (Freeman, 1983).

The interest of clinical psychologists in cross-cultural assessment first appeared in the early 60s. Torrance (1962) and Gowan and Torrance (1965) appear to have been the first researchers to publish articles on this subject. Their studies were followed by those that emphasized the development of norms for various personality and intellectual measures. However, only in the 1970s did clinicians and researchers attempt to incorporate these studies into a more coherent theoretical context. The end result was the emergence of a new field and a journal that reflected this orientation, the *Journal of Cross-Cultural Psychology*. Noteworthy during that period is the work of Anthony Marsella (see Marsella, 1987, for a review of this topic) on the cross-validation of self-report measures of depression among Asians as opposed to Europeans. Also of importance is the work of Gay and Abrahams (1973) who compared the assessment procedures of African American and Caucasian children.

Lonner (1980) reviewed 347 articles that were published in the *Journal of Cross-Cultural Psychology* between 1970 and 1979. He noted that 662 authors were from the United States and that the next two leading contributing countries were Israel (9%) and Canada (8%). These countries accounted for 52% of the publications. As many as 514 cultural groups were studied during this period. The most frequently studied groups were made up of individuals from the following origins: Canadian and U.S. Caucasian, Eastern or Central African, Indian, Israeli, U.S. Hispanic, Australian, New Zealand Caucasian, and Japanese.

During the 1970s and 80s the proliferation of articles in the field of cross-cultural psychology was mostly in the areas of personality and intellectual assessment. Aside from the work of Logue et al. (1973), who reported cross-cultural differences in symptomatology and organic signs found in Gilles de la Tourette's syndrome, few neuropsychological articles examining diverse populations had been published. This trend appears to have been a reflection of a fundamental lack of interest in this area by neuropsychological researchers.

In order to clarify trends in the literature regarding the importance of cultural background in neuropsychological testing, the author of this chapter conducted a thorough review of the literature. Articles that had been published during the past four decades were surveyed using Psychlit (Silverplatter, 1999). Figures 1 through 3 illustrate the absolute and relative numbers of neuropsychological studies published in this area. One sees that the aforementioned attitude continues to prevail. Namely, there appears to be a general notion within the field of neuropsychology that ethnicity and culture play a limited role in the evaluation of cognitive or physiological functioning (Cuèllar, 1998).

Articles that have been published often reflect major trends of the field during the period of publication. During the 1980s studies focused on the validity and utility of various neuropsychological batteries, reflecting the dominant "fixed battery" approach (Doerr & Storrie, 1982; Xu, Gong, & Matthews, 1987). During the 90s cross-cultural neuropsychological research started to emphasize the more flexible battery approach, focusing on the validity and utility of particular tests (Cuevas & Osterich, 1990; Boivin et al., 1995; Stanczak, Lynch, McNeil, & Brown, 1998). Parallel to these studies, researchers started to focus on cross-cultural differences in the expression of particular disorders (Lee, 1991), the development of culture-free test batteries (Rosselli, 1993), issues of illiteracy (Ardila, Rosselli, & Puente, 1994; Ardila, 1995; Cole & Engestroem, 1997), aging (Crook et al., 1993), memory (Mayfield & Reynolds, 1997), learning disabilities (Duane & Leong, 1985), and issues of self-awareness (Prigatano, Ogano, & Amakusa, 1997).

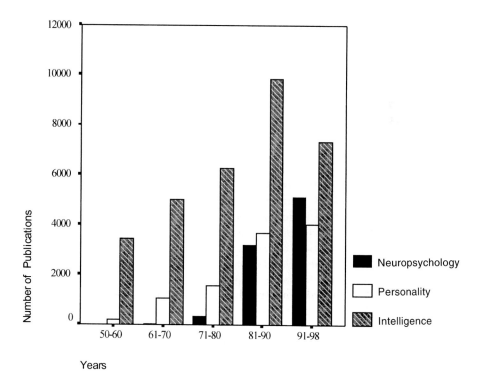

Fig. 1.   Raw number of publications in the past five decades categorized according to major psychological disciplines.

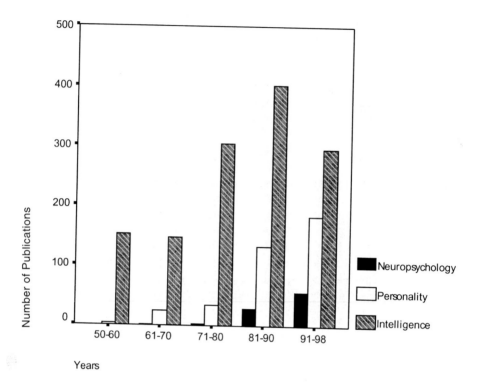

Fig. 2.   Raw number of cross-cultural publications in the past five decades categorized according to major psychological disciplines.

The Pitfalls of Cross-Cultural Neuropsychological Assessment

Cuèllar, Arnold, and González (1996) assessed the role of cultural elements
in the assessment process. Using the Brunswick Lens Model (see Murphy &
Davidshofer, 1994, for a review of the model) they attempted to locate the
sources of error in the diagnosis of intellectual and personality functioning.
The adaptation of this model to neuropsychological assessment is illustrated
in Fig. 4. One sees that the following issues are of importance when conducting neuropsychological assessment of minorities and bilinguals: (a) Illiteracy
significantly affects the validity of neuropsychological testing (Ardila, Rosselli, & Puente, 1994; Ardila, 1995; Cole & Engestroem, 1997); (b) Many
tests that have been translated do not have adequate representative samples
of subcultures within various ethnic subgroups (among Arabic speakers, for
example, Egyptians, Palestinians, and Lebanese each have their own dialect); (c) Scant research has been conducted on bilingualism and its effects on
language-based tests; and (d) Localization of injury as it pertains to language
areas.

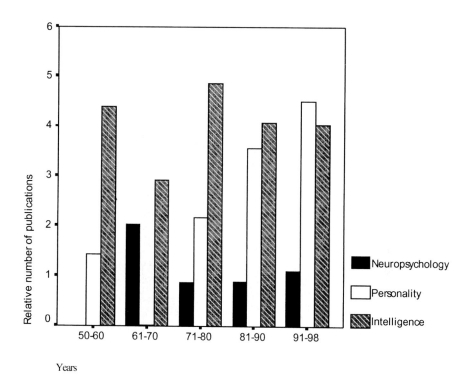

Fig. 3.   Relative number of cross-cultural publications in the past five decades categorized according to major psychological disciplines.

Cuèllar (1998) mentioned several guidelines regarding multicultural
assessment which may also be applied to neuropsychological assessment: (a)
Multicultural assessment does not advocate the deviation from standardized
procedures with ethnic minorities; (b) When "testing the limits" is conducted,
this should be done only after the entire test has been administered under
standard conditions; and (c) Psychologists need to gather information about
the patient's cultural background and motivations. Additional guidelines,
adopted from other sources, suggest the following: (d) Whenever the tests are
unable to control for specific cultural variables such as language or acculturation, one should consider evaluating patients differentially, using measures
that have been specifically adapted and renormed for a given population (see
also Lopez et al., 1989, for a review of this topic); and (e) Attempts should be
made to distinguish between various levels of acculturation (Cuèllar, Arnod,
& Maldonado, 1995). Following Dana (1996), a distinction between four
levels of acculturation is recommended: (a) Traditional, (b) Marginal, (c)
Bicultural, and (d) Assimilation. Using the latter distinctions and standard
scales such as the Acculturation Rating Scale for Mexican Americans (Cuèl-

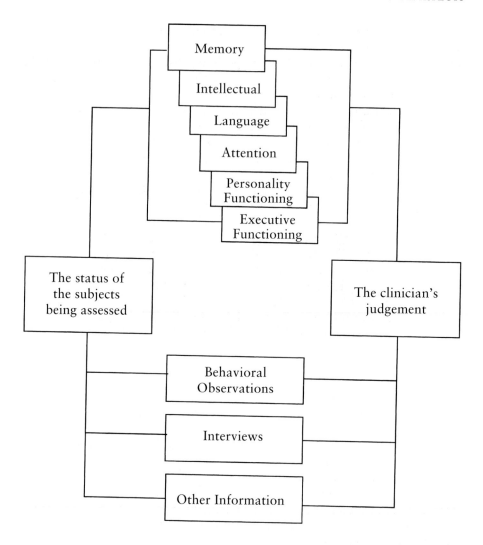

Fig. 4.   Brunswick Lens model applied to cross-cultural neuropsychological assessment.

lar, Harris, & Jasso, 1980), one is more likely to make valid diagnostic decisions regarding neuropsychological test performance (i.e., Manly et al., 1998c).

Service Delivery Guidelines

The wealth of data that has been accumulated in the past two decades regarding the importance of cultural variables on the perception, manifestation of symptoms, and base rates of disorders has led to the development of various service delivery guidelines. The American Psychiatric Association (APA) applied this notion to the DSM-IV specifying four areas that need to be addressed in a psychiatric evaluation (APA, 1994, pp. 843-844): (1) Cultural identification of the individual; (2) Cultural explanations of the individual's illness; (3) Cultural elements of the relationship between the individual and the clinician; and (4) An overall cultural assessment for diagnosis and care. The American Psychological Association (1991) came to similar conclusions. In their publication the importance of gathering socio-ethnic and background information is also emphasized.

To address the latter issue, the concept of "culturally competent assessment" was introduced. This concept attempts to clarify the application of service delivery to multicultural populations. The major components of this practice were illustrated by Dana (1996). These include: (a) Culturally specific styles of service delivery in the first language of the client; (b) An evaluation of cultural orientation; (c) Appropriate assessment methodology and tests; and (d) Guidelines for providing feedback to clients and their significant others.

Beyond the delivery of appropriate services, each clinician brings with her/him an interaction style. While some define the style across ethnic lines, arguing that a unique "Anglo-American" style exists (Dana, 1996), in my opinion, such a classification is a misnomer. Rather, each clinician brings into the setting his/her own clinical experience, which in turn shapes her/his cultural and personal service style (Artiola & Mullaney, 1998). This in mind, neuropsychologists should alter their expectations of individuals from other cultures and adapt their evaluation process accordingly. Various articles addressing the expectations of different cultural groups with regard to medical service delivery are available. These include, for example, the work of Gibbs (1985) among African Americans and the work of LaFromboise and Dixon (1981) among American Indians. Reading and familiarizing oneself with the attitudes and morales of the patients is likely to assist in the assessment process, particularly when evaluating "traditional" or "marginally assimilated" patients.

Assessment Guidelines for Bicultural Individuals

Neuropsychological testing emphasizes standardization and norm-referenced testing. However, it is widely accepted that the validity of such tests becomes weak when assessing individuals of low educational attainment (Ardila, Rosselli, & Puente, 1994). Also, during the past decade separate norms for assessing representative samples of American Hispanics, Asians, and African Americans have been developed (Lowenstein, Argueelles, & Argueelles, 1994). However, a review of the literature indicates that such efforts have been sparse, and the availability of such norms remains elusive. Table 1 summarizes the published norms for Hispanic and African-American persons on various measures. One sees that in many cases such norms were collected as part of research studies, not by the test publishers. As a result, many of the age groups within particular ethnic groups have no norm-based measures. Moreover, a review of the literature shows that norms for Asian Ameri-

Table 1. Articles and manuals that provide norms for common neuropsychological tests for African American and Hispanic Americans

Area of Cognition and Tests	African American	Hispanic American
General Intellectual Ability		
Mini Mental Status Exam	Ripich et al. 1997	Taussig & Ponton 1996
Wechsler Intelligence Test		
(WAIS-III, WISC-III)	–	Psychological Corp.
Achievement Tests		
Wide Range Achievement Test	–	–
Woodcock-Johnson Psycho-educational Battery- Revised	Payette & Clarizio 1994	Prewitt-Diaz & Rievera 1989
Executive Functions		
Design Fluency	–	Delgado et al. 1999
Stroop Test	–	–
Wisconsin Card Sorting	–	Artiola & Mullaney 1998
Attention		
Continuous Performance Test (CPT)		–
Paced Auditory Serial Addition Test	Diehr et al. 1999	Diehr et al. 1999
Symbols Digit Modalities Test	–	–
Memory		
California Verbal Learning Test	–	–
Wechsler Memory Scale – R	Manly et al. 1998b	Demsky et al. 1988
Rey Auditory Verbal Learning Test	Ripich et al. 1997	Ponton et al. 1996
Recognition Memory test	–	–
Language Tests		
Boston Naming Test	Manly et al. 1998b	Kohnert et al. 1998
Controlled Word Association Test	Gladsjo et al. 1999	Manly et al. 1998a
Token Test	Ripich et al. 1997	Psychological Corp.
Multilingual Aphasia Examination	Psychological Corp.	Psychological Corp.
Visual Perceptual Tests		
Hooper Visual Organization Test	Lewis et al. 1997	–
Trail Making Test	Manly et al. 1998b	Rosseli & Ardila 1996
Personality		
Beck Depression Scale	Psychological Corp.	Psychological Corp.
Geriatric Depression Scale	–	Zamanian et al. 1992
MMPI-2	National Computer Service	National Computer Service

cans and American Arabs, for example, are not available at all, although the national census shows that the proportion of these minority groups within the American population is growing.

A more complex issue occurs when assessing bicultural and bilingual individuals. Studies show that areas in the brain are differentially activated by native as opposed to second languages (see Kim, Relkin, Lee, & Hirsch, 1997, for a review of this topic). Additionally, recent studies show that neuropsychological measures that emphasize visual-spatial components do not necessarily produce less bias (Jacobs et al., 1997), perhaps due to the different communication strategies of various cultural groups (Puente et al., 1997; Yeo & Gallagher, 1996). Thus, in such cases, one should carefully distinguish between the various measures that are affected by such variables, and devise algorithms that could be used for corrections. Imagine, for example, an aging Italian immigrant who is referred for an evaluation following a car accident. How may we interpret her paraphasias? Should we test her or him in English or Italian? Studies show that assessing such individuals on separate occasions in each language may produce different results (Cuèllar, 1998).

One solution is to apply neuropsychological measures that were designed to minimize cultural bias. Such measures have been prepared for the WHO cross-cultural study on the neuropsychiatric aspects of HIV-1 infection and have been shown to "hold" sensitivity across different cultures (Maj et al., 1991, 1993). However, this solution has also been criticized. Greenfield (1997), for example, questions the assumption that one can develop ability tests that minimize cultural bias. Cultural variations in epistemology and test-taking attitudes may run contrary to traditions of the standardized assessment. The notion that a particular test may have right and wrong answers is a convention not shared by some cultures. At times, persons of a particular status within a particular culture, such as children, are not expected to express their views or solve problems. Thus, Greenfield argues that it is important to investigate each culture within its own terms, and whenever necessary, vary the particular testing procedures. Even then, she emphasizes, objectivity is not theoretically possible.

Malingering and Cross-Cultural Assessment

According to the APA (1994) malingering is "the intentional production of grossly exaggerated physical or psychological symptoms, motivated by external incentives such as avoiding military duty, avoiding work, obtaining financial compensation, evading criminal prosecution, or obtaining drugs." The techniques for the assessment of such behavior have been reviewed recently by Spreen and Strauss (1998). These authors distinguish between conventional measures, such as self-report inventories, and specific tests that were devised to detect malingering, such as the Portland Digits Recognition Tests.

Currently, the use of malingering tests is considered to be mainstream in forensic neuropsychological testing and has been incorporated into decision-making trees in neuropsychological assessment (Lucas, 1998; Lishman, 1998; Faust, 1996). Thus, whenever one conducts a forensic evaluation, the neuropsychologist needs to rule out motivational factors.

The role of malingering of minorities during forensic evaluations is extremely complicated. Although there are no published studies in this particular area, it is common in clinical practice to encounter cultures in which "making yourself be heard" is the only way to get proper compensation. Such behavior is characteristic of what Dana (1996) would have defined as "traditional" or "marginally assimilated" individuals. Such individuals have often experienced discrimination or have grown up in totalitarian regimes where "honest" behavior is rarely rewarded and the concept of "justice" is a misnomer. Whenever one encounters such patients, particularly immigrants, it is important to assess their behavior within the cultural explanations of their illness, and the interrelationship between the patient and the clinician.

Imagine, for example, an immigrant who falls from a stationary bus. He is transferred to the hospital, where MRI detects bilateral frontal lobe hematomas. He later stops working and divorces his wife. During the neuropsychological evaluation he exhibits difficulties on many measures, as well as on measures of malingering. While it would be foolish to assess the patient's disability level on the basis of his presenting symptoms alone, it would be equally foolish to completely discard his claims.

A careful review of the circumstances of the brain injury, the neuroradiological findings, and particularly the interaction of the patient's cultural background and type of injury is necessary. A consultation with a specialist regarding the immigrant's culture as it relates to his/her health and test-taking attitudes would be recommended in such a case.

Summary and Conclusions

Guidelines for the psychological and neuropsychological assessment of highly represented minorities have come of age, particularly in the United States, due to the extensive work of researchers, clinicians, and various professional organizations. However, a review of the literature shows that few neuropsychological measures have been adapted and normed for minority groups. As a result, North-American clinicians, as well as clinicians from other immigrant countries, have a limited number of measures available for the assessment of bicultural individuals. Moreover, whenever norms are available, they often fail to meet the quality of those published in the test manuals, and fail to distinguish between various levels of cultural orientation of the members of particular ethnic groups (Dana, 1996).

When considering the various guidelines for conducting neuropsychological assessment of minorities, one should differentially adopt the guidelines for each cultural group. For example, when assessing Hispanics, one should take into consideration both the general guidelines published by the APA and those published for this particular group (i.e., Ardila et al., 1994). Additionally, whenever possible, it has been recommended that the neuropsychologist should refer clients for whom English is a second language to a colleague who is fully fluent in their native language (Artiola & Mullaney, 1998).

As we head toward the twenty-first century, an increase in bicultural or even tricultural populations is expected. Keeping this in mind, more sophisticated methodologies will need to be developed. Such methodologies should incorporate the traditional guidelines listed earlier, as well as emphasize the multidimensional and diverse characteristics of many of the ethnic groups. This is best illustrated in immigrant societies, such as Israel, where a recent study of older adults identified as many as 30 different linguistic and cultural backgrounds (Poreh, 1999). In such cases, algorithms and indexes that evaluate the interaction between immigration, age of language acquisition, and cognitive functioning are necessary. This is illustrated, for example, in performance on the Controlled Oral Word Fluency Test. While native Hebrew speakers produce higher raw phonemic based output than their non-native countrypeople, the average switches between semantic categories is almost identical across various ethnic groups, and does not correlate with the age of language acquisition (Poreh, 1999).

In conclusion, understanding both the cultural and psychosocial functioning of patients who are referred for neuropsychological assessment is of the utmost importance for both diagnostic and care-planning purposes. Although it is often assumed that performance on cognitive tasks, personality measures, and measures of malingering and motivation offer an adequate estimation of functioning on daily living activities, little research has addressed this assumption. There is reason to believe that cultural and linguistic factors play an important role during the standardized examination. Continued research is needed to clarify these relationships so as to maximize the most reliable information concerning the assessment and rehabilitation techniques best suited for multicultural patients.

References

American Psychological Association (1991). *Service guidelines for ethnic, linguistic and culturally diverse populations*. Washington D.C.: American Psychological Association.

American Psychiatric Association (1994). *Diagnostic and Statistical Manual of Mental Disorders* (DSM-IV 1st ed.). Washington D.C.: American Psychiatric Association.

Ardila, A. (1995). Directions of research in cross cultural neuropsychology. *Journal of Clinical and Experimental Neuropsychology, 17*, 143-150.

Ardila, A., Rosselli, M., & Puente, A. E. (1994). *Neuropsychological assessment of the Spanish speaker*. New York: Plenum Press.

Artiola-i-Fortuny L., & Heaton, R. K. (1996). Standard versus computerized administration of the Wisconsin Card Sorting Test. *Clinical Neuropsychologist, 10,* 419-424.

Artiola-i-Fortuny, L., & Mullaney, H. (1998). Assessing patients whose language you do not know: Can the absurd be ethical? *Clinical Neuropsychologist, 12,* 113-126.

Boas, F. (1911). *The mind of primitive man.* New York: Plenum Press.

Boivin, M. J., Giordani, B., & Bornefeld, B. (1995). The use of the Tactual Performance Tests for cognitive ability tesing with African children. *Neuropsychology, 9,* 409-417.

Cole, M., & Engestroem, Y. (1997). A cultural-historical approach to distributed cognition. In G. Salomon (Ed.), *Distributed cognitions: Psychological and educational considerations* (pp. 1-46). New York: Cambridge.

Crook, T. H., Lebowitz, B. D., Pirozzolo, F. J., Zappala, G., Cavarzeran, F., Measso, G., & Massari, D.C. (1993). Recalling names after introduction: Changes across the adult life span in two cultures. *Developmental Neuropsychology, 9,* 103-113.

Cuèllar, I. (1998). Cross-cultural clinical psychological assessment of Hispanic Americans. *Journal of Personality Assessment, 70,* 71-86.

Cuèllar, I., Arnold, B., & González, G. (1996). Cognitive referents of acculturation: Assessment of cultural constructs in Mexican Americans. *Journal of Community Psychology, 23,* 339-356.

Cuèllar, I., Arnold, B., & Maldonado, R. (1995). Acculturation rating scale for Mexican Americans-II: A revision of the original ARSMA scale. *Hispanic Journal of Behavioral Sciences, 17,* 275-304.

Cuèllar, I., Hairis, I. C., & Jasso. R. (1980). An acculturation scale for Mexican American normal and clinical populations. *Hispanic Journal of Behavioral Sciences, 2,* 199-2l7.

Cuevas, J. L. & Osterich, H. (1990). Cross-cultural evaluation of the booklet version of the Category Test. *International Journal of Clinical Neuropsychology, 12,* 3-4.

Dana, R.H. (1996). Culturally competent assessment practice in the United States. *Journal of Personality Assessment, 66,* 472-487.

Delgado, P., Guerrero, G., Goggin, J. P., & Ellis, B. B. (1999). Self-assessment of linguistic skills by bilingual Hispanics. *Hispanic Journal of Behavioral Sciences, 21,* 31-46.

Demsky, Y. I., Mittenberg, W., Quintar, B., Katell, A. D., & Golden, C. J. (1998). Bias in the use of standard American norms with Spanish translations of the Wechsler Memory Scale Revised. *Assessment, 5,* 115-121.

Diehr, M. C., Heaton, R. K., Miller, W., & Grant, I. (1999). The Paced Auditory Serial Addition Task (PASAT): Norms for age, education, and ethnicity. *Assessment, 6,* 101.

Doerr, H. O., & Storrie, M. C. (1982). Neuropsychological testing in the People's Republic of China: The Halstead-Reitan Seattle/Changsha. *Clinical Neuropsychology, 4,* 49-51.

Duane, D. D., & Leong, C. K. (1985). *Understanding learning disabilities: International and multidisciplinary views.* New York: Plenum Press.

Faust, D. (1996). Assessment of brain injuries in legal cases. In B. Fogel, R. B., & Schiffer S. M. Rao (Eds.), *Neuropsychiatry.* Baltimore: Williams & Wilkins.

Freeman, D. (1983). *Margaret Mead and Samoa.* Cambridge: Harvard University Press.

Gay, G., & Abrahams, R. D. (1973). Does the pot melt, boil, or brew? Black children and white assessment procedures. *Journal of School Psychology, 11,* 330-340.

Gibbs, J. T. (1985). Establishing a treatment relationship with black clients: Interpersonal vs. instrumental strategies. In C. Germain (Ed.), *Advances in Clinical Social Work*. Silver Spring: National Association of Social Work, Inc.

Gladsjo, J. A., Schuman, C. C., Evans, J. D., Peavy, G. M., Miller S. W., & Heaton, R. K. (1999). Norms for letter and category fluency: Demographic corrections for age, education, and ethnicity. *Assessment, 6*, 147-178.

Gowan, J. C., & Torrance, E. P. (1965). An intercultural study of non-verbal ideational fluency. *Gifted Child Quarterly, 9*, 13-15.

Greenfield, P. M. (1997). You can't take it with you. Why ability assessments don't cross cultures. *American Psychologist, 52*, 1115-1124.

Jacobs, D. M., Sano, M., Albert, S., Schofield, P., Dooneief, G., & Stern, Y. (1997). Cross-cultural neuropsychological assessment: A comparison of randomly selected, demographically matched cohorts of English- and Spanish-speaking older adults. *Journal of Clinical and Experimental Neuropsychology, 19*, 331-339.

Kim, K. H., Relkin, N. R., Lee, K. M., & Hirsch, J. (1997). Distinct cortical areas associated with native and second languages. *Nature, 10*, 171-174.

Kohnert, K. J., Hernandez, A. E., & Bates, E. (1998). Bilingual performance on the Boston Naming Test: Preliminary norms in Spanish and English. *Brain and Language, 65*, 422-440.

LaFromboise, D. T., & Dixon, D. N. (1981). American Indian perception of trustworthiness in a counseling interview. *Journal of Counseling Psychology, 28*, 165-169.

Lee, S. (1991). Anorexia nervosa in adolescents of Asian extraction: Comment. *British Journal of Psychiatry, 158*, 284-285.

Lewis, S., Campbell, A., Takushi, C., Ruby, B. A., Dennis, G., Wood, D., & Weir, R. (1997). Visual organization test performance in an African American population with acute unilateral cerebral lesions. *International Journal of Neuroscience, 91*, 295-302.

Lishman, W. A. (1998). *Organic Psychiatry: The psychological consequences of cerebral disorder* (3rd ed.). Oxford: Blackwell Science Ltd.

Logue, P. F., Platzek, D., Hutzell, R., & Robinson, B. (1973). Neurological, neuropsychological and behavioral aspects of Gilles de la Tourette's syndrome: A case. *Perceptual and Motor Skills, 37*, 855-856.

Lonner, W. J. (1980). A decade of cross-cultural psychology: JCCP, 1970-1979. *Journal of Cross Cultural Psychology, 11*, 7-34.

Lopez, S. R., Grover, K. P., Holland, D., Johnson, M. J., Kain, C. D., Kanel, K., Mellins, S. A., & Rhyne, M. C. (1989). Development of culturally sensitive psychotherapists. *Professional Psychology: Research and Practice, 20*, 369-376.

Lucas, J. A. (1998). Traumatic brain injury and post concussive syndrome. In P. J. Snyder & P. D. Nussbaum (Eds.), *Clinical neuropsychology*. Washington, D.C.: American Psychological Association.

Maj, M., D'Elia, L., Satz, P., Janssen R., Zaudig, M., Uchiyama, C., Starace, F., Galderisi, S., Chervinsky, A. (1993). Evaluation of two new neuropsychological tests designed to minimize cultural bias in the assessment of HIV-1 seropositive persons: A WHO study. *Archives of Clinical Neuropsychology, 8*, 123-126.

Maj, M., Janssen, R., Satz, P., Zaudig, M., Starace, F., Boor, D., Sughondhabiram, D., Bing, E. G., Luabeya, M. K., Ndetei, D., Riedel, R., Schulte, G., & Sartorius, N. (1991). The World Health Organization's cross-cultural study on neuropsychiatric aspects of infection with the human immunodeficiency virus 1 (HIV-1): Preparation and pilot phase. *British Journal of Psychiatry, 159*, 351-356.

Manly, J. J., Jacobs, D. M., Sano, M., Bell, K., Merchant, C. A., Small, S. A., & Stern, Y. (1998a). Cognitive test performance among nondemented elderly African Americans and Whites. *Neurology, 50,* 1238-1245.

Manly, J. J., Jacobs, D. M., Sano, M., Merchant, C. A., Small, S. A., & Stern, Y. (1999). Effect of literacy on neuropsychological test performance in nondemented, education-matched elders. *Journal of the International Neuropsychological Society, 5,* 191-202.

Manly, J. J., Miller, S. W., Heaton, R. K., Byrd, D. D., Reilly, J., Velasquez, R. J., Saccuzzo, D. P., Grant, I., & the HIV Neurobehavioral Research Center (NHRC) Group (1998b). The effect of African-American acculturation on neuropsychological test performance in normal and HIV-positive individuals. *Journal of the International Neuropsychological Society, 4,* 291-302.

Marsella, A. (1987). The measurement of depressive experience and disorder across cultures. In A. J. Marsella, R. M. A. Hirschfeld, & M. M. Katz (Eds.), *The measurement of depression* (pp. 376-397). New York: Guilford Press.

Mayfield, J. W., & Reynolds, C. R. (1997). Black-White differences in memory test performance among children and adolescents. *Archives of Clinical Neuropsychology, 12,* 111-122.

Murphy, K. R., & Davidishofer, C. O. (1994). *Psychological testing: Principles and applications.* Englewood Cliffs: Prentice Hall.

Payette, K. A., & Clarizio, H. F. (1994). Discrepant team decisions: The effects of race, gender, achievement, and IQ on LD eligibility. *Psychology in the Schools, 31,* 40-48.

Ponton, M., Satz, P., Herrera, L., Ortiz, F., Urrutiia, C., Young, R., D'Elia, L., Furst, C., & Namerow, N. (1996). Normative data stratified by age and education for the Neuropsychological Screening Battery for Hispanics (NeSBHIS): Initial report. *Journal of the International Neuropsychological Society, 2,* 96-104.

Poreh, A. (1999). *Normative neuropsychological data stratified by age and education for Israeli older adults.* Unpublished manuscript.

Prewitt-Diaz, J., & Rivera, R. (1989). Correlations among scores on Woodcock-Johnson achievement subtest (Spanish), WISC--R (Spanish) and Columbia Mental Maturity Scale. *Psychological Reports, 64,* 987-990.

Prigatano, G. P., Ogano, M., & Amakusa, B. (1997). A cross-cultural study on impaired self-awareness in Japanese patients with brain dysfunction. *Neuropsychiatry, Neuropsychology, and Behavioral Neurology, 10,* 135-143.

Puente, A. E., Sol-Mora, M., Munoz C., & Juan, M. (1997). Neuropsychological assessment of Spanish-speaking children and youth. In C. R. Reynolds & E. Fletcher-Janzen (Eds.), *Handbook of clinical child neuropsychology: Critical issues in neuropsychology,* (2nd ed. pp. 371-383). New York: Plenum Press.

Ripich, D. N., Carpenter, B., & Ziol, E. (1997). Comparison of African-American and white persons with Alzheimer's disease on language measures. *Neurology, 48,* 781-783.

Rosseli, M., & Ardila, A. (1996). Cognitive effects of cocaine and polydrug abuse. *Journal of Clinical and Experimental Neuropsychology, 18,* 122-135.

Rosselli, M. (1993). Neuropychology of illiteracy. *Behavioural Neurology, 6,* 107-112.

Silver Platter Information, Inc. Silver Platter Information, Ltd., 100 River Ridge Drive, 10 Barley Mow Passage, Norwood, MA 02062.

Spreen, O., & Strauss, E. (1998). *A compendium of neuropsychological tests: Administration, norms, and commentary* (2nd ed.). New York: Oxford University Press.

Stanczak, D. E., Lynch, M. D., McNeil, C. K., & Brown, B. (1998). The Expanded Trail Making Test: Rationale, development, and psychometric properties. *Archives of Clinical Neuropsychology, 13,* 473-487.

Taussig, M. & Ponton, M. (1996). Issues in neuropsychological assessment for Hispanic older adults: Cultural and linguistic factors. In G. Yeo & T. D. Gallagher (Eds.), *Ethnicity and the dementias*. Washington D.C.: Taylor and Francis.

Torrance, E. P. (1962). Cultural discontinuities and the development of originality of thinking. *Exceptional Children, 29,* 2-13.

Xu, Y., Gong, Y., & Matthews, J. (1987). The Luria-Nebraska Neuropsychological Battery revised in China. *International Journal of Clinical Neuropsychology, 9,* 97-101.

Yeo, G., & Gallagher, T. D. (1996). *Ethnicity and the dementias*. Washington, D.C.: Taylor and Francis.

Zamanian, K., Thackrey, M., Starrett, R. A., Brown, L. G., et al. (1992). Acculturation and depression in Mexican American elderly. *Clinical Gerontologist, 11,* 3-4.

Chapter 18

MULTICULTURAL TRAINING IN CLINICAL NEUROPSYCHOLOGY

Philip S. Fastenau*, Jovier D. Evans,
Kathy E. Johnson and Gary R. Bond
Indiana University Purdue University Indianapolis
(IUPUI), Indianapolis, Indiana

Abstract

Throughout this volume, scholars have demonstrated the importance of ethnic and cultural issues in the practice of clinical neuropsychology and in neuropsychological research (Berry, 1994). We briefly describe a broad model for multicultural training and several specific models of curriculum development. From these models, we designed and tested several initiatives for improving multicultural training in an existing clinical neuropsychological training program. Our preliminary outcomes suggested that some of these initiatives hold promise and may be useful to other graduate programs in clinical neuropsychology, and perhaps to internships and postdoctoral fellowships. Based on these early experiences, we proffer 12 steps that we regarded to be most important to our progress. We also provide interested readers with a list of potential avenues (agencies and grant mechanisms) for funding such training initiatives.

---

*To whom correspondence should be addressed at: Department of Psychology (LD 124), Indiana University Purdue University Indianapolis (IUPUI), Indianapolis, Indiana, 46202-3275; e-mail: pfastena@iupui.edu. This chapter was supported by a training grant from the Rehabilitation Services Administration of the U.S. Department of Education (USDE # H129J970003).

Introduction

The development of cultural competence in the next generation of practicing psychologists has clearly become a national priority. The American Psychological Association has elevated multicultural training to a prominent position in its guidelines for accreditation, and at the National Multicultural Conference and Summit recommendations intended to promote cultural competence in all psychological endeavors were unanimously endorsed (APA, 1994; Sue, Bingham, Porché-Burke, & Vasquez, 1999). Entire volumes have been devoted to the role of ethnicity and cultural values in health care and education (e.g., De La Cancela & Guzman, 1991; Ferraro, 2001; Harrison, Thyer, & Wodarski, 1996; Jackson, 1991; Logan, 1996; Myers, Wohlford, Guzman, & Echemendia, 1991; Suzuki, Meller, & Ponterotto, 1996; Vacc, DeVaney, & Wittmer, 1995). The importance of training psychologists in multicultural issues has been increasingly recognized (De La Cancela & Guzman, 1991; Green, 1995; Jackson, 1991; Myers, Wohlford, Guzman, & Echemendia, 1991; Trimble, 1991; Zane & Sue, 1991). Yet, the training and practices of psychologists have lagged far behind the demographic trends of increasing diversity in the population (Hall, 1997).

These issues are especially relevant to the practices of neuropsychologists and rehabilitation psychologists working with neurological populations. For example, Friedman and Clayton (1996) argued that because African Americans are at increased risk for hypertension they are also much more vulnerable to strokes and other forms of chronic neurological disease. They also point out that there is a disproportionately high prevalence of lack of medical insurance coverage for people from ethnic minority backgrounds; this limits their access to health and rehabilitation services, with the adverse result of higher rates of chronic disabilities. People from ethnic-minority groups manifest disproportionately high rates of both disability and unemployment (Giordano & D'Alonzo, 1995). Three areas of disability seen frequently by neuropsychologists (mental illness, communication disorders, and substance abuse) show the most disproportionate representation by people from minority groups compared to many other disabilities (D'Alonzo, Giordano, & Oyenque, in press; Stewart, Anae, & Gipe, 1989).

The challenge for many programs today is to identify mechanisms for moving past simply discussing the importance of multicultural training in intervention, assessment, and teaching. While several excellent training models have been developed and published (Carter & Qureshi, 1995; Constantine & Gloria, 1999; Copeland, 1982; Myers, 1991a), few practical strategies have been offered for programs attempting to navigate towards those ideals. The effectiveness of specific strategies naturally will vary as a function of program characteristics such as size, training emphases, geographical location, and resource availability. However, we believe that broader dissemination of such strategies across programs could help to reduce the gap between current training practices and the published ideals. The purpose of the current chapter is to review the goals for cultural competence in the areas of assessment, intervention, and teaching in the area of clinical neuropsychology. We then will delineate one particular set of strategies recently adopted by our program that helped us to begin charting a path toward a model of training that is more culture-centered.

This chapter is divided into five main sections. First, we present our working definitions of terms that are integral to our discussion of multicultural training. We then focus on assessment issues related to neuropsychology, and highlight needs for additional research in certain key areas. In the third and fourth sections we present a model for improving multicultural training among psychologists, and then use this model as a framework to describe the specific strategies that our program has implemented to become more culture-centered. Finally, we introduce twelve key steps that neuropsychology training programs might implement to increase the diversity of their faculty and students, and to ensure that graduates are culturally competent.

Clarification of Terminology

A major factor that must be considered is the confounded and unclear notions of race, ethnicity, and culture. Researchers have argued that, if these variables have been considered at all, unclear definitions have been employed in research studies of cognitive ability tests, and the idea of examining them independently or in combination has been woefully lacking (Helms, 1995, 1997). For example, most studies attempt to control for these variables by characterizing groups based on race, but not examining relevant cultural and socioeconomic factors that may account for differences in performance on most cognitive assessments. The use of the term race has come under sharp criticism because it may convey a misleading sense of biological distinctiveness among different groups that might not even exist in any meaningful form (Betancourt & Lopez, 1995; Lin, Poland, & Nakasaki, 1993).

Ethnicity, however, connotes groups of individuals who typically share a common ancestry and culture as well as a sense of identity (McGoldrick, Pearce, & Giordano, 1982; Betancourt & Lopez, 1995). Ethnicity often is used interchangeably with both race and culture. Betancourt and Lopez (1995) suggest that ethnicity refers to the ethnic quality or affiliation of a group, which is normally defined in terms of culture. This affiliation is also bi-directional in the sense that cultural background can determine ethnic identity, and ethnic affiliation can also determine culture through specific means such as ethnic identification, perceived discrimination, and bilingualism. In summary, race, ethnicity, and culture are all interlinked, and future studies of cross cultural assessment approaches need to develop adequate modes of operationalizing these constructs to deal with a multicultural and multiethnic environment.

Socioeconomic status (SES) is another factor affecting the measurement of cognitive ability that should be considered more in studies examining racial or ethnic differences in neuropsychological performance (Grubb & Ollendick, 1986). SES connotes the degree of educational, vocational, and financial attainment, all of which are likely to be associated with differences in cognitive performance. For example, SES has a direct impact on the quality of educational opportunities, the financial resources necessary for adequate access to healthcare, and good nutritional standards. Controlling for the effects of SES, however, may not be sufficient to eliminate cultural or even biological (e.g. nutritional) differences seen in neuropsychological assessments.

Clearly, "race," "ethnicity," and "culture" are complex terms. In addition to the discussion above, there are other "cultural" differences that have not been addressed explicitly, such as gender, sexual orientation, and religion. For the purposes of this chapter, we will focus on race because it has been the focus of the chapters in this volume and because we regarded this to be an especially high priority in our own training program. Thus, the focus of the early initiatives that we describe in this chapter will be primarily addressing race. However, in all of our discussions, the terms "ethnicity" and "culture" can be regarded as proxies for the many dimensions across which human beings differ.

Multicultural Issues in Neuropsychological Assessment

Okazaki and Sue (1995) review several methodological problems inherent in research with ethnic minorities. One major issue is the appropriate selection and method of scientific study. This debate has led to the "etic-emic" controversy in psychological assessment. An emic approach to assessment views the construct under study from within the culture one is examining. This involves identifying a hypothesized construct within a particular culture and determining its meaning, operations, and consequences from within that culture. This is in contrast to an etic perspective, which seeks to identify "universals" from outside the culture under study (Berry, 1994, 1995; Dana, 1993). It is clear that culture does play a role in neuropsychological performance and that no test can be considered culture free (Anastasi, 1988; Manly, 1996).

Other researchers have noted various problems with bias and cultural equivalence in assessment instruments (van de Vijver, 1994; Helms, 1995). For example, van de Vijver (1997) notes that if instruments are differentially appropriate across groups, this represents bias in the test. Many tests assume a mastery of the language of the test, even when this language mastery is not equivalent across groups. In addition, previous exposure to psychological tests or similar tasks has a considerable effect on performance. Helms (1997) further states that tests themselves may be culturally biased and may not be measuring the same constructs across cultural groups. In other words, many ability tests fail to demonstrate cultural (i.e. racial, ethnic, or socioeconomic conditions of socialization) equivalence. Whether or not it is necessary to develop entirely new tests for use across cultures or, in some cases, to carefully translate and/or develop new, ethnicity-specific norms are important questions for future research.

In summary, problems inherent in cross-cultural research may have a profound impact on tests of cognitive ability when applied to different cultures. These dilemmas may emerge at the test development, normative, and validation stages due to one or all of the aforementioned problems. Issues of construct validity across cultures, problems with appropriate behavioral and cognitive operational definitions, and inherent sources of bias that have not been adequately controlled need to be examined in future research of cognitive abilities across cultures.

This brief overview, together with the issues raised throughout the present volume, highlights the impact of ethnic and cultural issues on all aspects of the practice of clinical neuropsychology, including assessment, psychotherapy, rehabilitation, program planning/evaluation, and research. One critical step toward addressing these issues is to train current and future neuropsychologists to be aware of the impact of ethnic factors on neuropsychological research and practice. In this chapter, we describe some first steps that can be taken toward improving multicultural training in a graduate clinical psychology/neuropsychology training program. To illustrate methods of implementing these initiatives, we describe specific strategies that we pursued to enhance the multicultural training within our program, together with preliminary results on the outcomes of our efforts (the successes and the frustrations). This self-review gives rise to recommendations for others who endeavor to enrich the multicultural training at their doctoral training sites.

A Model for Improving Multicultural Training

With the sponsorship of the National Institute of Mental Health, a national conference was convened in 1988 to address ethnic issues in clinical psychology training and service delivery. The panel was comprised of 47 scholars and students, who represented 28 training programs across the U.S. Summarizing the conclusions and consensus of the participants, Myers (1991b) delineated a series of recommendations, which can be distilled into four main priorities:
• Recruitment and development of minority faculty;
• Recruitment and training of minority students;
• Development and enrichment of training curricula;
• Funding and program evaluation.

These recommendations provided the model for the strategies implemented in our training program. These initiatives are described below. We are not proposing to have a definitive approach; rather, we are sharing our early experiences and insights from a "work-in-progress," now at the end of only three years into the challenge. It is hoped that this description of our early efforts might serve as a resource to other programs that wish to pursue similar changes in their training programs.

Infusing Multicultural Training Into An Existing Program: A Case Study at IUPUI

The multicultural training initiatives described in this chapter were implemented at Indiana University Purdue University Indianapolis (IUPUI). The program is APA-accredited in Clinical Psychology with advanced training available in clinical neuropsychology. Grounded in the Boulder Model (Belar & Perry, 1992) of clinical psychology (i.e., the "scientist-practitioner" approach to training in psychotherapy, assessment, psychopathology, and research), the IUPUI program is distinguished in its focus on adaptation to *chronic* health and psychiatric conditions (e.g., diabetes, heart disease, epilepsy, traumatic brain injury, schizophrenia, bipolar affective disorder).

The program has emphases in three specialty areas, one of which is clinical neuropsychology. Our neuropsychology training is modeled after the graduate training guidelines articulated by the American Psychological Association (APA) Division on Clinical Neuropsychology (Div. 40) and the International Neuropsychological Society (INS) in 1987 (Reports of the INS – Division 40 Task Force, 1987) and more recently in 1997 (Proceedings of the Houston Conference, 1998). These guidelines dictate that neuropsychology students complete training in a generic psychology core (e.g., statistics, methodology, learning/cognition, social, development), general clinical psychology (e.g., psychopathology, psychometrics, interview, assessment, intervention, ethics), foundations of brain-behavior relationships (e.g., neuroanatomy, neuroscience, developmental neuropsychology), and foundations for the practice of clinical neuropsychology (neuropsychological assessment, research, and professional issues). Two faculty completed postdoctoral fellowships and are eligible for ABPP-CN board certification; in addition, two adjunct faculty supervising students on practicum are board-certified (ABPP-CN).

With regard to the multicultural status of our program prior to implementing multicultural training initiatives, all of our core clinical faculty were White/Non-Hispanic males (0% ethnic minority), and only two other faculty (non-clinical psychologists) in the department were faculty of color (8%). Only four faculty (15%) in the department were women; all were White/Non-Hispanic, and only one (non-clinical) was a support member for the clinical program (making up 9% of our combined core and support faculty). Prior to the training initiatives, 7% of the students in our master's and doctoral programs were from ethnic minority backgrounds (all Asian). There was no course on cultural issues in our clinical curriculum, and a review of graduate course syllabi prior to the multicultural training initiatives showed little evidence of multicultural concepts and principles. During a preliminary site visit by the APA at that same time, these were identified as limitations to our graduate clinical psychology training program. At that same time, the faculty had identified an increased multicultural emphasis as a priority for the department as a whole. It was in this context of cultural homogeneity (faculty, graduate students, and curriculum) that we explored strategies for improving multicultural training in our program.

The multicultural training initiatives were funded by a training grant from Rehabilitation Services Administration (RSA) of the Department of Education. The project had five objectives, modeled after the NIMH model summarized above: (1) Recruit a tenure-track faculty member from an ethnic background who had expertise in cultural competency and who could help advance clinical practices and research with traditionally underrepresented groups. (2) Energetically recruit strong graduate students from ethnic minority groups for the clinical psychology program. (3) With the input of an advisory board (consisting of graduate students, health care professionals from the community, and consumers of clinical services), design a training program for addressing the current and future needs of the field. (4) Provide intensive training in multicultural knowledge and skills for 15 graduate students (five per year for three years) in three areas of critical need, which included clinical neuropsychology. (5) Provide continuing education opportunities for practicing psychologists.

Formation of the Multicultural Training Committee
Three of the authors of this chapter (GB, PF, and KJ) penned the greater part of the RSA grant; when the grant was funded, we formed the Multicultural Training Committee and took responsibility for seeing the initiatives carried out. In addition, as a function of the grant, a new faculty member (JE on this chapter) and a coordinator were hired. These two individuals joined the Multicultural Training Committee.

Recruitment and development of minority faculty
As part of the goal to increase multicultural competency, we had proposed to hire a scholar with expertise in cultural diversity, especially with regard to the role of ethnic factors in health psychology and clinical neuropsychology. There was a preference for a research program addressing African-American issues because that group comprises two-thirds of the minority population in Central Indiana, where the university is located. In addition, we had hoped to hire someone who was from an underrepresented ethnic background, so that this individual would serve as a role model to prospective applicants and students from minority ethnic cultures. Our faculty search process was carefully planned; we took advantage of many excellent resources that had emerged in recent years with regard to recruiting and retaining faculty from underrepresented ethnic backgrounds (American Psychological Association Commission on Ethnic Minority Recruitment, Retention and Training in Psy-

chology, 1996a, 1996b, 1997; American Psychological Association Office of Ethnic Minority Affairs, 1997; Clay, 1997; Murray, 1997). This resulted in an energetic and innovative faculty search to hire a candidate who would be optimally matched to the goals of the multicultural training initiative. We assembled a large, multidisciplinary Search and Screen Committee, 40% of whom were African American. We also sought ongoing input and consultation with Dr. Herman Blake, a nationally recognized African-American scholar in the area of achieving excellence and diversity in academia.

The Search and Screen Committee used numerous methods and media for disseminating information about the position. In the event that our methods may be useful examples to other search committees, we have included a listing of our major approaches in Appendix A. Mailings included a copy of the position announcement; a letter describing the RSA training objectives and appealing to colleagues to post/distribute the information for all prospective candidates for the faculty position; statistics on the faculty and students; and a description of the department, university, and metropolitan area, including ethnic composition and the availability of cultural activities for diverse groups. In addition, members of the Search and Screen committee invested many hours contacting potential applicants by phone to discuss the position with them and to encourage them to apply. Finally, during phone interviews and on-site interviews, candidates were contacted by faculty of color to give them an opportunity to learn more about the department, university, and metropolitan area, especially with regard to the degree to which faculty of color are welcomed and supported and with regard to the cultural climate of the community.

In addition to having the generous support of this interdisciplinary search committee, we also received strong support from the university. First, an administrator from the IUPUI Office of Faculty Development and Retention joined the search committee to provide input and resources for minority recruitment. Second, the university provided matching funds in the amount of $150,000 to subsidize a portion of the salary and fringe benefits for the new faculty hire during the first three years (the duration of the training grant). Finally, both the department and the school approved the creation of the new permanent, tenure-track position and agreed to fund that position indefinitely after the grant expired.

At the beginning of the first year of our multicultural training initiative, during which the faculty search took place, we hired a temporary project coordinator until a full tenure-track search could be conducted. We were fortunate to retain an African-American clinical psychologist who had 15 years experience consulting with national organizations and health care agencies on diversification of their work force. In his first year on the RSA project, he prepared and taught a course in multicultural psychotherapy, organized and convened an advisory board, spearheaded the recruitment of students, presented colloquia in the department, and presented workshops in the community. More importantly, he was vigilant during program and department meetings to remind the faculty and staff of the renewed commitment to multiculturalism and to identify more opportunities to advance this initiative throughout the department and curriculum.

During the first year, we conducted the full search described above. Because we already had roughly equal numbers of faculty in our specialty areas of neuropsychology, health psychology, and severe/persistent mental illness, the search was not limited to any one specific area. Four very strong candidates (all people of color, two of whom were female) came to interview. All had research activities and interests in the area of cultural factors and health. In spite of the narrow focus of the search (i.e., requiring a research focus in multicultural issues and health), we received an exceptional pool of applications that rivaled, if not exceeded, prior department searches that had fewer restrictions. From this competitive pool, we hired an African-American neuropsychologist with expertise in ethnic factors in neuropsychological assessment (author JE on this chapter). He joined the temporary project coordinator as co-coordinator on the multicultural training project, and he assumed responsibility for teaching the multicultural psychotherapy course.

In the third year of the grant, the department was conducting a search for another tenure-track opening in health psychology. Although there was no imperative to hire someone with expertise in cultural issues, the faculty expressed considerable appreciation for the cultural focus that pervaded the research program of one of the candidates, who was hired into the position. This is a testimony to the impact of these training initiatives on the climate of the department, changing the attitudes and values of the faculty with a resulting impact on hiring behavior. We were also fortunate that this candidate was a female scholar from a Hispanic background. In addition to bringing to the department her expertise and commitment to studying cultural factors in health care, she further enhances the diversity of our clinical faculty and provides an additional role model for students from minority backgrounds, especially for women of color.

Recruitment of students

We adopted a two-pronged approach for recruiting students of color to the graduate program. First, we more energetically identified and pursued minority students who were applying to graduate school. Second, we identified and recruited talented undergraduate students of color in their junior year *prior* to applying to graduate school.

Graduate applicants

The first focus was on minority students applying to graduate school. The project coordinators held several meetings with the Assistant Dean in charge of minority recruiting for the university, who represented the Department of Psychology on several university recruiting trips to Historically Black Colleges and Universities (HBCUs). We encouraged him to target students interested in clinical psychology, and we pursued the leads he developed in his recruitment. Also, we reviewed lists of students seeking doctoral programs from the APA Minority Fellowship Program (MFP). Sixty-four applications and information packets were mailed to minority undergraduates from several lists. In addition, we attended the annual "African American Student Summit," a campus student conference, to discuss opportunities in our program and to distribute recruitment literature.

Prior to the initiation of our recruiting, two of our graduate students were from ethnic minority backgrounds. After two years of recruiting, our ethnic representation rose from 7% (two students, both Asian heritage) to 16% (two Asian, two Pacific Islander, and one Hispanic). All students who were admitted to the program on a training fellowship have continued to be funded in full by the same mechanisms as other students (primarily by research assistantships in the department).

Undergraduate students

The second strategy entailed active recruitment of students of color earlier in the educational pipeline. We targeted talented undergraduate students of color who were in their junior year of college, capitalizing on the Committee on Institutional Cooperation (CIC) *Summer Research Opportunities Program (SROP)*. In that program, minority undergraduates are invited to apply for a summer experience designed to prepare them for graduate study and faculty careers. Through the SROP, students work on a research project guided by a faculty mentor and have the opportunity to explore a topic of interest at one of fifteen host CIC universities. Special educational enrichment activities, such as workshops, are also scheduled during the summer. Participants are expected to devote full time to the program during the eight-to-ten week summer session.

In our first year of SROP recruitment, six candidates from various colleges and universities across the U.S. were selected and offered funding to participate in the SROP at IUPUI. All had research interests that complemented the work of some of our faculty. Faculty in our program made telephone calls and sent electronic mailings to these students to provide a more personal aspect to our recruitment efforts. Unfortunately, these students were also heavily recruited to other summer programs; only one of the six accepted our offer for the SROP.

Our first attempt at using the SROP for recruitment led us to believe that early recruitment is vital. In the following year, we recruited earlier. As a consequence, three SROP candidates accepted fellowships in our department for that summer.

Integration of multicultural concepts into the curriculum

A common approach to multicultural training is the *separate course model*, which entails adding a single specialized course to the curriculum (Copeland, 1982). The *separate course model* offers several advantages but carries some liabilities, as well. The main advantage is that a separate course is relatively easy to implement into a training program and finding an expert in multi-cultural issues is more feasible than attempting to increase the multicultural competency of the entire faculty at once. In addition, if a separate course is on the class schedule, it ensures that this material will be covered within the program and students will gain exposure to issues of multiculturalism within a training context. If there are no available faculty members to develop this course, a department might hire adjunct or associate faculty to fulfill this role as an interim solution.

A major disadvantage to this approach is its brevity and lack of depth (Reynolds, 1995). An additional drawback is a lack of exposure to these topics outside of the course. There is also the danger of these issues being perceived as unimportant by the rest of the program faculty, which would convey a lack of commitment to the development of multicultural counseling competencies. Furthermore, a separate course may place a high level of burden on the faculty member assigned to teach the course (Reynolds, 1995; Ridley et al., 1997).

Ridley, Mendoza, and Kanitz (1994) proposed a hierarchical framework for the placement of a multicultural course within the core curriculum of a graduate counseling program. Each stage, or level of this hierarchy builds upon successful mastery of the preceding stage. The *first stage* is the development of a training philosophy. Faculty must clarify the theoretical framework underlying a multicultural emphasis, with the idea of defining the goals and scope of training. The *second stage* involves the development of learning objectives. Examples may include having counselors display culturally responsive behaviors, ethical knowledge and practice, cultural empathy, and an understanding of basic cultural self-awareness, as well as the limits of standard theoretical orientations. In the *third stage*, instructional strategies are designed to achieve these learning objectives. This involves didactic methods, experiential exercises, modeling, practicum experiences, and research, to name a few. The *fourth stage* involves program designs, ranging from one separate course on multicultural counseling to integrating these multi-cultural concepts across the curriculum. Finally, at the *fifth stage* the program is evaluated to ensure quality with regard to the program structure (Ridley et al., 1997; Ridley et al., 1994).

Boutte (1999) maintains that curricular modifications should entail both a reexamination and a redefinition of what is considered "accepted knowledge," and that simply adding a multicultural course or multicultural supplements to existing courses is not enough. In order for a training program to successfully prepare students to serve diverse populations, multicultural training must be infused throughout coursework, practica, and research experiences (Sue et al., 1999). Guzman (1991) notes that commitment is the most critical ingredient for training programs to successfully foster cultural competence. If faculty members are not unified in their commitment to ensuring that multicultural training is a high priority, training responsibilities will likely be shouldered by a small number of overburdened instructors. Furthermore, when multicultural issues are addressed solely within one course, students may infer that multicultural issues are ancillary to other aspects of training (Guzman, 1991).

We decided to use a multi-pronged strategy, adding a mandatory specialized course while increasing the emphasis on multiculturalism throughout the rest of the curriculum. We now turn to a discussion of some of the specific curriculum changes in areas of assessment, intervention, practicum training, research, ethics, general psychology, and training in teaching.

Assessment

General psychological assessment. In the general assessment sequence, multicultural issues are incorporated as a regular part of the didactic and experiential components of the course. For instance, when students learn about individually administered IQ tests, they discuss other instruments that have been developed to be "culture fair." Moreover, the class discusses attempts at making tests more interpretable for other cultural groups, such as the System Of Multicultural Pluralistic Assessment (SOMPA; Oakland & Shermis, 1989). As another example, the class discusses the appropriateness of test interpretation when an instrument is normed on another culture (e.g., use of a test that was normed on 2,000 White children in rural Kentucky for immigrant screening). Finally, the reading materials for the course have sections that specifically address diversity issues.

Neuropsychological assessment. The course on neuropsychological assessment presents all of the pertinent issues discussed previously in the chapter with regard to the unclear notions of race, ethnicity, culture and SES and how these affect performance on most tests of cognitive function. Furthermore, we discuss the lack of appropriate normative data for most neuropsychological tests and examine any research which seeks to address this problem from a multicultural framework. In addition, we discuss practical and appropriate strategies for addressing these limitations in the context of a clinical neuropsychological evaluation. To date, these discussions have broadened the students' awareness of these issues as they relate to the practice of clinical neuropsychology and began the discussion of possible research studies to address these issues.

Intervention

Multicultural counseling course. Our specialized course on multicultural psychotherapy explores the ways in which increasing diversity in the population requires adjustments in the delivery of mental health services. The focus is on different racial, ethnic and minority groups, their customs and values, and the impact these can have on the delivery of therapy. Consistent with the recommendations of Ridley and his colleagues (1997), this course covered the following topics: rationale for focusing on multicultural issues; racism, power, and prejudice; psychological assessment and diagnosis; therapy process variables and outcome goals; intervention strategies; multicultural counseling research; racial identity development; ethical issues in multicultural counseling; and information regarding normative samples. The course featured a combination of lecture and group participation exercises designed to expand on the written information presented in class.

At the first offering of the course, not only did graduate students in clinical psychology enroll, but also students from other areas of campus (e.g., social work, education). It has now been added to the set of required core courses in the clinical psychology program. Unexpectedly, undergraduate students began expressing interest in the topic, leading to a new undergraduate elective in multicultural counseling.

Intervention sequence. In addition to this specialized course, multicultural concepts are presented and discussed in the year-long psychotherapy sequence in the students' first year of training. Multicultural issues are embedded in the discussions throughout the course. For example, when addressing attending skills, we discuss body awareness, body space comfort zones, and tolerance for sustained eye gaze and how these behaviors differ by sex and culture. When we discuss reflection of feelings we explore cultural display rules and cultural differences in emotional responding. Some aspect of multicultural differences is addressed in virtually every class meeting. In supervision, multicultural issues are always assessed and addressed whenever the clients are not from the majority culture. Even if they are from the majority culture, we still often address issues of sensitivity to religious differences (e.g., conservative Christian), SES, and other human differences.

Psychiatric rehabilitation course. Finally, because our program focuses on chronic health conditions, we have a course surveying psychosocial and community rehabilitation interventions for people with severe and persistent mental illness, focusing on empirically validated practices. Multicultural issues are discussed throughout the seminar, based on both research evidence and clinical experience. The instructor draws on his own research (e.g., Salyers & Bond, 2001) and involves community service providers to describe the role of cultural competency in practice. Each program model is examined from the perspective of their adaptations in different communities and cultural groups.

Practicum training

Through the RSA grant, students have been funded to spend a summer (10 - 15 weeks) at nationally recognized medical centers to work with neuropsychologists and other clinical professionals who have been dedicated to translating neuropsychological procedures and services to multicultural communities. The RSA grant provided travel funds and a stipend to the students who were selected for "summer institutes"; there was no cost to the site, except the supervisor's/mentor's time.

Five students went to settings serving an ethnically diverse clientele (e.g., Los Angeles County Harbor – UCLA Medical Center, University of Chicago Medical Center, the Department of Veterans' Affairs Medical Center in New

Orleans). As the RSA grant comes to a close, however, we will need to identify alternative sources of funding, such as creative partnerships with the host
sites, if we wish to continue this initiative.

Research
Adding multicultural concepts and principles into an intervention course and
in practicum training are perhaps the most apparent changes to make in a
clinical curriculum because the earliest multicultural literature focused on
counseling and therapy, and more current literature is addressing assessment.
Other courses, however, may pose more of a challenge and may require more
innovation and creativity from instructors until more written and multimedia
resources are available.

  With regard to research training, multicultural concepts were integrated
into our graduate seminar on research methods. The major course requirement is to write a research proposal that is intended to serve as a draft of the
master's thesis proposal. Several changes were made to that course as part of
the RSA multicultural initiative. Here are some examples:

• Race was used as an independent variable in illustrative examples during
  lectures and during question-and-answer periods. Design issues can often
  be illustrated with many different case examples, but the instructor deliber-
  ately chose to use race as a variable to highlight this variable as a potential
  research subject.
• The instructor drew attention to the failure to include ethnic minorities in
  the vast majority of published studies in clinical psychology, neuropsychology, and rehabilitation.
• In the lecture on human subjects, the class examined the Tuskegee Syphilis
  Study, in which African Americans were left untreated (and uninformed)
  for four decades after penicillin became widely available and widely used
  (Dooley, 1984). We discussed the role of this incident on the deeply-held
  suspicion of many African Americans toward research.

  In addition to making changes to the formal coursework in research methodology, we took steps to increase our emphasis on cultural issues in research
training in other ways. First, we increased the exposure of students to ethnic
minority groups in research study sites. Second, we invited colloquium speakers who were experts in cultural issues and who were actively conducting
research on relevant topics. Finally, we hired a postdoctoral fellow of color.
Both the new faculty hire discussed above and the postdoctoral fellow had
research interests in cultural issues. These new hires provided role models for
students and contributed their expertise to students conducting theses and
dissertations on multicultural research topics.

  Since the initiation of the RSA multicultural training initiative, several
students have pursued theses and other research studies with multicultural
issues as their primary focus. One student is pursuing a thesis and presented
a paper on the role of ethnicity and socioeconomic status in medication
adherence among children with epilepsy. Another student has been exploring

ethnic factors in adolescent health. In addition, several students have been working with neuropsychology faculty in the department and at the medical center on multicultural projects. Examples include a normative assessment study with ethnic minorities; a study of the rates of severe mental illness and cognitive deficits in indigent populations; a study testing cognitive interventions among elderly African-Americans; and a study examining rates of dementia in African-Americans in the U.S. in comparison to native Africans in Nigeria and Kenya.

Ethics
The course on ethics was expanded to include the topic of cultural diversity, which is subsumed under the broad ethical imperative to respect human differences. The syllabus was revised such that approximately 20% of the discussion, readings and presentations were devoted to cultural diversity explicitly. The readings systematically addressed women's issues, gay and lesbian issues, issues that are more unique to the aging population, and ethnic issues. In addition, the issues of ethnicity and cultural differences were incorporated into other topics, discussions, and vignettes throughout the remainder of the course.

General psychology courses
Although issues of diversity may be readily infused into clinical and neuropsychological coursework and research, integration may pose more of a challenge for courses that provide breadth of training across other areas of psychology. Instructors of courses such as social and personality psychology can select textbooks to ensure that a multicultural emphasis is present or augment deficient texts with supplemental readings. Furthermore, instructors can select classroom activities such as debates and discussions to facilitate exploration of diversity issues and use techniques such as journaling to promote self exploration. Heppner and O'Brien (1994) evaluated the effectiveness of graduate training in multicultural issues. Students reported that the most important factor in helping them to become more sensitive to multicultural issues was the interpersonal exchanges that took place in class. Heppner and O'Brien (1994) recommend that multicultural courses be taken early on in students' training so that multiculturalism could most effectively be incorporated into classroom discussions during subsequent coursework. This appears to be a necessary prerequisite for promotion of cultural competence in general psychology courses. We also recommend that non-clinical faculty attend developmental workshops on multiculturalism in order to ensure that they can be effective facilitators and moderators of classroom discussions.

In addition to core curriculum courses designed to provide training in research, assessment, and intervention, students at IUPUI are required to take five additional specialty courses (e.g., family and disability seminar, psychopharmacology) and four courses in general psychology (psychobiology, cognitive development, social psychology, and psychopathology). Instructors of these courses have experienced mixed levels of success in incorporating issues of diversity in their content. While faculty agree on the importance of training all students to be aware of and sensitive to multicultural issues, course syllabi and selected textbooks reflect this commitment to varying degrees. Several instructors report that they assign supplementary readings related to multicultural issues and focus class debates on issues related to ethnic diversity. In the psychopathology course, similarities and differences across cultures in the incidence and natural histories of particular disorders are covered through the textbook and constitute a continuous theme in lectures and discussion. However, instructors grapple with the problem that the literature in the field of minority mental health may not always be easily accessible (Myers, 1991a). This problem is exacerbated in general psychology courses such as cognitive development, where researchers often lament the preponderance of studies focused on White, middle-class children who all too often attend university preschools (Medin & Atran, 1999). Until the research base becomes more representative in non-clinical areas of psychology, instructors may continue to struggle to adequately represent multicultural perspectives in core course offerings.

Training in teaching
Perhaps the most effective proactive step towards establishing the centrality of multicultural issues in both undergraduate and graduate level training is to make it a focal point in the training of new instructors. As part of their requirements, our clinical doctoral students are expected teach a minimum of one semester. Courses taught include Introductory Psychology, Life-Span Development, and Abnormal Psychology. In preparation for this teaching experience, students complete a seminar on the teaching of psychology. The Teaching Seminar covers practical aspects of teaching such as assessment and syllabus construction. However, two principal themes concern the preparation to teach a diverse student body and the importance of incorporating issues of diversity into course content. Teaching seminars can provide ideal opportunities for graduate students to reflect upon stereotypes and biases that they may have absorbed, and to reevaluate their pedagogical methods for teaching students from diverse ethnic groups (Davis, 1993). For example, some instructors tend to respond favorably to students who are extremely vocal during class discussions, and who demonstrate critical thinking by questioning the assumptions and points of view expressed by others. It is important that new teachers recognize that some students are brought up to perceive such behaviors as disrespectful or rude, and to be prepared to assess student performance through a variety of means.

Training new teachers is an ideal forum for cultivating faculty responsibility and tolerance more broadly. In the Teaching Seminar, the importance of instructors as role models for addressing diversity issues is stressed. Novice teaching assistants frequently express concern that they might not respond effectively to insensitive comments expressed in class. In the Teaching Seminar students have the opportunity to role play situations in which an instructor must confront prejudice in the classroom, and to discuss means by which cultural sensitivity and acceptance may be modeled during lectures and other classroom activities (Cannon, 1994; Reyes & Halcón, 1996). In sum, teacher training in predoctoral programs provides an opportunity to establish the importance of multicultural training in higher education, provide beginning teachers with information on pedagogical methods appropriate for diverse settings, and to promote the modeling of behaviors indicative of cultural competence in the classroom.

Continuing education for existing practitioners
Although not specific to neuropsychologists, continuing education workshops were designed to combine didactic and experiential training. As a function of our multicultural initiatives, these workshops were conducted through several different agencies, including the State Department of Mental Health, the State Department of Vocational Rehabilitation, and Indiana University Medical School.

Initial evaluation of the IUPUI initiatives

Indicators of progress
As part of our multicultural enterprise, we have taken an early look at the utility of various initiatives for increasing cultural competency among emerging clinical neuropsychologists. After three years of developing this multicultural training program, we have enjoyed some early successes:

- We convened a core group of faculty committed to enhancing multicultural training in our program and department.
- We have seen an increase in the ethnic diversity of our clinical faculty, expanding from none (0%) to two (33%) of the six core clinical faculty. We have seen an increase in women on the clinical faculty also, expanding from none (0%) to one (17%) of the six core clinical faculty, although this is still far below the proportion in the general population.
- We have added both undergraduate- and graduate-level courses in multicultural issues and have expanded other courses to integrate these concepts into the broader curriculum, although a more systematic review of all of our courses is in order.
- Multicultural issues have become frequent topics in our program and departmental seminars and colloquia.
- Faculty and students are pursuing research on multicultural topics and are considering the impact of ethnicity and cultural factors on research where multicultural issues are not the focus of the study.
- Multicultural practica during the summers have given students an opportunity to train with national scholars who have expertise in providing clinical services to diverse populations and in conducting research on multicultural issues.

- The proportion of students from underrepresented ethnic backgrounds has increased from two (7%) to four (16%).
- A total of 14 students completed an intensive traineeship program in multicultural training as part of their graduate studies in clinical psychology. Seven of the trainees (50%) were pursuing additional specialization in neuropsychology; of those seven, three trainees (42%) were ethnic minorities (two of Pacific Islander origin, one of Hispanic origin). Five of the trainees (36%) completed an additional three-month full-time summer training experience at a nationally reputed site serving diverse ethnic populations; of those five summer trainees, three (60%) were ethnic minorities specializing in neuropsychology.
- We have begun systematically recruiting undergraduates from minority backgrounds into summer research mentorships.

Future directions
Although we are encouraged by the progress we have seen, this is only a beginning. There are some initiatives that did not realize their potential:
- Our minority enrollments still lag far behind the national proportions of ethnic minorities in the general population of the U.S. In particular, African-American and Hispanic-American students continue to be grossly underrepresented in our program.
- We have yet to demonstrate that multicultural issues are addressed throughout our entire curriculum.
- We do not have a systematic plan to ensure adequate training in cultural sensitivity in our practicum training.
- We do not have a systematic plan to assess the extent to which students and faculty are internalizing these principles or to which their overt behavior is changing.

First Steps Toward a Multicultural Neuropsychology

The challenge of building a new, ethnically diverse neuropsychology will not be easy. Recruiting more ethnic minorities into neuropsychology training is not a matter of simply offering a supplemental stipend in postdoctoral fellowships, or even in graduate training programs. Students from ethnic minority backgrounds are more encouraged to pursue a career when they see other minorities in that profession. Currently, ethnic minorities comprise only 7% of the APA Division of Clinical Neuropsychology (American Psychological Association Research Office, 1998).

This raises the question of how we increase the number of academic neuropsychologists. To succeed in an academic appointment in many Ph.D. programs in clinical neuropsychology, new faculty must produce quality research and publish in scholastic journals. These skills are not acquired overnight, which brings us back in circular fashion to recruiting and retaining more graduate students from ethnically diverse backgrounds, who are not as inclined to enter graduate programs unless they see ethnic diversity in the faculty. Furthermore, the research skills required for succeeding in an academic appointment are not acquired at all if someone does not have the vision of an academic career early in their training.

Undergraduate recruitment and preparation

We propose that the diversification of neuropsychology must begin with involving more ethnic minority *undergraduate* students in neuropsychological research. At a minimum, this can be done informally by current neuropsychologists on faculty at clinical psychology training programs and at medical centers that are near graduate training programs. More formal programs like the SROP described earlier in this chapter offer the advantages of (1) formulating discrete training goals and structured training experiences to help students develop their skills in scientific reasoning and methods and (2) creating a community of ethnically diverse researchers. Ethnic minority scholars could be invited to talk about their research activities and careers with these young developing scholars. When such programs can be linked among a network of multiple institutions, the community grows. Teleconferences during the year can provide a cost-effective method for bringing in guest speakers, and an annual conference can bring all of these ethnically diverse students together to experience the community in a more tangible, visible way. In that setting, the excitement and vision of what the field could look like becomes clearer, and the role that each of those students can play in making the vision a reality becomes evident.

Other programs also exist for recruiting undergraduates. The Division of Minority Opportunities in Research of the National Institute of General Medical Sciences (NIGMS) contains two sections aimed at increasing the number of minority biomedical scientists: *Minority Access to Research Careers (MARC)* and *Minority Biomedical Research Support* (MBRS) Branch. The latter subdivision offers several funding mechanisms, such as the Initiative for Minority Student Development (IMSD) Program, the Support of Continuous Research Excellence (SCORE) Program, and the Research Initiative for Scientific Enhancement (RISE) Program. All of these programs and funding mechanisms support research training opportunities for students and faculty from minority groups who are underrepresented in biomedical research and encourage the development and/or expansion of innovative programs to improve the academic and research competitiveness of underrepresented minority students and to facilitate their progress toward careers in biomedical research.

As yet another and more formal approach, our advisory council has recommended forging links between undergraduate institutions with large ethnic minority enrollments and graduate programs in clinical neuropsychology. Undergraduate students with great potential could be identified early in their undergraduate careers. At the end of their sophomore year, they could be recruited into a program like the SROP where they would start working with faculty in the neuropsychology training program directly. Given the questions raised about the predictive validity of GRE scores for ethnic minority applicants (Dollinger, 1989), this would give students an opportunity to demonstrate their knowledge, competency, and aptitude in a real-world setting. Clinical programs might even offer admission to a special BS/Ph.D. program to the students who show the most aptitude for neuropsychological research; college juniors could be admitted into a joint program and begin working more intensively on research in the graduate neuropsychology program while completing their Bachelor's degree. A similar model is in place for medical training at University of Missouri – Kansas City (UMKC), and federal agencies have recently issued requests for proposals to develop these undergraduate – graduate institutional links for promoting minority scholarship development in particular.

Internship and postdoctoral training
Although the multicultural training initiatives described here are being tested in a graduate program, many of these same initiatives could be implemented in internships and postdoctoral fellowships. Postdoctoral fellowships, in particular, can play a unique role in recruitment, namely through respecialization. For example, postdoctoral faculty might identify and recruit minority clinicians who have shown interest in and potential for research and mentoring; such neuropsychologists who may have pursued primarily practitioner roles after graduation could pursue advanced research training to prepare them for academic roles. Similarly, minority psychologists who trained as general clinical psychologists or in another specialty such as health psychology (or even developmental neuropsychology or neurophysiology) could be recruited into postdoctoral fellowships to respecialize in clinical neuropsychology.

Continuing education
This chapter – and our training initiatives – strongly emphasized formal training in graduate school, with the suggestion that many of these strategies could apply to internships and postdoctoral fellowships. As another component of our project, we provided continuing education training to clinicians throughout Indiana by bringing colloquium speakers to campus and by sponsoring workshops at focal points in the community (e.g., Division of Mental Health, State Vocational Rehabilitation Services). All neuropsychologists require continuing education to stay abreast of changes and innovations in the field. The majority of clinicians would likely benefit from workshops and continuing education courses specifically designed to address multicultural issues and state-of-the-art practices with patients from culturally different backgrounds. Such courses could keep the clinician current on new research, propose new models, and review widely used neuropsychological instruments (and those coming out on the market) with regard to cultural appropriateness.

Twelve steps to a multicultural neuropsychology

In this volume, many scholars have described the impact of ethnic and cultural factors on the science and practice of clinical neuropsychology. Clearly, there are many issues to address, and there is much work to be done. But we stand a better chance of getting this work accomplished and of maintaining a contemporary and informed multicultural agenda if there are more neuropsychologists of color among our ranks. This points to the importance of recruitment, training, and retention of people of color in the field. In this chapter, we implemented training initiatives derived from an NIMH model and provided initial empirical data in support of their efficacy. If more programs will consider pursuing such multicultural initiatives, we can build a more diverse field of neuropsychology. In our experience thus far, we would emphasize the following twelve steps toward developing a multicultural training program in neuropsychology:

1. *Establish a Multicultural Training Committee (MTC).* While multicultural training cannot rest solely on the shoulders of a few faculty, we believe that it is helpful and essential for a core group of faculty (a Multicultural Training Committee) to spearhead program changes and to oversee multicultural training initiatives. Members of this committee could pursue seats on other strategic committees in the department and university to help provide ongoing input into the development of policies and curricula. One way to ensure that a multicultural focus is actively maintained is to schedule "Multicultural Issues" to appear on the program and department meeting agendas at least once per semester, if not at every meeting.

2. *Establish connections with higher administration.* Securing a commitment for the multicultural training initiatives from higher administration is essential for any innovations to succeed. It is unlikely that our hiring initiatives would have succeeded if we had not had the commitment from the higher administration to create the position, to provide part of the bridge monies to support the position during the grant period, and to fund the salary line permanently after the grant expired. Furthermore, it was critical for the prospective faculty members from minority backgrounds to see that the academic community (especially the administration) is receptive to diversity and even committed to supporting diverse faculty and student populations. Furthermore, the introduction of new courses must meet with acceptance from the administration, perhaps tolerating low enrollments initially until a new multicultural course draws the attention of a larger student constituency.

3. *Recruit and retain faculty from diverse backgrounds.* Faculty from diverse backgrounds are critical to systemic change, not only serving as role models to students but also to provide essential input into program, departmental and university policies and to help foster increasing respect for cultural differences. Matching the U.S. census (projected to be 28% ethnic minorities in 2000; U. S. Bureau of the Census, 1996) would be a laudable

goal. If there is not a current faculty opening, training programs could consider hiring an adjunct faculty member in the interim.

4. *Promote the cultural climate in program materials.* Program announcements and materials should describe the cultural climate of the program, department, university, and community (e.g., proportion of students, faculty, and population of color; history of retention and graduation rates of students of color).

5. *Recruit undergraduates early.* To help guide strong scholars into the field of neuropsychology, promising undergraduate students from underrepresented backgrounds should be identified early in their undergraduate careers and should be involved in neuropsychological research under a faculty member's mentorship.

6. *Show a commitment to multicultural training on all syllabi.* Multicultural training is more than adding a single course – it requires an integration of multicultural concepts throughout the entire curriculum, including courses, research, and clinical practica. Ideally, all course syllabi would explicitly address multicultural issues (e.g., in course objectives, schedule of topics).

7. *Schedule multicultural colloquia regularly.* Multicultural topics appear regularly on departmental seminars, colloquia, and weekly clinical rounds or "Brown Bag" seminars.

8. *Recruit creatively and energetically.* Every year, faculty must energetically recruit students of color, drawing on innovative resources such as list serves, web pages, and personal contacts with undergraduate institutions where there is a significant proportion of students of color.

9. *Take risks in admissions.* Successful recruitment of students from ethnic minority backgrounds requires admissions committees to redefine the predictors of and potential for success in graduate school; this introduces some risk, but we are confident that some calculated risks are necessary. Furthermore, recruiting efforts must be proactive and energetic.

10. *Involve minority students.* Getting students of color involved in multicultural training initiatives (e.g., serving on the Multicultural Training Committee or leading a "journal club" in multicultural research) can infuse energy and excitement into the process and can help promote the students' leadership skills for continuing these initiatives when they graduate and go to new institutions.

11. *Reach out to new minority students.* To ensure the retention and success of minority students, mentorship might involve more energetic outreach (such as identifying a mentor for the student right away and getting the student linked up with a research group right away).

12. *Diversify practica training.* Practicum sites should offer substantial experience with diverse clients under the supervision of psychologists who are experienced in working with those populations.

Funding Multicultural Training Initiatives

Implementing sweeping changes in a program that lacks cultural diversity in its curriculum, faculty, and students is sure to be time- and labor-intensive. These initiatives can also be expensive, especially in the early stages. For example, bridge monies may be necessary to subsidize new faculty hires until the permanent positions can be approved or fully funded by the institution. Additional stipends and tuition remissions may be needed to increase the incentives for strong minority student applicants. Ultimately, fellowships might come from university budget lines after the training program has demonstrated success at recruiting strong students from diverse backgrounds; furthermore, individual students should be encouraged to compete externally for fellowships. Summer training experiences (either bringing in undergraduates from other institutions or sending graduate students or postdoctoral fellows to other training sites) are virtually unlimited if provision can be made for the trainee's expenses. These initiatives may ultimately be funded by the training institutions involved, but pilot funds can be helpful to demonstrate the utility and feasibility of these joint ventures. Honoraria for guest speakers may be greater in the early years of the multicultural initiatives, especially if the department hosts workshops and colloquia to enhance multicultural awareness and competency among the entire faculty. All of these examples demonstrate that additional funding can be very useful when a program is attempting to make ambitious changes, particularly during the early years. There are many resources that are available. Although these may vary from year to year, we have compiled a list of funding sources that may help to guide the search for external funding for initiatives such as these (see Appendix B).

Summary

Throughout this volume, scholars in neuropsychology have identified the complex multicultural issues that are emerging in our field. In this chapter, we have emphasized the importance of multicultural training for addressing these issues in clinical neuropsychological research and practice. We briefly described a broad model for multicultural training and several specific models of curriculum development. From these models, we designed and tested several initiatives for improving multicultural training in an existing clinical neuropsychological training program. Our preliminary outcomes suggested that some of our initiatives hold promise (two and a half years after initiating the program) and may be useful to other programs, and perhaps to internship and postdoctoral fellowship programs. Based on these early experiences, we proffered twelve steps that we regarded to be most important to our progress. We also provided interested readers with a list of potential avenues (agencies and grant mechanisms) for funding such training initiatives. It is our hope that this exchange of experiences and practical suggestions will facilitate the further diversification of the field of neuropsychology.

References

American Psychiatric Association (1994). Executive summary and recommendations. In American Psychiatric Association (Ed.), *Ethnic minority elderly: A task force report of the American Psychiatric Association* (pp. 1-19). Washington, D.C.: American Psychiatric Association.

American Psychological Association Commission on Ethnic Minority Recruitment, Retention and Training in Psychology (1996a). *How to recruit and hire ethnic minority faculty.* Washington, D.C.: American Psychological Association.

American Psychological Association Commission on Ethnic Minority Recruitment, Retention and Training in Psychology (1996b). *Valuing diversity in faculty: A guide.* Washington, D.C.: American Psychological Association.

American Psychological Association Commission on Ethnic Minority Recruitment, Retention and Training in Psychology (1997). *Visions and transformations: The final report.* Washington, D.C.: American Psychological Association.

American Psychological Association Office of Ethnic Minority Affairs (1997). Recruitment, Retention, and Training of Psychologists of Color. In APA Office of Ethnic Minority Affairs (Ed.), *Communiqué* (pp. 38-54). Washington, D.C: American Psychological Association.

American Psychological Association Research Office (1998). *1997 APA Directory Survey, with new member updates for 1998.* Washington, D.C.: American Psychological Association.

Anastasi, A. (1988). *Psychological testing.* New York: Macmillan.

Belar, C. D., & Perry, N. W. (1992). The National Conference on Scientist-Practitioner Education and Training for the Professional Practice of Psychology. *American Psychologist, 47,* 71-75.

Berry, J. W. (1994). Acculturation and psychological adaptation: An overview. In A. M. Bouvy, F. van de Vijver, Boski, P. & Schmitz, P. (Eds.), *Journeys into cross-cultural psychology* (pp. 129-141). Berwyn: Swets & Zeitlinger.

Berry, J. W. (1995). Psychology of acculturation. In N. R. Goldberger & J. B. Veroff (Eds.), *The culture and psychology reader* (pp. 457-488). New York: New York University Press.

Betancourt, H., & Lopez, S. R. (1995). The study of culture, ethnicity, and race in American psychology. In N. R. Goldberger & J. B. Veroff (Eds.), *The culture and psychology reader* (pp. 87-107). New York: New York University Press.

Boutte, G. (1999). *Multicultural education: Raising consciousness.* New York: Watsworth.

Cannon, L. W. (1994). Fostering positive race, class, and gender dynamics in the classroom. In K. A. Feldman & M. B. Paulsen (Eds.), *Teaching and learning in the college classroom* (pp. 301-306). Needham Heights, MA: Ginn Press.

Carter, R. T., & Qureshi, A. (1995). A typology of philosophical assumptions in multicultural counseling and training. In J. G. Ponterotto, J. M. Casas, L. A. Suzuki, & C. M. Alexander (Eds.), *Handbook of multicultural counseling* (pp. 239-262). Thousand Oaks: Sage.

Clay, R.A. (1997). Attracting minorities to biomedical sciences. *APA Monitor, 28*(5).

Constantine, M. G., & Gloria, A. M. (1999). Multicultural issues in predoctoral internship programs: A national survey. *Journal of Multicultural Counseling and Development, 27,* 42-53.

Copeland, E. J. (1982). Minority populations and traditional counseling programs: Some alternatives. *Counselor Education and Supervision, 21,* 187-193.

D'Alonzo, B. J., Giordano, G., & Oyenque, W. (in press). American Indian vocational rehabilitation services: A unique project. *American Rehabilitation.*

Dana, R. H. (1993). *Multicultural assessment perspectives for professional psychology.* Boston: Allyn & Bacon.

Davis, B. G. (1993). *Tools for teaching*. San Francisco: Jossey–Bass Publishers.

De La Cancela, V., & Guzman, L. P. (1991). Latina mental health service needs: Implications for training psychologists. In H. F. Myers, P. Wohlford, L. P. Guzman, & R. J. Echemendia (Eds.), *Ethnic minority perspectives on clinical training and services in psychology* (pp. 59-64). Washington, DC: American Psychological Association.

Dollinger, S. J. (1989). Predictive validity of the Graduate Record Examination in a clinical psychology program. *Professional Psychology, 20,* 56-58.

Dooley, D. (1984). *Social research methods*. Englewood Cliffs: Prentice-Hall.

Ferraro, F. R. (2001). *Minority and cross-cultural aspects of neuropsychological assessment*. Lisse: Swets & Zeitlinger.

Friedman, C. A., & Clayton, R. J. (1996). Multiculturalism and neuropsychological assessment. In L. A. Suzuki, P. J. Meller, & J. G. Ponterotto (Eds.), *Handbook of multicultural assessment: Clinical, psychological, and educational applications* (pp. 291-318). San Francisco: Jossey-Bass Publishers.

Giordano, G., & D'Alonzo, B. J. (1995). Challenge and progress in rehabilitation: A review of the past 25 years and a preview of the future. *American Rehabilitation, 21*(3), 14-21.

Green, J. W. (1995). *Cultural awareness in the human services: A multi-ethnic approach* (2nd ed.). Boston: Allyn & Bacon.

Grubb, H. J., & Ollendick, T. H. (1986). Cultural-distance perspective: An exploratory analysis of its effect on learning and intelligence. *International Journal of Intercultural Relations, 10,* 399-414.

Guzman, L. P. (1991). Incorporating cultural diversity into psychology training programs. In H. F. Myers, P. Wohlford, L. P. Guzman, & R. J. Echemendia (Eds.), *Ethnic minority perspectives on clinical training and services in psychology* (pp. 67-70). Washington, DC: American Psychological Association.

Hall, C. C. I. (1997). Cultural malpractice: The growing obsolescence of psychology with the changing U. S. population. *American Psychologist, 52,* 642-651.

Harrison, D. F., Thyer, B. A., & Wodarski, J. S. (1996). *Cultural diversity and social work practice* (2nd ed.). Springfield: Charles C. Thomas, Publisher.

Helms, J. E. (1995). Why is there no study of cultural equivalence in standardized cognitive ability testing? In N. R. Goldberger & J. B. Veroff (Eds.), *The culture and psychology reader* (pp. 674-719). New York: New York University Press.

Helms, J. E. (1997). The triple quandary of race, culture, and social class in standardized cognitive ability testing. In D. P. Flanagan, J. L. Genshaft, & P. L. Harrison (Eds.) *Contemporary intellectual assessment* (pp 517-532). New York: Guilford Press.

Heppner, M. J., & O'Brien, K. M. (1994). Multicultural counselor training: Students' perceptions of helpful and hindering events. *Counselor Education and Supervision, 34,* 4-18.

Jackson, J. S. (1991). The mental health service and training needs of African Americans. In H. F. Myers, P. Wohlford, L. P. Guzman, & R. J. Echemendia (Eds.), *Ethnic minority perspectives on clinical training and services in psychology* (pp. 33-42). Washington, D.C.: American Psychological Association.

Lin, K. M., Poland, R. E., & Nakasaki, G. (1993). Introduction: Psychopharmacology, psychobiology, and ethnicity. In K. M. Lin, R. E. Poland, & G. Nakasaki (Eds.), *Psychopharmacology and psychobiology of ethnicity* (pp. 3 - 10). Washington, DC: American Psychiatric Press.

Logan, S. L. (1996). *The Black family: Strengths, self-help, and positive change*. Boulder: Westview Press.

Manly, J. J. (1996). *The effect of African American acculturation on neuropsychological test performance*. Unpublished doctoral dissertation, University of California – San Diego and San Diego State University.

McGoldrick, M., Pearce, J. K, & Giordano, J. (1982). *Ethnicity and family therapy*. New York: Guilford Press.

Medin, D. L., & Atran, S. (1999). *Folkbiology*. Cambridge: MIT Press.

Murray, B. (1997). Educators share tips on recruiting minorities. *APA Monitor*, March, 53.

Myers, H. F. (1991b). Summary and Conclusions. In H. F. Myers, P. Wohlford, L. P. Guzman, & R. J. Echemendia (Eds.), *Ethnic minority perspectives on clinical training and services in psychology*. Washington, D.C.: American Psychological Association.

Myers, H. F., Wohlford, P., Guzman, L. P., & Echemendia, R. J. (1991). *Ethnic minority perspectives on clinical training and services in psychology*. Washington, D.C.: American Psychological Association.

Oakland, T., & Shermis, M. D. (1989). Factor structure of the Sociocultural Scales. *Journal of Psychoeducational Assessment, 7*, 335-342.

Okazaki, S., & Sue, S. (1995). Methodological issues in assessment research with ethnic minorities. *Psychological Assessment, 7*, 367-375.

Proceedings of the Houston Conference on Specialty Education and Training in Clinical Neuropsychology (1998). *Archives of Clinical Neuropsychology, 13*, 157-250.

Reports of the INS – Division 40 Task Force on Education, Accreditation, and Credentialing (1987). *The Clinical Neuropsychologist, 1*, 29-34.

Reyes, M. L., & Halcón, J. J. (1996). Racism in academia: The old wolf revisited. In C. Turner, M. Garcia, A. Nora, & L. E. Rendón (Eds.), *Racial and ethnic diversity in higher education* (pp. 337-348). Needham Heights: Simon & Schuster.

Reynolds, A. L. (1995). (1995). Challenges and strategies for teaching multicultural counseling courses. In J. G. Ponterotto, J. M. Casas, L. A. Suzuki, & C. M. Alexander (Eds.), *Handbook of multicultural counseling* (pp. 312-330). Thousand Oaks: Sage Publications.

Ridley, C. R., Espelage, D. L., & Rubinstein, K. J. (1997). Course development in multicultural counseling. In D. B. Pope-Davis & H. L. K. Coleman (Eds.), *Multicultural counseling competencies: Assessment, education and training, and supervision*, Vol. 7 (pp. 131-158). Thousand Oaks: Sage Publications.

Ridley, C. R., Mendoza, D. W., & Kanitz, B. E. (1994). Multicultural training: Reexamination, operationalization, and integration. *Counseling Psychologist, 22*, 227-289.

Salyers, M. P., & Bond, G. R. (2001). An exploratory analysis of racial factors in staff burnout among assertive community treatment case managers. *Community Mental Health Journal, 37*, 393-404.

Stewart, J. L., Anae, A. P., & Gipe, P. N. (1989). Pacific Islander children: Prevalence of hearing loss and middle ear disease. *Topics in Language Disorders, 9*(3): 76-83.

Sue, D. W., Bingham, R. P., Porché-Burke, L., Vasquez, M. (1999). The diversification of psychology: A multicultural revolution. *American Psychologist, 54*, 1061-1069.

Suzuki, L. A., Meller, P. J., & Ponterotto, J. G. (1996). *Handbook of multicultural assessment: Clinical, psychological, and educational applications*. San Francisco: Jossey-Bass Publishers.

Trimble, J. E. (1991). The mental health service and training needs of American Indians. In H. F. Myers, P. Wohlford, L. P. Guzman, & R. J. Echemendia (Eds.), *Ethnic minority perspectives on clinical training and services in psychology* (pp. 43-48). Washington, D.C.: American Psychological Association.

U. S. Bureau of the Census (1996). *Current Population Reports, Series P25-1130, "Population Projections of the United States by Age, Sex, Race, and Hispanic Origin: 1995 to 2050"*. Washington D.C.: U.S. Bureau of the Censor.

Vacc, N. A., DeVaney, S. B., & Wittmer, J. (1995). *Experiencing and counseling: Multicultural and diverse populations* (3rd ed.). Bristol: Accelerated Development.

Van de Vijver, F. (1994). Bias: Where psychology and methodology meet. In A. M. Bouvy, F. van de Vijver, P. Boski, & P. Schmitz (Eds.), *Journeys into cross-cultural psychology* (pp. 111-126). Berwyn: Swets & Zeitlinger.

Van de Vijver, F. (1997). Neuropsychology from a cross cultural perspective. *INSNET, Spring,* 3-4.

Zane, N., & Sue, S. (1991). Culturally responsive mental health services for Asian Americans: Treatment and training issues. In H. F. Myers, P. Wohlford, L. P. Guzman, & R. J. Echemendia (Eds.), *Ethnic minority perspectives on clinical training and services in psychology* (pp. 49-58). Washington, D.C.: American Psychological Association.

Appendix A

Major Approaches Used for Faculty Recruitment

- Electronic mailings were sent to list servers, organizations, universities and centers of research and training that focus on cultural and ethnic issues, rehabilitation, severe mental illness, and/or neurological populations.
- Directors of multicultural research centers were contacted individually.
- Faculty personally contacted colleagues at clinical and counseling psychology programs at universities with predominantly ethnic minority enrollments (e.g., Howard University).
- Faculty personally contacted colleagues at clinical and counseling psychology programs, internship sites, and postdoctoral fellowship sites, especially in cities with large and diverse ethnic populations such as Washington, D.C.; Philadelphia, PA; New York, NY; Chicago, IL; Detroit, MI; Miami, FL; Los Angeles, CA.
- We obtained lists of doctoral candidates in Psychology who were graduating or who had recently graduated (e.g., McKnight Fellowship recipients; participants in the Committee on Institutional Cooperation [CIC] programs). Eligible candidates were contacted by phone, and phone calls were followed with informational mailings.
- A focused search of the literature was conducted to identify over 200 experts in cultural and ethnic issues in mental health and rehabilitation. A letter and copy of the position announcement were sent to all of them, asking them to consider the position themselves and to forward the announcement to all of their colleagues who might be interested in the position.
- Advertisements were placed in the professional newspapers and newsletters, especially those targeting minority populations (e.g., newsletter for APA's Division on Minority Issues).
- Faculty recruited at national meetings throughout the year.

Appendix B

Funding Sources for Multicultural Training Initiatives

A. Specific Grant Mechanisms
   1. Rehabilitation Services Administration (RSA) Long-Term Training Grants (Pre- and Post-doctoral)
   2. National Institutes of Health (NIH) Minority Supplements (Pre- and Post-doctoral)
   3. National Research Service Awards (NRSA) Minority Fellowships (Pre- and Post-doctoral)
   4. American Psychological Association (APA) Minority Fellowships (Predoctoral only)
   5. McKnight Fellowship (Pre-doctoral, for Florida residents)

6. Committee on Institutional Cooperation (CIC) Summer Research Opportunities Program (SROP) (Pre-doctoral)

B. Agencies and Organizations with General Information and/or People to Contact
   1. National Institutes of Health (www.nih.gov)
   2. National Institute of Mental Health (www.nimh.nih.gov)
   3. National Institute of Neurological Disorders and Stroke (www.ninds.nih.gov)
   4. National Institute of General Medical Sciences (www.nigms.nih.gov)
   5. Department of Education (www.ed.gov/offices/OSERS)
      a. Rehabilitation Services Administration (RSA)
      b. National Institute on Disability and Rehabilitation Research (NIDRR)
   6. American Psychological Association (www.apa.org)

C. Specific Interest Groups – Consult agencies and organizations within the mentor's and trainee's specific interest areas (e.g., American Epilepsy Society, National Alliance for Research on Schizophrenia and Affective Disorders). Often, these organizations will have dissertation grants and fellowships for pre-baccalaureate and/or post-doctoral training, earmarked for trainees and scholars from ethnically diverse backgrounds.

D. State Agencies – Individual states may have special scholarships and grants designated to assist ethnic minorities in collegiate and graduate education.

E. Institutional resources
   1. Your host unit (e.g., School of Science, College of Social Sciences)
   2. Graduate School
   3. Department of Graduate Medical Education (for medical schools and training hospitals)
   4. Office of Financial Aid
   5. Office of Minority Affairs (may be called Ethnic Affairs, Diversity Management, etc.)
   6. Office of Grants and Sponsored Programs/Research

Chapter 19

BASE RATE ANALYSIS IN CROSS-CULTURAL CLINICAL PSYCHOLOGY:
DIAGNOSTIC ACCURACY IN THE BALANCE

Wm. Drew Gouvier, James B. Pinkston,
Michael P. Santa Maria and Katie E. Cherry
Department of Psychology, Louisiana State University,
Baton Rouge, Louisiana

Abstract

Most clinicians would agree that an accurate diagnosis of psychological disorders depends upon sound clinical judgment, combined with the outcome of reliable and valid diagnostic tests. Another, often overlooked factor that has a direct influence on accuracy of diagnosis is the base rate of the disorder type in the population. Base rates are defined as the number of people with the condition divided by the number of people in the reference population, and are a statistic reflecting current population prevalence. In this chapter, we consider the influence of base rates on diagnostic accuracy, with special emphasis on the effect of differential base rates in minority and specialty groups on the diagnostic enterprise. In the first section, we discuss base rates from a historical and practical perspective. To illustrate the influence of base rates on diagnostic accuracy in special populations, we consider the differential diagnosis of Alzheimer's disease (AD) and multi-infarct dementia (MID) in Caucasian and African-American populations. Next, we present information on differential diagnosis of schizophrenia among persons with and without mental retardation (MR). These examples are used to demonstrate how base rate information can be used to aid in the selection of diagnostic measures, and also to show the dramatic impact that differing base rates can have on overall diagnostic accuracy. The chapter concludes by revisiting the issues of differential base rates in cross-cultural psychology.

Introduction

When using psychological tests to detect or diagnose mental disorders, reliability and validity of the test instruments are offered as crucial concepts necessary to ensure that the diagnostic enterprise is a worthwhile pursuit. With reliability setting a theoretical upper limit on validity, replicable consistency of measurement (reliability) helps to ensure that, provided the test measures what it purports to measure (validity), the diagnostic enterprise is likely to yield better results than we would expect to obtain by chance alone. When a test's results are known to correlate with its ultimate diagnostic classification outcomes, the test is thought to be a valid test (Faust & Nurcombe, 1989).

A casual review of the neuropsychological research literature on test reliability and validity reveals a high proportion of studies that compare the test performance of N people with condition X versus N controls without condition X. Under such circumstances, where the proportion of people with condition X is the same as the proportion of people without condition X, the reliability and validity of the test are the sole determinants of the test's diagnostic accuracy in detecting condition X. We were all trained to think this way, and this scenario describes the prototypical situation in which the professor asks the graduate students to look at a problem, "holding all other things equal," or when the student reads research papers on the diagnosis of X that use balanced or equal N designs. Under these conditions, where reliability and validity rule the roost because the N's of the diagnostic categories are equal, and the efficacy of the test is determined by its validity coefficient alone, when the validity coefficient (which is inherently constrained by the reliability coefficient) is .9, more of the classifications are accurate than when it is .7, or .5, and so on. As we approach the range where a test's validity in identifying condition X becomes increasingly marginal, the situation changes. When differentiating between members of two groups of equal numbers (half with the condition and half without the condition), using a test that is accurate only 50% of the time would be of no value to the diagnostic enterprise as its results would be no better than those obtained by chance alone. However, this same test, showing 50% accuracy in identifying persons with or without condition X, could still have some diagnostic value for use in classifying people who were distributed proportionally among FOUR different groups, only one of which is composed of persons with condition X. Classification of this sample by chance alone, or by using base rate information alone, would be accurate 25% of the time, while classification using the test would be twice as accurate at 50%. This example demonstrates how the base rate of the condition being diagnosed exerts an influence on the diagnostic accuracy of the test being used to diagnose the condition.

Base rates can be mathematically defined as the number of persons with the condition divided by the number of persons in the reference population. They are a statistic reflecting current population prevalence of the condition of interest.

The relationship between condition base rate and diagnostic accuracy is affected by the base rate itself, as well as by the classification accuracy (based on reliability and validity) of the test or measure being used (Meehl, 1954). The effect of base rates operates to skew diagnostic accuracy in favor of predictions to the more prevalent category, and to reduce accuracy of predictions to the less prevalent category (Faust & Nurcombe, 1989). These effects are depicted in Table 1, which shows the resultant diagnostic accuracy under conditions where base rates vary from 5% to 50%, and test accuracy (under ideal circumstances of BR = 50%) varies from 60% to 90%.

Referring to Table 1, under conditions where the test is 80% accurate, but the base rate of the condition is only 15%, diagnostic judgments that the condition is present based solely on the test results are, more probably than not, wrong. This principle applies whether considering the results of a single test with 80% accuracy, or a battery of tests which, taken in composite, yield an overall 80% accuracy rate. The previous example clearly demonstrates how a test can be reasonably reliable and valid, but still not add to diagnostic accuracy. This introduces the concept of test effectiveness. Test effectiveness is in the same league as reliability and validity in determining diagnostic accuracy, but has received relatively little attention in the psychological literature. The effectiveness of a test is established by whether the overall diagnostic accuracy achieved by using the test exceeds

Table 1. The relationship between condition base rate and diagnostic accuracy.

	Condition State	Base Rate of Condition X		
		.50	.15	.05
Test Accuracy = 80%				
Likelihood of Correct	Present	80%	41%	17%
Identification	Absent	80%	96%	99%
Test Accuracy = 60%				
Likelihood of Correct	Present	60%	21%	07%
Identification	Absent	60%	89%	97%
Test Accuracy = 90%				
Likelihood of Correct	Present	90%	61%	32%
Identification	Absent	90%	98%	99%

Note. "Present" means the condition is truly there, "Absent" means it is not.

the accuracy achieved by using base rates alone in making diagnostic judgments (Faust & Nurcombe, 1989; Gouvier, Hayes, & Smiroldo, 1998). For
any test, there is a range of base rates within which the test is effective,
but when base rates go below or exceed the effectiveness range of a test,
diagnostic accuracy using base rate prediction alone exceeds that achieved
by using the test (Meehl, 1954).

A test is effective only when the base rate of the condition being diagnosed
exceeds the combined false positive and false negative error rate of the test
when base rates are below 50%. When base rates are above 50%, the test is
effective only when 1 minus the base rate exceeds the combined false positive
and false negative error rate. Stated mathematically:

> For base rates below 50%, test is effective when BR>FP+FN errors.
> For base rates above 50%, test is effective when 1-BR>FR+FN errors.

These considerations have potentially very significant implications when
using psychological tests to evaluate individuals who come from groups
which are known to have varying base rates for the disorders being diagnosed. Under some circumstances, where the base rate for the disorder is relatively lower for members of the group to which the individual being evaluated
belongs, tests which may be effective among individuals from groups which
have a higher base rate for the condition, may be ineffective. Conversely,
tests which are generally ineffective for diagnosing a condition because the
disorder is so infrequent in the general population, may become effective
when used with members of a sub-group which shows a generally higher base
rate for the condition. The following examples using differential diagnosis
in dementia among persons from different racial categories, and differential
diagnosis of schizophrenia among individuals with and without mental retardation will exemplify these two different sets of circumstances.

Differential Diagnosis in Dementia

Dementia is characterized by a generalized loss of cognitive functioning
which is sufficient enough in magnitude to impair social or occupational
performance (APA, 1994). It has been estimated that as many as 10% of
individuals over age 65, and as many as 50% of those over age 85 may
suffer from dementia (Heilman & Valenstein, 1993). While these values are
significant in their own right, they take on greater importance when one
considers the increasing number of older persons in today's society.

Dementia can result from a myriad of causes, such as: brain degeneration,
cerebrovascular disease, toxic exposure, metabolic disturbances, trauma,
infections, etc. Two of the most common causes are Alzheimer's Disease
(AD; a primary degenerative dementia) and multi-infarct dementia (MID;
cerebrovascular disease; Heilman & Valenstein, 1993; Lezak, 1995). For the

purposes of this example, we will concern ourselves with only AD and MID, as they account for the majority of the dementia cases seen.

Reaching an accurate diagnosis in suspected cases of dementia is a challenging problem, especially in its early stages. As its onset is often insidious, dementia may be mistaken for normal aging processes (Cherry & Smith, 1998). It may also be associated with social isolation and even shame, which further complicate its detection. At least one report indicates that up to 50% of dementia cases go unrecognized until the individual is quite severely impaired (Yeo & Gallagher-Thompson, 1996).

Advanced age is clearly tied with the presence of dementia. Race plays a role in its manifestation as well. There is strong evidence that genetics play a role in the risk of developing AD (Amaducci, Lippi, & Bracco, 1992; Terry & Katzman, 1983). Factors linked with the risk of developing MID (e.g., hypertension, diabetes) are also genetically linked and differ across races (Yeo & Gallagher-Thompson, 1996). In Caucasian populations within the United States, AD accounts for as many as 90% of all dementia cases (Evans et al., 1989). By contrast, in African-American populations within the United States, MID accounts for approximately 50% or more of dementia cases (Wallace, 1993). Correctly distinguishing between types of dementia is important for prognosis. For example, it has been reported that length of survival following diagnosis with MID is shorter than for other dementias (Lezak, 1995).

Knowing and understanding the importance of the differing base rates for the dementias will assist the clinician in making accurate diagnoses of either AD or MID (Faust, 1986). The values reported above indicate that up to 90% of Caucasian individuals over age 65 who show the clinical symptoms of dementia (e.g., general decline in cognitive functioning with memory impairment) are likely to suffer from AD (or even more if the person is quite old), though they may suffer from other causes of cognitive decline as well. The other 10% of demented Caucasians are likely to be suffering from another form of dementia, usually MID. Furthermore, if the same clinical symptoms of dementia are seen in an African-American individual, the likelihood that the cause is primarily AD is no more than 50%, as 50% or more of such cases are due to MID.

If a diagnostician were to only use the base rates for AD versus MID in Caucasians to differentiate between AD and MID in persons over age 65, he or she would do best to decide all demented Caucasians presenting to him or her had AD. The diagnostic decision of AD would be quite accurate, as the base rate for AD in Caucasians over age 65 is approximately 90%. Doing this would make the clinician correct 90% of the time, yielding only 10 misdiagnoses out of 100. Therefore, if one wishes to use a test finding or symptom to differentiate between AD and MID in a population of Caucasians over age 65, this finding must be better than 90% accurate in making this differentiation. Otherwise, it will add nothing to the classification accuracy obtained based on using the base rates for the diagnosis alone (Meehl, 1954;

Meehl & Rosen, 1955). This is necessarily true, as using a diagnostic sign with a combined error rate higher than the base rate of the condition to be diagnosed is inherently less accurate than adhering to base rate prediction alone (Faust & Nurcombe, 1989).

In the case of differentiating between AD and MID in African Americans the situation is somewhat different. Approximately 50% of dementia cases among African Americans are due to MID (Wallace, 1993). Thus, a test sign or clinical symptom which is correct 70% of the time in discriminating AD from MID will add significantly to diagnostic accuracy over base rate classification alone. Using just the base rates to differentiate between AD and MID in African Americans would essentially leave the clinician to flip a coin, as the base rates for MID, and other dementing conditions together, are split at 50%. Any method of diagnosis using a test finding or clinical symptom which is more accurate than a 50%, chance level, will add to diagnostic accuracy over base rate adherence alone in this situation. Improved diagnostic accuracy in identifying cases with MID has clear implications for treatment. For example, it provides the physician with greater confidence in making the decision to pursue a course of treatment to promote enhanced cerebral perfusion, and a fact based justification for accepting the associated risks thereof.

This example illustrates the effect a population's base rate has on the utility of a given test finding or clinical symptom in prediction. If, as in the case of persons who are Caucasian, demented, and over age 65, one finds a test finding or clinical symptom which is reasonably accurate at distinguishing between AD and MID (e.g., 80% accurate), the usefulness of this test finding or symptom is diminished when one realizes that the base rates for AD in this population is 90%. Simply going by the base rate odds and deciding to call all demented persons in this population AD will yield only ten errors out of a 100. Using the 80% accurate test sign or clinical symptom will yield 20 errors out of a hundred, a 100% increase in errors. Conversely, this same test finding or clinical symptom which yields an "unacceptable" 20% error rate among demented Caucasians over 65, still offers a noticeable improvement over base rate prediction alone among demented AfricanAmericans over 65 where the rate of AD and MID are both approximately 50%. In this situation, using the same clinical symptom produces a noticeable (250%) decrease in the error rate over base rate adherence alone and becomes quite valuable in diagnostic prediction.

Diagnosis of Schizophrenia in Mental Retardation

The second example illustrates the effect of base rates on differential diagnosis involving schizophrenia among individuals with and without mental retardation (MR). As with any disorder, patients diagnosed with schizophrenia are more likely to have received an accurate diagnosis as a function of the prevalence of the disorder in the population. The incidence of schizophrenia in the general population is 1 per 1,000 (Keith, Regier, & Rae, 1991). The point prevalence for schizophrenia spectrum disorders in the general population was reported as 1.4 per 1000 in an Italian case register study (de Salvia, Barbato, Salvo, & Zadro, 1993). A British inner-city health authority study provided general population prevalence estimates for schizophrenia of 4.7 per 1,000 for 1986 and 5.1 per 1,000 for 1991 (Jeffreys et al., 1997).

In a multi-center study involving a psychiatric population, sensitivity of the Structured Clinical Interview for the DSM-III-R (SCID-III-R; Williams et al., 1992) was .89 and specificity was .97 (Faraone et al., 1996). The study demonstrated that as the prevalence (base rate) of schizophrenia in a population goes up, one can have more faith in the accuracy of a diagnosis of schizophrenia by DSM criteria – sensitivity increases as a function of prevalence of the condition. The more persons with schizophrenia there are in a population, the more confident one can be that a diagnosis of schizophrenia is accurate. However, one should have increasing faith in a diagnosis of "not schizophrenia" by DSM criteria as a function of decreasing prevalence of the condition in a population. The less common schizophrenia is in a group of people, the more likely it becomes that a diagnosis of "not schizophrenia" will be accurate.

Consider, for example, that a large (n=2000) sample of psychiatric patients is available and the prevalence of schizophrenia in this sample is 19%, the same prevalence as reported in the Faraone et al. (1996) study. In this case our base rate squares would look like those in Table 2. Sensitivity (true positives / true positives + false negatives) = 338 / (338 + 42) = .89. Specificity (true negatives / true negatives + false positives) = 1571 / (1571 + 49) = .97. Of the 387 cases in which a diagnosis of schizophrenia is made (true positives + false positives), the diagnosis of schizophrenia is accurate in 338 of 387 cases, or 87.3% of the time.

Let us assume for the moment that the diagnostic accuracy of the SCID-III-R for schizophrenia achieved with the inpatient psychiatric sample (Faraone et al., 1996) is applicable to the general population. If a large (n=2,000) epidemiological study were conducted and the sole criterion for the diagnosis of schizophrenia were the SCID-III-R, we might find something like what appears in Table 2. Table 3 assumes the same sensitivity of .89 and specificity of .97, but employs the lower and computationally more conserva-

Table 2. A base rate example for diagnosing schizophrenia.

Person's actual condition		SCZ	not SCZ
Test says:	SCZ	338	49
	not SCZ	42	1571

Note. N=2000. SCZ=schizophrenia.

Table 3. A second base rate example for diagnosing schizophrenia.

Person's actual condition		SCZ	not SCZ
Test says:	SCZ	9	60
	not SCZ	1	1930

Note. N=2000. SCZ=schizophrenia.

tive prevalence of 5.1 per 1,000 which was reported in the Jeffreys et al. (1997) study. Sensitivity (true positives / true positives + false negatives) = 9 / (9 + 1) = .89. Specificity (true negatives / true negatives + false positives) = 1930 / (1930 + 60) = .97. In this case, of the 39 cases in which a diagnosis of schizophrenia is made (true positives + false positives), the diagnosis is accurate in 9 of 39 cases, or 23.1% of the time.
Insert Table 3 about here

Why is there such a disparity in accurate diagnoses of schizophrenia between the two examples? The higher prevalence of schizophrenia in the inpatient sample facilitated higher diagnostic accuracy. In the general population, false positives for a diagnosis would likely occur among: 1) persons with a history of substance abuse, 2) people who have been prescribed prescription drugs with significant psychotropic side effects, 3) people who have experienced psychotic features consistent with severe major depression, or 4) demented persons who
frequently report perceptual disturbances and possibly decreased personal hygiene or social interest.

The SCID-III-R is different from pure self-report instruments [e.g. Scale 8 (Schizophrenia) of the Minnesota Multiphasic Personality Inventory - 2 (MMPI-2; Butcher, Dahlstrom, Graham, Tellegen, & Kaemmer, 1989)] in that the skill of the examiner is important to diagnostic accuracy. Lay examiners, as are often employed in large population-based epidemiological studies, would be more prone to make the aforementioned misdiagnoses *when working with both members of the general population and psychiatric inpatient samples.* In clinical settings, diagnostics is generally facilitated by the luxury of combining standardized assessment instruments with a wealth of background information and clinical and collateral interview data. The preceding examples assume that sensitivity and specificity are constant across disparate prevalence rates, though this may not necessarily be the case (Kraemer, 1992). Nonetheless, for instruments which are not affected by level of examiner skill, diagnostic accuracy necessarily changes as a function of the prevalence of a condition.

To carry the schizophrenia example one step further, consider making a diagnosis of schizophrenia in an MR population. The US Department of Education database for children 6 to 17 years of age reports the nationwide rate for MR at 11.4 per 1,000 (King et al., 1997). Even with advances in medical science, the prevalence of MR has remained relatively constant over the past 50 years. This is the case as reductions in the incidence of MR of preventable etiologies has been roughly matched by decreased mortality of high-risk infants, increased longevity of persons with MR, and the emergence of new diseases (King et al., 1997; Pulsifer, 1996). Also, by definition, persons with MR must have an IQ which is in the bottom 2.5% of the population, and since any population will have a fairly constant number of persons with an IQ in the bottom 2.5%, statistics dictate a reasonably stable prevalence for MR, though its diagnosis also requires documented impairments in adaptive functioning (APA, 1994).

Base rates for psychiatric disturbance differ between persons with and without MR. The prevalence of psychiatric disturbance in mentally retarded (MR) persons has been conservatively estimated at five times higher than that of non-retarded persons (Rutter, Tizar, Yule, Graham, & Whitmore, 1976). Reid (1972) reported a point prevalence of schizophrenia in MR adults of 32 per 1,000. Bregman (1991) quoted a more conservative figure of 20-30 per 1000. Heaton-Ward (1977) reported the incidence of schizophrenia in MR adults to be 34 per 1,000 per year. The higher prevalence of psychopathology in MR populations can provide a basis to illustrate how base rates factor into an instrument's diagnostic accuracy.

In MR populations, the diagnosis of psychiatric conditions by traditional means has been criticized on the grounds that traditional techniques are of low validity and lead to improper treatment decisions (Boshes, 1987; Hill, Balow, & Bruininks, 1985; Linaker & Helle, 1994; Moucha, 1985). Thus, more recently, brief behavior checklists for the screening of psychiatric conditions in MR populations have been developed and validated. The Schizophrenia scale of the Psychopathology Instrument for Mentally Retarded Adults (PIMRA; Senatore, Matson, & Kazdin, 1985) is a brief, simple, seven-item yes/no checklist. A modified version of the PIMRA has been demonstrated to correctly classify 75.5% of MR adults as schizophrenic versus non-schizophrenic (sensitivity=68.4%, specificity=93.3%; Linaker & Helle, 1994). Although the diagnostic accuracy of the PIMRA with MR clients is lower than that of traditional instruments such as the SCID-III-R and the Research Diagnostic Criteria (RDC; Spitzer, Endicott, & Robins, 1978) for the diagnosis of schizophrenia in non-MR adults (Faraone et al., 1996), there are two primary considerations which, in combination, make the simple checklist-type instruments such as the PIMRA superior to traditional instruments for the assessment of schizophrenia in MR adults. The difficulty associated with MR patients' verbal comprehension of traditional instruments yields low validity for these instruments (Boshes, 1987; Hill et al., 1985; Linaker & Helle, 1994; Moucha, 1985). This fact combined with the higher base rate of psychiatric conditions (e.g. schizophrenia) in MR populations permits the use of an alternate assessment protocol for psychopathology in MR individuals. The use of shorter, simpler diagnostic instruments, which do not posses the level of discriminant validity needed to be effective when used for diagnostic purposes within the low base rate general populace, can still be appropriate for the diagnosis of comorbid psychopathology in persons with MR.

Summary and Conclusions

The preceding examples demonstrate that certain symptoms or test findings that are shown to be useful, appropriate, and effective tools in some circumstances, may reduce diagnostic accuracy in others. Conversely, measures that appear less useful in low base rate situations become useful diagnostic tools when the base rate increases. Thus, some measures that have utility in aiding clinical diagnoses may not be useful in population screening situations, because the error rates of the tests may be much higher than the population base rate for the disorder being screened, resulting in an unacceptably high number of false positive errors.

These considerations compel a reexamination of the method by which psychologists render clinical diagnoses. Despite our doctoral-level training, human capacity for making accurate judgments remains severely limited and constrained by a multitude of factors of which most are wholly unaware (Faust, 1984). The classroom examples and equal-N research reports we are all exposed to have inadvertently trained members of our profession to ignore the effect of base rates on diagnostic accuracy. It is a poor match to the real world when psychologists make judgments as if our test's accuracies were as good as the reliability and validity coefficients cited in our journal articles. We can no longer hold our heads in the sand and act like our clients have a 50/50 chance of having condition X. We can no longer rely on our published reliability and validity statistics as sufficient justification for using any particular test, because if the base rate of the condition being diagnosed is lower than the test's combined error rate (as is very frequently the case), more probably than not, our diagnostic conclusion will be wrong. As clinicians, we become obligated to take base rate considerations into account when interpreting test findings, and we must recognize that the diagnostic skew introduced by the base rates must sometime claim the lion's share of the variance in our diagnostic judgment.

Nonetheless, base rates should guide diagnostic judgments, and not rule them (Faust & Nurcombe, 1989), and the problems presented by base rate influence are not insurmountable (Gouvier et al, 1998). As diagnosticians, knowing about these effects compels us to become responsible in managing and accounting for them, and this forces us to follow the advice of Emirel Lagasse and "kick it up a notch" in our diagnostic practice. Failure to do so, by each and every one of us, will doom our profession to continue to knowingly engage in incompetent practice, and will possibly lead to the practice of clinical psychology being delegated to the dustbin of "junk science" (Gouvier, 1999).

References

Amaducci, L., Lippi, A., & Bracco, L. (1992). Alzheimer's disease: Risk factors and therapeutic challenges. In M. Bergener (Ed.), *Aging and mental disorders: International perspectives*. New York: Springer.

American Psychiatric Association (1994). *Diagnostic and statistical manual of mental disorders: DSM-IV* (4th ed.). Washington, D.C.: American Psychiatric Association.

Boshes, R. A. (1987). Pharmacotherapy for patients with mental retardation and mental illness. *Psychiatric Annals, 17,* 627-632.

Bregman, J. D. (1991). Current developments in the understanding of mental retardation part II: Psychopathology. *Journal of the American Academy of Child Adolescent Psychiatry, 30,* 861-872.

Butcher, J. N., Dahlstrom, W. G., Graham, J. R., Tellegen, A., & Kaemmer, B. (1989). *Minnesota Multiphasic Personality Inventory-2 (MMPI-2): Manual for administration and scoring*. Minneapolis: University of Minnesota Press.

Cherry, K. E., & Smith, A. D. (1998). Normal memory aging. In M. Hersen & V.B. Van Hasselt (Eds.), *Handbook of clinical geropsychology* (pp. 87-110). New York: Plenum Press.

de Salvia, D., Barbato, A., Salvo, P., & Zadro, F. (1993). Prevalence and incidence of schizophrenic disorders in Portogruaro: An Italian case register study. *Journal of Nervous and Mental Disease, 181,* 275-282.

Evans, D. A., Funkenstein, H. H., Albert, M. S., Scherr, P. A., Cook, N. R., Chown, M. J., Hebert, L. E., Hennekens, C. H., & Taylor, J. O. (1989). Prevalence of Alzheimer's disease in a community population of older persons. *Journal of the American Medical Association, 262,* 2551-2556.

Faraone, S. V., Blehar, M., Pepple, J., Moldin, S. O., Norton, J., Nurnberger, J. I., Malaspina, D., Kaufmann, C. A., Reich, T., Cloninger, C. R., DePaulo, J. R., Berg, K., Gershon, E. S., Kirch, D. G., & Tsuang, M. T. (1996). Diagnostic accuracy and confusability analyses: An application to the Diagnostic Interview for Genetic Studies. *Psychological Medicine, 26,* 401-410.

Faust, D. (1984). *The limits of scientific reasoning*. Minneapolis: University of Minnesota Press.

Faust, D. (1986). Leaning and maintaining rules for decreasing judgment accuracy. *Journal of Personality Assessment, 50,* 585-600.

Faust, D., & Nurcombe, B. (1989). Improving the accuracy of clinical judgment. *Psychiatry, 52,* 197-209.

Gouvier, W.D. (1999). Baserates and clinical decision making in neuropsychology. In J. Sweet (Ed.), *Forensic neuropsychology: Fundamentals and practice*. New York: Elsevier.

Gouvier, W. D., Hayes, J., & Smiroldo, B. (1998). The significance of baserates, test sensitivity, test specificity, and subjects' knowledge about symptoms in assessing TBI sequelae and malingering. In C. Reynolds (Ed.), *Detection of malingering during head injury litigation*. New York: Plenum Press.

Heaton-Ward, A. (1977). Psychosis in mental handicap. *British Journal of Psychiatry, 130,* 525-533.

Heilman, K. M., & Valenstein, E. (1993). *Clinical neuropsychology* (3rd ed.). New York: Oxford University Press.

Hill, B. K., Balow, E. A., & Bruininks, R. H. (1985). A national study of prescribed drugs in institutions and community residential facilities for mentally retarded people. *Psychopharmacology Bulletin, 25,* 279-284.

Jeffreys, S. E., Harvey, C. A., McNaught, A. S., Quayle, A. S., King, M. B., & Bird, A. S. (1997). The Hampstead Schizophrenia Survey 1991: I. Prevalence and service use comparisons in an inner London Health Authority, 1986-1991. *British Journal of Psychiatry, 170,* 301-306.

Keith, S.J., Regier, D.A., & Rae, D.S. (1991). Schizophrenic disorders. In L.N. Robins & D.S. Rae (Eds.), *Psychiatric disorders in America: The epidemiological catchment area study.* New York: The Free Press.

King, B. H., State, M. W., Shah, B., Davanzo, P., & Dykens, E. (1997). Mental retardation: A review of the past 10 years. Part I. *Journal of the American Academy of Child and Adolescent Psychiatry, 36,* 1656-1663.

Kraemer, H. C. (1992). *Evaluating medical tests: Objective and quantitative guidelines.* Newbury Park: Sage Publications.

Lezak, M. D. (1995). *Neuropsychological assessment* (3rd ed.). New York: Oxford University Press.

Linaker, O. M., & Helle, J. (1994). Validity of the schizophrenia diagnosis of the Psychopathology Instrument for Mentally Retarded Adults (PIMRA): A comparison of schizophrenic patients with and without mental retardation. *Research in Developmental Disabilities, 15,* 473-486.

Meehl, P. E. (1954). *Clinical versus statistical prediction: A theoretical analysis and review of the evidence.* Minneapolis: University of Minnesota Press.

Meehl, P. E., & Rosen, A. (1955). Antecedent probability and the efficiency of psychometric signs, patterns, or cutting scores. *Psychological Bulletin, 52,* 194-216.

Moucha, S. (1985). Issues in pharmacology with the mentally retarded. *Psychopharmacology Bulletin, 21,* 262-267.

Pulsifer, M. B. (1996). The neuropsychology of mental retardation. *Journal of the International Neuropsychology Society, 2,* 159-176.

Reid, A. H. (1972). *The psychiatry of mental handicap.* Oxford: Blackwell Scientific Publications.

Rutter, M., Tizard, J., Yule, W., Graham, Y., & Whitmore, K. (1976). Research report: Isle of Wight studies, 1964-1974. *Psychological Medicine, 6,* 313-332.

Senatore, V., Matson, J. L., & Kazdin, A. E. (1985). An inventory to assess psychopathology of mentally retarded adults. *American Journal of Mental Deficiency, 89,* 459-466.

Spitzer, R. L., Endicott, J., & Robins, E. (1978). Research diagnostic criteria: Rationale and reliability. *Archives of General Psychiatry, 35,* 773-782.

Terry, R. D., & Katzman, R. (1983). Senile dementia of the Alzheimer type. *Annals of Neurology, 14,* 497-506.

Wallace, G. L. (1993). Neurological impairment among elderly African-American nursing home residents. *Journal of Health Care for the Poor and Underserved, 4,* 40-50.

Williams, J. B. W., Gibbon, M., First, M. B., Spitzer, R. L., Davies, M., Borus, J., Howes, M. J., Kane, J., Poper, H. G., Rounsaville, B., & Wittchen, H. (1992). The structured clinical interview for DSM-III-R (SCID). II. Multisite test-retest reliability. *Archives of General Psychiatry, 49,* 630-636.

Yeo, G., & Gallagher-Thompson, D. (1996). *Ethnicity and the dementias.* Washington D.C.: Taylor & Francis.

Chapter 20

LOOKING FOR THE THREADS:
COMMONALITIES AND DIFFERENCES*

Rosalie J. Ackerman, Ph.D., and
Martha E. Banks, Ph.D.
ABackans Diversified Computer Processing, Inc.,
Akron, Ohio

Abstract

This chapter provides a brief review of the foci and recommendations from the other contributors to this book. Specific focal points include:
- Nature, purpose, and cultural implications of assessment
- suggestions for test administrators
- approaches to empirical normative database development
- demographic concerns beyond ethnicity
- impact of psychiatric disorders on neuropsychological function
- repercussions of misdiagnosis/mistreatment/idiosyncratic errors

The final portion of the chapter is an overview of the development of the Ackerman-Banks Neuropsychological Rehabilitation Battery for use with African-American and European-American adults.

---

*The authors contributed equally to this chapter. Throughout the chapter, the terminology used for various ethnic groups reflects that used by the authors of the original articles.

Commonalities and Differences (and Omissions)

Nature, purpose, and cultural implications of assessment

Testing has very different meanings for people with various cultural experiences. Banks (2000b) observed that:

> 'Good neuropsychological assessment leads to a set of functional strengths and weaknesses which can be used to develop effective treatment planning. If a person is evaluated with a test that was normed on a group of people who are significantly different from that person, the test results should not be considered valid. In neuropsychology, the tests are generally normed on middle to upper class white men who experienced societal advantages, including social values, similar to those of the test developers. As a result, many African Americans perform relatively poorly on neuropsychological tests even in the absence of neurological impairment. That is because the tests assume a certain level of baseline function, some of which is based on experiences which are not available to many African Americans. Therefore, it is possible for African Americans to be considered as having more functional weaknesses and fewer strengths than they actually have. If they are not evaluated as having adequate strengths to benefit from rehabilitation, they are unlikely to be referred for treatment. In this way, neuropsychological assessment is used as a gatekeeping mechanism to determine who will and who will not enter rehabilitation.'

Poreh (2001) observed that the meaning of neuropsychological assessment is determined by the cultural identity of the individual, the cultural meaning of the illness, and cultural elements of the relationship between the individual and the clinician. The vast majority of neuropsychologists are European-American. Members of ethnic minority cultures are likely to be reluctant to engage in neuropsychological assessment due to a long history of European-American exploitation of ethnic minorities (Allen, 1994; Ferraro, Bercier, Holm, & McDonald, 2001; Gardiner, Tansley, & Ertz, 2001). It is critical to consider that the meaning of brain dysfunction is informed on an individual basis by religious and/or spiritual beliefs (see Escandell, 2001, for examples of cultural implications of seizure disorders). As a result, such dysfunction can be perceived, for example, as a challenge to be overcome, a deserved punishment, or fate.

In addition to the perception of the assessment process from the perspective of the clients, one must examine the perceptions of the neuropsychologist. As Lamberty (2001) noted, the use of neuropsychological assessment has evolved over the last 50 years. Early assessments, which took five to seven hours to administer, were designed to determine the presence or absence of brain dysfunction and/or to differentiate between 'organic' and psychiatric problems. Later, two- to four-hour neuropsychological assessment focused on the localization of brain damage; that application is still critical for assessment prior to neurosurgery. Current applications involve identification of patient strengths and weaknesses in order to develop recommendations for rehabilitation, psychotherapy, and family interventions. This shift is particularly important for members of many cultures in which assessment without treatment is unconscionable. While traditional neuropsychologists perceive the field as including only assessment with an emphasis on testing, assessment is only part of a treatment process. Rehabilitation psychologists and other medical treatment staff use the results of neuropsychological assessment for the development of treatment plans and the monitoring of clients' progress during and after formal rehabilitation. Poreh (2001) observed that there is a need for multicultural rehabilitation. The treatment following neuropsychological assessment should clearly be as culturally relevant as the assessment.

Lamberty also described the positive and negative aspects of fixed and mixed batteries. A major consideration, which Gardiner et al. (2001) noted, is the lack of established neuropsychological assessment procedures which has resulted in poor service to many American Indians.

Suggestions for test administrators

There are several concerns about the ways in which neuropsychological tests are administered. Some of these include the culturally appropriate amount of time used to develop rapport, giving or exchanging of culturally relevant gifts, and limited time frames for actual testing.

Comfortable and respectful seating arrangements vary among cultural groups. Traditional European-American training involves placing a test table or desk between the test administrator and the client, so that they face each other. Bylsma, Ostendorf, and Hofer (2001) suggest sitting beside clients, using food as a reinforcer, and provision of childcare in Guam. Gardiner et al. (2001) recommend avoiding direct eye contact and sitting at a corner of a table with the American-Indian client seated at the narrow end of the table, with ready access to the door.

Personal contacts, especially the initial approach, are important first steps in developing rapport (Gardiner et al., 2001). Their suggestions also include observing the eye contact and grip of the handshake to determine the amount of time to spend establishing a working relationship with the client. Ferraro et al. (2001) emphasize the respect that must be demonstrated to elders through initial approach and an offering of gifts, prior to requesting participation in the assessment. They also note that looking American-Indian clients directly in the eyes is considered disrespectful.

None of the other authors specifically addressed gender concerns in the development of rapport. In some patriarchal cultures, it would be inappropriate to attempt to assess a woman without first building rapport with and getting permission from her husband, father, or the family patriarch. In Saudi Arabia, for example, decisions about participation in assessment are not made by the individuals being assessed, but are actually family decisions with which identified patients might agree or disagree (Escandell, 2001). The gender of the person conducting an assessment is an important consideration in terms of the appropriate level of eye or other physical contact.

An additional consideration is involvement of multiple people in the assessment process. Bylsma et al. (2001) describe the openness and concern of the community and a seeking of information about the results of assessment which are contrary to the European notions of confidentiality. They also note that sometimes it is appropriate to include families in the assessment sessions. Echemendia and Julian (2001) address the importance of developing rapport with parents prior to formal assessment with Latino children; they recommend scheduling one or two hours of pretest interview in order to maximize family cooperation and test performance.

Time is a critical variable with meaning that varies significantly among cultures. Many neuropsychological tests include an emphasis on speed of response, consistent with a Eurocentric perception of the importance of quick accuracy. In many other cultures, however, the emphasis is placed on quality of responses, rather than speed. For many people, the concept of quickness is incompatible with good quality.

One consideration of the testing situation involves the goal of assessment. If the goal is to determine strengths under the best circumstances, assistive devices can be used with a recommendation that such devices be made available to the client outside of the assessment session. For example, clients who are hard of hearing might benefit from amplification during testing. Fillenbaum, Unverzagt, Ganguli, Welsh-Bohmer, and Heyman (2001), however, recommend that amplification be used for directions, but not for tasks involving repetition of spoken phrases.

Approaches to development of culturally relevant norms

As Poreh (2001) noted, most neuropsychological test norms for ethnic minorities are developed by independent researchers after the tests are marketed; such norms are not provided by test developers. The funding for the independent researchers usually involves a hypothesis-based research design, rather than exploration to generate hypotheses. In addition, the populations are narrowly circumscribed, so that, for example, people with psychiatric diagnoses are excluded (e.g., Dick, Teng, Kempler, Davis, & Taussig, 2001). The outcome of this approach is that it is not clear that the tests being developed are appropriate for the patients who present with multiple medical conditions.

Lamberty (2001) indicated that there is a need for empirically based approaches to neuropsychological assessment (see also American Educational Research Association (AERA), American Psychological Association (APA), & National Council on Measurement in Education (NCME), 1999). Wolfe (2001) outlined three approaches to empirically developing culturally relevant neuropsychological assessment measures:

1. Modification of existing tests was the approach used by Ardila, Rodriguez-Mendendez, and Rosselli (2001); Dick et al. (2001); Echemendia and Julian (2001); and Murai, Hadano, and Hamanaka (2001).
2. Development of new tests was demonstrated by Ackerman and Banks (1989, 1992b, 1994a); Banks and Ackerman (1991); and Gutierrez (2001).

3 Norm development of existing tests was conducted by Bylsma et al. (2001);
   Ferraro et al., (2001); Fillenbaum et al., (2001); Gardiner et al., (2001);
   Lichtenberg, Ross, Youngblade, and Vangel (1998); Salmon, Galasko, and
   Wiederholt (2001); Strickland, D'Elia, James, and Stein (1997); and Wolfe
   (2001).

Demographic concerns beyond ethnicity

Several contributors indicated that it is inappropriate to conduct comparisons of ethnic groups without regard to examining the diversity within those
groups or the consideration of qualitative differences between groups. This
section is subdivided into some of the variables which should be considered
in culturally relevant neuropsychological assessment. It is important to note
that many of the variables interact with each other and serve as confounding
variables in the determination of causation of symptoms. As a result, it is
incumbent upon neuropsychologists to always include examination of the
patients' perceptions of changes in function, with a specific focus on loss or
degradation of premorbid functioning, *even in areas which are not currently
included in traditional neuropsychological tests.*

Manly and Jacobs (2001) clearly stated that group comparisons do not
explain or examine reasons for differences. Gutierrez (2001) added that it is
inadequate to merely measure the cultural distance between groups; qualitative examination should determine whether or not a specified function is
actually being measured in all groups involved in comparative studies. Dick
et al. (2001) indicated that intragroup differences are usually greater than
intergroup differences.

One emphasis is on the need to move beyond antiquated notions of biological 'race' to an acknowledgment that assessment of people must include
attention to cultural factors. The concept of ethnicity is a first step in this
process, but, as Manly and Jacobs (2001) observed, consideration of immigration status from Africa or the West Indies is seldom examined in studies
of African Americans. Federal classification schemes (prior to the 2000 U.S.
Census) ignore 'cultural, socioeconomic, educational, or racial experiences'
(Manly & Jacobs, 2001, p. 83). Furthermore, there is minimal attention paid
to cultural status of African Americans relative to urban or rural U.S. or
Canadian African Americans or members of other ethnic groups. Ardila et
al. (2001) and Echemendia and Julian (2001) note similar diversity among
Latinos/Hispanics, whose cultures are based in different countries and dia-
lects of Spanish.

Gender

Lamberty (2001) noted that gender concerns in neuropsychological assessment need to be addressed. Fillenbaum et al. (2001) observed that women
performed better than men on the Word List Learning. Strickland et al.
(1997) found that African-American women performed better than African-
American men on Stroop Color Naming and Word Reading. Miles (2001)

noted that African-American women are at greater risk for stroke than African-American men up to age 75 years. The above research supports the concern that ethnicity should be disaggregated by gender; similar to the ethnic comparative research, however, it does *not* provide an explanation for the gender differences.

Age

There are two primary groups for which age is considered a major concern in neuropsychology: children and elderly adults. For children, the primary issue is determination of developmental progression, whereas, for elderly adults, the focus is on differentiating between normal aging and dementia (see Bylsma et al., 2001; Dick et al., 2001; Fillenbaum et al., 2001; Salmon et al., 2001; Wolfe, 2001). Williams and Bowman (2001) noted that there were differences in cognitive functioning between rural and urban children in the United States and Nigeria until they reached eleven years of age; beyond that age, cognitive functioning was equivalent.

Escandell (2001) noted that the concept of age as used by United States pediatric neuropsychologists is quite different from that in the Saudi Arabian culture. Age in Saudi-Arabia is linked to general historical events so that children's ages are accurate to within two years. As a result, the U.S. practice of developmental norms based on months or days is not applicable for this population.

One issue which is seldom addressed is cohort effect. In addressing the concerns of older women, Banks (2000a) noted that:

> 'In the 1970s, programs were developed in gerontologic psychology, focusing on healthy aging. The 1980s and early 1990s saw a funding shift to geriatric psychology, with an emphasis on the assessment and treatment of dementia...This change in focus of training funds has resulted in some interesting cohort effects. Psychologists with a positive health focus have information on people born before World War One and whose early middle age was during the Depression. Psychologists trained to examine the negative side of aging trained with people whose childhoods were during the Depression and whose young adulthood was during World War Two. In other words, our strongest knowledge about aging involves two generations who lived through very different times.'

In Guam, Bylsma et al. (2001) observed that the older indigenous people typically had only two or three years of formal education. Ferraro et al. (2001) found a cultural cohort effect in that 80-89 year old Native Americans had more education than their Non-Native counterparts, whereas 60-79 year old Non-Natives had more education than their Native counterparts.

Education

Education accounts for high proportions of variance in performance on neuropsychological tests (Dick et al., 2001; Escandell, 2001; Fillenbaum et al., 2001; Salmon et al., 2001). This is reflected in part in the literacy of ethnic minorities and bilinguals (Poreh, 2001). It is inappropriate to equate education across cultures (Dick et al., 2001; Fastenau, Evans, Johnson, & Bond, 2001; Manly & Jacobs, 2001).

Lamberty (2001) described education as a 'protective factor' in the evaluation of dementia in older adults. There is a concern, however, that rather than being a 'protective factor', education can actually mask early dementia in highly educated people, functioning as a 'cloaking device' rather than a 'neuroprotective poultice'. Miles (2001) noted that African Americans with less than eight years of formal education showed greater cognitive decline across twelve years than those with more education.

Wolfe (2001) found that less educated people sometimes perform like some brain-injured patients on neuropsychological tests. Echemendia and Julian (2001) documented the impact of education on a variety of language functions as well as calculation, fine visual motor movements, and finger alternation.

Socioeconomic status

There is often an assumption that People of Color are living in poverty as much of the psychological research involving People of Color uses convenience sampling through public facilities used by poor people. This gives a very distorted picture, ignoring the impact of the social environment; as Manly and Jacobs (2001) noted, socioeconomic status is often confounded with race and ethnicity (see also Williams & Bowman, 2001). Fillenbaum et al. (2001) indicated that socioeconomic factors prevented African Americans from participating in the one year followup of their research. It is critical to examine the lifelong history of socioeconomic status. As Echemendia and Julian (2001) discussed, socioeconomic status (SES) is not static. For immigrants, it is important to examine both pre- and post-immigration SES. It should be noted that education is often an important predictor of future SES. People with poor educational backgrounds have difficulty obtaining employment which leads to high income (Ardila et al., 2001).

Low socioeconomic status results in poor nutrition and limited access to quality health care (Echemendia & Julian, 2001; Fastenau et al., 2001). Poor nutrition leads to metabolic deficiencies which are reflected in poor attention and concentration, poor memory, visual degradation, and attenuation of sensorimotor function.

Language

Ardila et al. (2001) observed that poor education in either English or Spanish results in no language mastery. Murai et al. (2001) noted that reading performance in aphasic patients was influenced by the grade levels at which they were taught morphemes and phonemes. Echemendia and Julian (2001) addressed specific impact of education on language comprehension, phonological discrimination, naming, repetition, verbal fluency, buccofacial movements, and ideomotor praxis. Therefore, language mastery and education are highly correlated and have considerable impact on neuropsychological test performance.

Lamberty (2001) and Escandell (2001)wrote that it is inappropriate to merely translate tests without attention to culture or good understanding of the second language's morphology and syntax. Gutierrez (2001) applied this concept through a combination of translation based on idiomatic, rather than literal, meanings, followed by backtranslation (see also Wolfe, 2001). The original Luria-Nebraska Neuropsychological Battery (Golden, Purisch, & Hammeke, 1985) failed to take this into consideration; some of the test items are taken from literal English translations of Luria's Russian texts (Luria, 1973 (p. 293), 1980 (p. 476)). Phonemic relationships among the words in Russian are lost in the literal English translations.

One linguistic consideration involves the actual structure of the language and the amount of energy required to speak individual words. Escandell (2001) described the impact of such simplistic translation as changing the difficulty of test items as Arabic grammar changes the lengths of sentences. Furthermore, the actual language used by an Arab patient is socially specific, similar to the differential uses of familiar and formal French. In the development of Cross-Cultural Neuropsychological Assessment Battery, Dick et al. (2001) translated and backtranslated an English, American-based test into Chinese, Vietnamese, and Spanish. They noted that the Chinese and Vietnamese members of the research pool had the best performances on Digit Span Forward; in Chinese and Vietnamese, the words for the numbers one through nine are monosyllabic, whereas in Spanish, the words for seven of those numbers are multisyllabic. Similarly, in Arabic, the words for colors and numbers are all multisyllabic (Escandell, 2001). People speaking Spanish had worse performance than those speaking other languages. Murai et al. (2001) provided case examples of aphasia in bilingual speakers of Japanese and Korean. Due to the agglutination approach to syntax in Japanese, it is possible to assess dissociation of phonemes (discrete sounds) from morphemes (meaningful groups of sounds). The authors found that there were significant differences in the processing of Japanese and Korean; as aphasics recovered, they regained different aspects of the two languages.

Level of language knowledge and formality of language impact on the ability to perform well on neuropsychological tests. Manly et al. (1998) demonstrated that the use of Black English, clearly a cultural and not a neurological factor, impacted negatively on performance of Trail Making Test – Part B and the WAIS-R Information subtest. Bylsma et al. (2001) found that, although people in Guam spoke English and several native and other foreign languages, their English was often casual and spoken at a level below the formal education of the speakers. Ardila et al. (2001) suggested that receptive language ability be tested in both languages for bilingual children and older people; the neuropsychological assessment should be conducted in the stronger language. Echemendia and Julian (2001), on the other hand, suggest testing in both languages, if possible.

Within languages, there are a variety of dialects. Manly et al. (1998) described the impact of Black English on neuropsychological test performance. Ardila et al. (2001) detail some critical differences among the Spanish dialects from various countries. They provided examples of words which have very different meanings from one country to another as well as the combining of languages into combinations which have only specific local meaning. It is critical to develop normative samples for each subculture (Ardila et al., 2001; Echemendia & Julian, 2001; Manly & Jacobs, 2001; Poreh, 2001).

Bilingualism (and by extension, multilingualism) creates a special set of problems in neuropsychological assessment. There is a continuum of language mastery in bilingualism. Some people speak one language well both formally and informally and another language well informally; whereas others speak both languages only passably both formally and informally. There are differences in mastery depending upon the contexts and ages at which each language is learned. For example, in some areas of the United States, immigrant adults speak a native language in the home, in community activities, and in religious settings, but speak English while attending school and/or working. Children in such homes learn to use the native language informally and English relatively formally, especially if all of their exposure to English is in school. Many Europeans are multilingual due to their proximity to other countries. Upon immigration, many speak some English, but it is modified by other languages used in a variety of settings. In Africa, a similar pattern of multilingualism is noted, due to small community-based languages and the development of intercommunity languages, as well as those imposed by Europeans. In terms of neuropsychological assessment, Ardila et al. (2001) cited research indicating that bilingual people perform worse on tests than monolingual people. Ardila et al. (2001) indicated that it is critical that neuropsychological reports contain specific statements about degree of bilingualism of people being tested.

There are several ethical concerns involved in the use of translators and the handling of translation. Ardila et al. (2001) indicated that simultaneous translation is unethical. Echemendia and Julian (2001), while acknowledging that there are few bilingual neuropsychologists, caution against using family members as translators due to violation of confidentiality and bias in the translations. They also warn that it is not appropriate to use untrained paraprofessionals as translators.

Acculturation

Several authors address the issue of acculturation as movement away from ethnic traditions and toward the dominant European American culture (Ardila et al., 2001; Echemendia & Julian, 2001; Manly & Jacobs 2001). However, many researchers examining ethnic identity consider ties to ethnic traditions and biculturalism in which people are able to function well both within ethnic and dominant cultures (Cross, 1994; Helms & Piper, 1994; Markstrom-Adams & Adams, 1995).

Neurotoxic exposure

In Guam, Salmon et al. (2001) observed that people were exposed to cycads and aluminum through the manufacture of food products and that the diets were low in calcium and magnesium. Although Guam has been the site of considerable military activity for more than 60 years, there is no mention by Salmon et al. (2001) or Bylsma et al. (2001) of the possible exposure to toxic waste byproducts of military weapons and equipment (Hartman, 1995, 1998). This problem has recently been noted in Hawaii and Puerto Rico with serious health impact on indigenous people (Trask, 2000). The biodegradation of military waste could account in part for the high rates of amyotrophic lateral sclerosis in the 1950s and the decrease since then.

Stress

Manly and Jacobs (2001) address stereotype threat as a stressor for African Americans. Echemendia and Julian (2001) described acculturation stress, similar to stereotype threat. While the research on stereotype threat has been used to provide an explanation of score differences between African Americans and European Americans, it is seldom placed in perspective with the impact of unrelenting racism, in part manifested through differential quality of education, experienced by African Americans (Whaley, 1998). Bylsma et al. (2001) noted that high work pressure leads to strokes and heart attacks. Williams and Bowman (2001) described the impact of economic uncertainty on stress and socioeconomic status for rural populations. Fastenau et al. (2001) observed the high rate of hypertension in African Americans; the lack of medical coverage and limited access to rehabilitation put them at risk for disabling conditions resulting from chronic hypertension.

Rural living conditions

Williams and Bowman (2001) addressed the unpredictable weather conditions which impact on agricultural economics. Other neuropsychological issues include exposure to neurotoxins (e.g., pesticides, hormones, fertilizers, lead-based petroleum products) (Ackerman, 1998) and traumatic brain injuries sustained in farm accidents (Bylsma et al., 2001).

Impact of psychiatric disorders on neuropsychological function

Dick et al. (2001) excluded people with histories of psychiatric problems from their research, yet many patients with neurological problems have experienced psychiatric difficulties, including substance abuse and alcohol dependence. For example, Bylsma et al. (2001) noted that there is a high frequency of depression leading to suicide and a high prevalence of schizophrenia in Guam. Older American Indians tend to be less depressed than their European-American counterparts (Ferraro et al., 2001); that might be due, in part, to the difference in social status accorded older people. In traditional American-Indian cultures, older people are treated with considerable respect, whereas European-American cultures tend to disrespect older people. Gardiner et al. (2001) documented the impact of depression, substance abuse, and other psychiatric disorders on neuropsychological test performance. It is important to appreciate the prevalence rates of psychiatric disorders among members of populations, as neuropsychological assessment should include at least screening for such disorders (Gouvier, Pinkston, Santa Maria, & Cherry, 2001).

Misdiagnosis

Dick et al. (2001) cautioned about the potential of misdiagnosis in the absence of appropriate tests or adequate normative data. Echemendia and Julian (2001) further noted that if there is any language comprehension and/or expression difficulty, there is high risk for misdiagnosis. It is critical that there be consonance among the language of the test, the language of the test taker, and the language of the test administrator. For rural populations, the Bender often misclassified patients as brain damaged if they had low levels of education, were African-American, or older (Williams & Bowman, 2001). Miles (2001) indicated that disparities from the dominant culture (middle-class European American young to middle adulthood males) increase the risk of misdiagnosis.

Escandell (2001) directly addresses one of the most important cultural variables that leads to misdiagnosis. Behaviors and beliefs that are acceptable in one culture are considered symptoms of illness in another. The examples of responses to hexing, evil eye, and Zar or Gin are considered normal behavior in some cultures, but would be misdiagnosed as psychosomaticism, paranoia, and dissociation by U.S. trained health professionals. Similar misdiagnoses have occurred with the misinterpretation of slang from one culture to another. Normal expressions of spiritual beliefs in some cultures are misperceived as symptoms of religiosity.

Echemendia and Julian (2001) found that highly educated adults with traumatic brain injury scored at the same level as noninjured members of low SES groups. However, for people in Guam, Salmon et al. (2001) found that socioeconomic status had no impact on MMSE performance after controlling for education.

Poreh (2001) cautioned that the use of measures of malingering can lead to misdiagnosis in cross-cultural applications. The decision-tree approach to neuropsychological assessment which includes assessment of malingering can quickly lead to misdiagnosis of minorities. In European-American cultures, especially for males, physical/medical distress is minimized as a cultural norm. Behaviors which are culturally appropriate for other cultures, such as not hiding one's discomforts from others, are apt to be misinterpreted on malingering measures based on the European-American concept. As a result, there is a risk that ethnic minority people are perceived as exaggerating real problems, whereas they are sincerely *not minimizing* those problems, deserve to have their symptoms taken seriously, and are in need of appropriate culturally relevant treatment.

There has been a long-standing problem of lack of neuropsychological assessment for victims of violence despite evidence of open- and closed-head injuries, extended loss of consciousness, and concussion (Abbott, 1997; Ackerman, 1996; Ackerman and Banks, 1994b, 1996, 2000; Ackerman, Banks, & Corbett, 1998; Banks, 1999, 2000b; Banks & Ackerman, 1996a, 1996b; Banks, Ackerman, & Corbett, 1995; Campbell & Soeken, 1999; Covington, Maxwell, Clancy, Churchill, & Ahrens, 1995; Escandell, 2001; Koss, Ingram, & Pepper, 1997; Kyriacou et al., 1999; Monahan & O'Leary, 1999; Muelleman, Lenaghan, & Pakieser, 1996). Such victims have been diagnosed as having posttraumatic stress disorder, with no further psychological evaluation. The professionals who work with victims are seldom sophisticated about neuropsychology. As a result, they do a disservice to victims by not providing or referring them for neuropsychological assessment which could lead to rehabilitation. This is particularly a problem for women and girls of all ethnicities and for ethnic minority men and boys, as they are more likely to be victims of interpersonal violence than European American men. Greenfeld et al. (1998) noted that 'rates of nonlethal intimate violence are highest among black women' (p. 11) (see also Dennis, Key, Kirk, & Smith, 1995; Marsh, 1993; Raj, Silverman, Wingood, & DiClemente, 1999).

Development of the Ackerman-Banks Neuropsychological Rehabilitation Battery

Nature, purpose, and cultural implications of assessment

The 85-item Ackerman-Banks Neuropsychological Rehabilitation Battery was developed to provide a valid, efficacious screening instrument, for the rehabilitation setting, with minimal assessment time (45 to 90 minutes) and cost for patients. Unlike other neuropsychological tests which are designed to determine the presence and/or actual site(s) of brain injury, the Ackerman-Banks Neuropsychological Rehabilitation Battery serves to reflect neurobehavioral strengths and weaknesses of patients in order to quickly develop treatment plans and generate referral questions for in-depth assessment and treatment by specialists. The battery can also be used to monitor progress during and after treatment and to contribute to determination of competence.

The Ackerman-Banks Neuropsychological Rehabilitation Battery is designed to be administered to patients suspected of or previously diagnosed as having neurological or neuropsychological impairment. Unlike traditional neuropsychological tests designed for differential diagnosis of neuropsychological impairment and/or localization of brain dysfunction, the Ackerman-Banks Neuropsychological Rehabilitation Battery is specifically designed for the determination of levels of functioning/disability, development of rehabilitation recommendations, and the monitoring of progress in treatment.

Feedback for patients and their families after formal assessment is facilitated through multimedia software which demonstrates the interrelationships among neurobehaviors and neuroanatomy (Banks & Ackerman, 1995). The Ackerman-Banks Neuropsychological Rehabilitation Battery has been used in rehabilitation inpatient and outpatient, medical inpatient, and psychiatric inpatient and outpatient settings. It is anticipated that research using the Ackerman-Banks Neuropsychological Rehabilitation Battery will lead to broader applications.

The test includes items for tasks controlled by the left and right hemispheres in relatively equal balance. Items were added to include emotionality, such as anxiety, depression, impulsivity, and frustration tolerance. The test evolved across twelve years and was refined in response to questions generated by multidisciplinary treatment teams during the development of individual treatment plans and discussions of the rehabilitation process.

In the Ackerman-Banks Neuropsychological Rehabilitation Battery, several neuropsychological concepts are assumed. Brain functioning is based on Lurian (Luria, 1973, 1980) principles. As a result, brain-injured patients are regarded as having functional strengths and weaknesses. It is expected that each patient can serve, to a certain extent, as her or his own baseline. As a group, therefore, brain injured patients present a wide range of strengths and weaknesses. In addition, rehabilitation treatment staff compare current patients to past patients in order to assess performance and prognosis. The range of abilities of people without known brain injury adds little to the information about the widely diverse brain-injured population.

Based on this philosophy, it is appropriate to use this population as its own normative sample for evaluation of functioning. The Ackerman-Banks Neuropsychological Rehabilitation Battery was developed using such a normative sample. This test was developed with a normative sample consisting exclusively of brain-injured patients. This is consistent with the notion that brain-injury is not a unitary concept, but that brain-injured patients have strengths and weaknesses based on the location, causes, and severity of their injuries. In addition, as the test is intended for use with patients referred for rehabilitation, it was deemed appropriate to use that population as the normative sample.

Important features of the battery include the use of large print, alternative modes of providing instruction, and enlarged visual stimuli which are especially appropriate for the assessment of geriatric patients. Information from test scales can be made directly available to rehabilitation staff for the development of treatment plans utilizing strengths and weaknesses reflected in the patients' profiles.

In keeping with the foresight of Matarazzo (1992, p. 1013), the Ackerman-Banks Neuropsychological Rehabilitation Battery is designed to '...validly measure the following: (a) Efficiency in receiving information through different sense modalities, (b) ability to hold that information in immediate storage (capacity for attention and concentration), (c) efficiency in processing that information, and (d) ability to execute the verbal or motor operations required to complete one's response to the item presented.' Right hemisphere functions are also included as recommended by Diller (1992) in his Centennial Lecture on 'Stroke and Rehabilitation'.

The Ackerman-Banks Neuropsychological Rehabilitation Battery has consistency and validity to measure neuropsychological functioning relevant to strengths useful for rehabilitation, activities of daily living, monitoring of progress in rehabilitation, and reentry in vocational endeavors. The utility of this test is demonstrated through the use of a clinical normative population as opposed to extrapolation from a 'normal' sample. A clinical population provides a more accurate basis for generalization and prediction than does extrapolation from an unrelated population. Clinical and statistical maxima were not reached on the summary scales (Attention/Concentration, Left Hemisphere, Right Hemisphere, and Neuropsychological Status) by any of the patients (see Table 1); this reflects the clinical nature of the normative sample.

Suggestions for test administrators

The goal of the Ackerman-Banks Neuropsychological Battery is to determine the best possible function of the client. Both aural and visual amplification are encouraged. There is a certain amount of testing of limits built into the test. For example, all timing is designed to encourage quality performance, rather than neurophysiological reaction time.

Assessment is considered the duty of the psychologist. As a result, most of the work involved in the administration and scoring depends on the psychologist who must attend to multiple aspects of client responses. For example, a task such as the writing of one's name is scored for legibility, size of letters, spelling, the need for visual instructions in addition to or instead of auditory instructions, and the time taken to write the name. Each of those discrete scores loads on one or more of the neuropsychological function scales which are listed below.

Makeup and impact of the Ackerman-Banks Neuropsychological Rehabilitation Battery

Forty-three scales were formulated to provide detailed information about different aspects of neuropsychological performance. Each of the 85 test items is scored on positive dimensions with various levels to generate a representative measure of the patients' skills with 462 scoring dimensions. The scoring involves multiple facets of each test item. For example, items which are administered orally all load on the auditory input scale, whereas all those administered visually load on the visual input scale. Some items are administered in more than one modality and load on all appropriate scales. The types of approaches used by the patient and errors encountered for each test item are taken into account in the development of the scoring protocol. There is a strong emphasis on assessing the abilities of the patient, with a focus away

Table 1. Normative scores for the A-BNRB scales (N=300).

	Mean	(SD)	SEM	Minima	Maxima	Highest Possible
Alertness						
Attention/Concentration	592.98	(156.55)	9.04	111	897	1020
Prosody						
Receptive Prosody	13.90	(5.92)	0.34	0	26	26
Expressive Prosody	26.62	(7.59)	0.44	0	37	37
Memory						
Long-term Memory	20.52	(5.74)	0.33	1	28	28
Short-term Interference Memory	58.88	(17.35)	1.00	9	104	116
Short-term Input Memory	82.95	(24.01)	1.39	11	127	129
Short-term Retrieval Memory	66.13	(19.84)	1.15	5	108	114
Sensorimotor						
Auditory Input	114.30	(28.29)	1.63	17	156	166
Auditory Discrimination	92.56	(22.85)	1.32	18	133	137
Tactile Input	29.89	(10.67)	0.62	0	46	46
Tactile Output	76.66	(19.49)	1.13	20	113	118
Visual Input	123.16	(33.29)	1.92	31	186	197
Visual Discrimination	80.15	(23.91)	1.38	12	127	134
Visual-spatial Construction	70.36	(16.54)	0.96	12	104	113
Proprioception	68.46	(18.79)	1.09	12	101	102
Motor Quality	150.06	(36.36)	2.10	47	222	247
Motor Writing	39.56	(15.53)	0.90	2	72	83
Speech						
Speech Production	176.30	(41.74)	2.41	37	240	251
Dysarthria	68.96	(27.75)	1.60	7	98	98
Dysnomia, Neologisms	63.29	(16.23)	0.94	1	79	79
Confabulation	33.72	(5.57)	0.32	10	40	40
Perseveration	19.93	(6.20)	0.36	0	27	27
Lisping	7.91	(0.57)	0.03	1	8	8
Academic Abilities						
Mathematics	43.91	(16.01)	0.92	0	74	78
Reading	51.53	(16.46)	0.95	0	73	74
Writing	53.18	(17.55)	1.01	2	81	82
Cognitive Problem Solving						
Concreteness	17.89	(7.01)	0.41	0	34	34
Integration	178.07	(51.72)	2.99	25	288	342
Judgment	33.48	(10.27)	0.59	5	55	61
Speed	64.29	(24.96)	1.44	0	115	135
Organic Emotions						
Depression	59.16	(20.63)	1.19	4	103	110
Anxiety	46.64	(14.73)	0.85	5	79	84
Impulsivity	16.27	(2.24)	0.13	8	20	20
Laterality						
Left-Right Confusion	8.96	(3.54)	0.20	0	15	15
Left-Brain Controlled Balance	40.61	(12.64)	0.73	0	64	64
Right-Brain Controlled Balance	39.42	(14.57)	0.84	0	65	65
Left Hemisphere	410.10	(100.15)	5.78	75	575	619
Right Hemisphere	335.83	(88.34)	5.10	97	512	547
Neuropsychological Status	129.60	(36.29)	2.10	17	195	221
Treatment Problems						
Peripheral Control	13.36	(1.88)	0.11	0	14	14
Awareness of Deficits	69.13	(10.04)	0.58	0	85	85
Socially Inappropriate Comments	83.35	(3.53)	0.20	54	85	85
Frustration Tolerance	79.02	(7.24)	0.42	38	85	85

from the deficit model that is the foundation of many psychological tests. This is consonant with rehabilitation philosophy.

Neuropsychological functions include Alertness (Attention/Concentration), Memory (Long-term, Short-term Interference, Short-term Input, and Short-term Retrieval Memory), Sensorimotor (Auditory Input, Auditory Discrimination, Tactile Input, Tactile Output, Visual Input, Visual Discrimination, Visual-spatial Construction, Proprioception, Motor Quality, and Motor Writing), Speech (Speech Production, Dysarthria, Dysnomia and Neologisms, Confabulation, Perseveration, and Lisping), Academic Abilities (Mathematics, Reading, and Writing), Cognitive Problem Solving (Concreteness, Integration, Judgment, and Speed), and Laterality (Left-Right Confusion, Left-Brain Controlled Balance, Right-Brain Controlled Balance, Left Hemisphere, Right Hemisphere, Neuropsychological Status). Organic Emotions (Depression, Anxiety, and Impulsivity), Prosody (Receptive and Expressive Prosody), and Treatment Problems (Peripheral Control, Awareness of Deficits, Socially Inappropriate Comments, and Frustration Tolerance), functions seldom included in neuropsychological batteries, are used to determine patients' behavioral approaches to stressful tasks and to predict how well patients will respond in rehabilitative programs. Normative scores for all of the scales in the battery are provided in Table 1. Details of the validity and reliability studies are provided in the professional and training manuals for the test (Ackerman & Banks, 1994a, 2000).

In response to the criticisms of Lezak (1995) and other neuropsychologists (e.g., Matarazzo, 1992), this test does not give one overall score for all dimensions of neuropsychological functioning; it provides multiple sampling of behavior across an interval of test time rather than limiting the patient to only one opportunity to score correctly or incorrectly. Lezak (1995) noted that 'Only by treating each patient as a unique individual can the neuropsychological examiner hope to address the variety of issues and patient needs that prompted the examination and the enormous variations in patients' capacities and characteristics...' (p. 4).

The test scales were developed clinically, rather than statistically through the use of factor analysis. As each test item loads on multiple scales, there is high intercorrelation among the scales. This is consistent with the observation by Gutierrez (2001) that all cognitive functions of the brain can be seen as overlapping.

Approaches to development of culturally relevant norms

Most neuropsychological batteries are normed on nonclinical populations composed primarily of middle to upper SES European American men with at least 12 years of education. The Ackerman-Banks Neuropsychological Rehabilitation Battery was normed on a clinical population that included 47% women and 17% African Americans. This approach addresses the concern of Poreh (2001) that test developers should provide information about the performance of ethnic minorities as part of the original material included with the test, rather than merely marketing a test normed on a homogeneous population or failing to disaggregate test results.

As the battery is electronically scored by the publisher, an electronic record exists for all administered tests (Banks & Ackerman, 1991). It is easy, therefore, to develop local norms when an adequate number of batteries are administered. With slightly larger samples, more precise local norms, based on specific demographic subgroups, can be calculated. It is strongly recommended that other test publishers consider using this approach to updating normative samples and providing test administrators with norms relevant to their clinical populations.

The Ackerman-Banks Neuropsychological Rehabilitation Battery was developed with the intent that a person with a fifth-grade education could easily complete all items without error and in a short period of time. Adults without brain injury would be expected to attain maximal scores with little meaningful variation; such performance by members of that population would not provide a reasonable comparison standard against which to measure performances of brain-injured people.

The test developers recognized that overlooked populations in need of neuropsychological assessment and rehabilitation include victims of interpersonal violence some of whom (such as victims of intimate partner violence) suffer repeated brain injuries (Abbott, 1997; Campbell & Soeken, 1999; Covington et al., 1995; Monahan & O'Leary, 1999) similar to those found in athletes playing contact sports (Collins et al., 1999; Kelly, 1999; Matser, Kessels, Jordan, Lezak, & Troost, 1999; Matser, Kessels, Lezak, Jordan, & Troost, 1999; Powell & Barber-Ross, 1999). In addition, several patients in the normative sample had experienced exposure to neurotoxins, such as cleaning chemicals, pesticides, and solvents (Hartman, 1995; Lezak, 1995; Reidy, Bowler, Rauch, & Pedroza, 1992; Valciukas, 1991). This is a problem for people who work in housekeeping, agricultural, and dry-cleaning jobs, as well as those working in or living near refineries or toxic-waste dumps. Members of lower socioeconomic classes, overrepresented by People of Color, are at highest risk for exposure to neurotoxins.

Use of tests for various forms of brain dysfunction
The normative sample included both outpatients and inpatients with a variety of brain compromises, including head injuries, strokes, and neurodegenerative diseases (Ackerman, 1998; Ackerman & Banks, 1992a, 1995; Banks & Ackerman, 1997). The goal was to develop an assessment procedure normed on typical neuropsychological rehabilitation patients. Unlike localization-focused batteries, the normative sample included patients with multiple sites and sources of brain injury. Many patients had multiple diagnoses reflective of progressive health compromise, such as nicotine use, substance abuse, hypertension, and heart attacks.

Demographic concerns

The normative sample for the Ackerman-Banks Neuropsychological Battery consisted of 300 inpatients and outpatients on the rehabilitation units of two private medical centers and a federal government medical and domiciliary hospital program. The group consisted of adults (age range of 17 to 91 years) with an average age of 60.8 ± 17.0 years and 11.8 ± 2.8 years of education. Formal, classroom education was used to determine level of education; people who obtained GEDs were only credited with the years in which they attended school. The authors noted, however, that using years of classroom education did not address the quality of that education.

It should be noted that the majority (63.6%) were 60 years old or older. Seventeen percent of the participants were African American and 82.6% were European American; members of other ethnic groups were not referred for assessment during the eight years of data collection. The normative sample was 47.3% female and 92.9% right-handed. Thirteen percent were single, 45.5% married, 17.7% separated or divorced, and 23.7% widowed. Twenty percent were disabled prior to evaluation, 40.1% were retired, 1.7% were employed part time, 23.6% were employed or in school full time, and 9.8% were homemakers. Professionals made up 17.9% of the sample, business people 15.9%, blue collar/clerical/farmer 50.7%, homemakers 13.5%, students 1%, unemployed 0.7%, and disabled 0.3%. Seventy-eight percent of the sample population wore glasses and 53.3% wore them at the time of the evaluation. Five percent usually wore hearing aids and 6.3% wore them during their evaluations; some of the people who wore hearing aids and/or amplifiers during the evaluation preferred not to wear them most of the time or had received them shortly before assessment.

Detailed demographics including marital status, usual occupation, occupational status, and use of glasses and hearing aids are in Table 2.

Performance on the Ackerman-Banks Neuropsychological Rehabilitation Battery poorly discriminated between genders (75.7%, Wilks' $\Lambda = .68$, $p < .01$; see Table 3), African Americans and European Americans (70.2%, Wilks' $\Lambda = .86$, $p < .01$; see Table 4), combined ethnic-gender groups (56.2%, Wilks' $\Lambda = .87$, $p < .01$; see Table 5), and did not discriminate among age groups (44.0%, Wilks' $\Lambda = .96$, n.s.; see Table 6), education levels (52.4%, Wilks' $\Lambda = .96$, n.s.; see Table 7), and combined age-education groups (45.6%, Wilks' $\Lambda = .77$, n.s). It should be noted that age and education were not significantly correlated ($r = 0.03$, n.s.)

These results provide support for the utility of this battery with a variety of people without penalty for low education level or advanced age. For ethnicity and gender, although the discrimination was statistically significant, the level of correct classification was too low to be considered a clinical concern. Test performance was examined to determine if there were ethnic, gender, and/or combined ethnic and gender differences in performance. Significant group differences were found in age, education, and six of the test scales (see Table 8).

Table 2. Normative sample demographics (N=300).

	Mean	Standard Deviation	Minimum	Maximum
Age	60.8	17.0	17	91
Education	11.8	2.8	2	21
Age				
17 – 19 years		1.0%		
20 – 29 years		4.7%		
30 – 39 years		10.7%		
40 – 49 years		10.0%		
50 – 59 years		10.0%		
60 – 69 years		24.3%		
70 – 79 years		30.3%		
80 – 91 years		9.0%		
Education				
Elementary		4.3%		
Some high school		25.0%		
High school graduate		41.3%		
More than high school		28.7%		
Ethnicity				
African-American		17.4%		
European-American		82.6%		
Gender				
Female		47.3%		
Male		52.7%		
Ethnicity and Gender				
African-American female		7.0%		
African-American male		10.4%		
European-American female		40.1%		
European-American male		42.5%		
Marital Status				
Single		13.0%		
Married		45.5%		
Separated/divorced		17.7%		
Widowed		23.7%		
Handedness				
Right		92.9%		
Left		5.4%		
Mixed		1.7%		
Glasses				
Usually wear		77.7%		
Myopia correction		54.0%		
Presbyopia correction		66.3%		
Wearing at evaluation		53.3%		
Hearing Aid(s)				
Usually wear		5.0%		
Wearing at evaluation		6.3%		
Usual Occupation				
Professional		17.9%		
Business		15.9%		
Blue collar/clerical/farmer		50.7%		
Homemaker		13.5%		
Student		1.0%		
Disabled		0.3%		
Unemployed		0.7%		
Occupational Status				
Retired		40.1%		
Disabled		19.9%		
Full-time employed/school		23.6%		
Homemaker		9.8%		
Unemployed		4.7%		
Part-time Employment		1.7%		

Table 3. Gender classification. ($N = 300$).

	Predicted Group Membership	
	Female	Male
Actual Group Membership		
Female	105	37
Male	36	122

Correct classification 75.67%.

Table 4. Ethnicity. ($N = 300$).

	Predicted Group Membership	
	African American	European American
Actual Group Membership		
African American	37	15
European American	74	173

Correct classification 70.23%.

Table 5. Ethnicity and gender combined. ($N = 300$)

	Predicted Group Membership			
	African American		European American	
	Female	Male	Female	Male
Actual Group Membership				
African American female	13	2	2	4
African American male	4	21	4	2
European American female	24	13	65	18
European American male	7	29	22	69

Correct classification 56.19%.

Ethnicity
There were two differences between ethnic groups. The African Americans ($M = 57.87$ year) were, on average, younger than the European Americans ($M = 61.74$ years) ($F_{(1, 296)} = 4.06$, $p < .05$). African Americans had better Left-Brain Controlled Balance than European Americans ($F_{(1, 296)} = 4.14$, $p < .05$).

Gender
Gender accounted for differences in both demographics and test performance. Women ($M = 64.93$ years) were significantly older than men ($M = 54.68$

Table 6. Age. ($N = 300$)

	Teens	20s	30s	40s	50s	60s	70s	80s+

| | | | | Predicted Group Membership | | | | |

Actual Group Membership

	Teens	20s	30s	40s	50s	60s	70s	80s+
17 - 19 years old	2	1	0	0	0	0	0	0
20 - 29 years old	0	12	0	2	0	0	0	0
30 - 39 years old	1	5	19	2	1	1	1	2
40 - 49 years old	0	1	5	11	7	2	3	1
50 - 59 years old	1	2	2	2	14	1	2	6
60 - 69 years old	1	6	2	5	8	24	12	15
70 - 79 years old	0	2	5	6	7	14	37	20
80 - 91 years old	0	0	2	1	3	3	5	13

Correct classification 44.00%.

Table 7. Education. ($N = 300$).

		Predicted Group Membership		
	Elementary	Some high school	High school graduate	More than high school
Actual Group Membership				
Elementary	8	3	2	0
Some high school	6	44	14	11
High school graduate	10	34	46	34
More than high school	3	11	14	58

Correct classification 52.35%.

years) ($F_{(1, 296)} = 16.04$, $p < .001$). Similarly, women ($M = 12.45$ years) had significantly more education than men ($M = 11.46$ years) ($F_{(1, 296)} = 5.14$, $p < .05$). Men exhibited better Tactile Input ($F_{(1, 296)} = 4.56$, $p < .05$), better Proprioception ($F_{(1, 296)} = 9.97$, $p < .01$), less Dysarthria ($F_{(1, 296)} = 4.14$, $p < .05$), less Left-Right Confusion ($F_{(1, 296)} = 6.94$, $p < .01$), and better Left-Brain Controlled Balance ($F_{(1, 296)} = 11.20$, $p < .001$) and Right-Brain Controlled Balance ($F_{(1, 296)} = 22.48$, $p < .001$) than women.

Ethnicity and gender
The combination of ethnicity and gender also revealed some group differences. African American women ($M = 13.00$ years) had significantly more education than any other ethnic-gender group ($F_{(1, 296)} = 4.03$, $p < .05$). African American men had significantly better Proprioception ($F_{(1, 296)} = 4.80$, $p < .05$) and Right-Brain Controlled Balance ($F_{(1, 296)} = 4.31$, $p < .05$) than members of the other ethnic-gender groups. African-American women

Table 8. Ethnic-gender means for the Ackerman-Banks Neuropsychological Rehabilitation Battery (N = 300).

	African-American		European-American		Group Differences
	Women	Men	Women	Men	
Age	65.57	50.16	64.29	59.20	G***, E*
Education	13.00	11.13	11.90	11.79	G*, G&E*
Alertness					
Attention/concentration	589.37	610.06	586.03	596.03	
Prosody					
Receptive prosody	14.38	12.58	13.95	14.09	
Expressive prosody	27.19	26.46	26.52	26.65	
Memory					
Long-term memory	21.05	20.97	20.68	20.17	
Short-term interference memory	59.86	61.32	58.35	58.62	
Short-term input memory	86.49	84.42	81.93	82.98	
Short-term retrieval memory	69.67	68.74	65.09	65.90	
Sensorimotor					
Auditory input	119.24	116.26	114.76	112.57	
Auditory discrimination	94.43	95.84	91.93	92.06	
Tactile input	27.20	32.94	29.07	30.36	G*
Tactile output	77.38	82.39	74.87	76.85	
Visual input	116.57	131.16	121.27	124.09	
Visual discrimination	76.52	83.94	79.99	79.98	
Visual-spatial construction	71.48	71.94	70.34	69.81	
Proprioception	61.67	77.03	66.55	69.32	G**, G&E*
Motor quality	149.48	159.84	145.66	151.95	
Motor writing	41.95	40.65	38.41	40.01	
Speech					
Speech production	176.33	185.45	175.24	175.06	
Dysarthria	63.81	79.52	67.21	68.91	G*
Dysnomia, neologisms	65.24	67.03	63.51	61.85	
Confabulation	34.90	32.58	33.95	33.59	
Perseveration	18.52	19.94	19.12	20.94	
Lisping	7.95	8.00	7.93	7.86	
Academic Abilities					
Mathematics	40.43	43.10	41.56	46.91	
Reading	52.05	51.81	52.91	50.07	
Writing	57.95	54.03	53.61	51.77	
Cognitive Problem Solving					
Concreteness	19.81	17.16	18.19	17.46	
Integration	173.48	178.32	176.96	179.83	
Judgment	34.62	32.19	33.93	33.18	
Speed	62.38	67.23	62.71	65.39	
Organic Emotions					
Depression	62.14	59.42	58.53	59.21	
Anxiety	44.52	47.00	45.19	48.27	
Impulsivity	16.14	15.42	16.14	16.62	

Table 8, continued.

	African-American		European-American		Group Differences
	Women	Men	Women	Men	
Laterality					
Left-right confusion	7.81	10.03	8.59	9.24	G^{**}
Left-brain controlled balance	39.00	48.26	37.98	41.50	G^{**}, E^{*}
Right-brain controlled balance	32.10	46.94	36.13	41.94	$G^{***}, G\&E^{*}$
Left hemisphere	405.21	427.58	406.50	410.08	
Right hemisphere	321.35	358.78	328.93	339.20	
Neuropsychological status	129.35	134.71	127.39	130.60	
Treatment Problems					
Peripheral control	13.48	13.26	13.60	13.13	
Awareness of deficits	68.38	69.03	68.35	70.02	
Socially inappropriate comments	83.67	84.16	82.83	83.59	
Frustration tolerance	80.77	78.10	78.45	79.49	

G = Gender.
E = Ethnicity.
G&E = Ethnicity and Gender Combined.
* $p < .05$.
** $p < .01$.
*** $p < .001$.

patients were older, more educated, more likely to be widowed, and much more physically and neuropsychologically disabled than other patients. African-American men patients were younger, had less education, were more impulsive, more likely to be divorced or separated, and did not wear their glasses for reading or watching television. These data support the hypothesis that African Americans, particularly African-American women, are more disabled than other people before being referred for rehabilitation. It also appears that African-American men become severely ill and need comprehensive rehabilitation at younger ages than other people.

Age
Important features of the battery include the use of large print, alternative modes of providing instruction, and enlarged visual stimuli which are especially appropriate for the assessment of geriatric patients. Rehabilitation strategies can be formulated for young, middle-aged, and older adults. Although the format of the Ackerman-Banks Neuropsychological Rehabilitation Battery is ideal for the development of individual educational plans, the battery has not yet been normed for use with children.

Education
The Ackerman-Banks Neuropsychological Rehabilitation Battery was developed with the intent that a person with a fifth grade education could easily complete all items without error and in a short period of time. Therefore, the test is less sensitive to education effects than other neuropsychological batteries (see Table 7).

Socioeconomic status
Patients in the normative sample included private payers as well as people receiving Medicare and Medicaid. Family income information was not available for many of the patients. Employment status and levels of employment are included in Table 2.

Language
The Ackerman-Banks Neuropsychological Rehabilitation Battery was developed in English, with consideration of vocabulary that would be appropriate for members of several ethnic groups. In addition, the language is specifically geared to a fifth grade or lower reading level to minimize interference for people with poor educational backgrounds.

Acculturation
Acculturation was not measured in the development of the battery. In the first author's testing experience, there were a number of clients who had American-Indian names and/or parents, but who did not identify as American Indians; this included clients from North and South Carolina, Pennsylvania, New York, West Virginia, and Ohio. Out of respect for their wishes, they are included as either African American or European American in the normative sample.

Impact of psychiatric disorders on neuropsychological function
Most of the patients had multiple diagnoses on Axes I and III, using DSM-III-R criteria (American Psychiatric Association, 1987). This population is representative of the types of patients referred for rehabilitation. Test items include measures of anxiety, depression, impulsivity, and frustration tolerance. It is considered the duty of the neuropsychologist to address the psychiatric concerns as part of the overall recommendations for further assessment and treatment.

Summary

This chapter reviewed neuropsychological testing which has a variety of meanings for both patients and neuropsychologists. Culturally relevant neuropsychological assessment should be the first step in the rehabilitation process. The need for the development of culturally relevant norms is increasingly evident due to population projections which indicate increasing proportions of People of Color. Due to the proliferation of computer technology, it is possible to share, exchange, and add to data sets in cooperative efforts to build increasingly specific norms. Within ethnic groups, whether imposed by federal guidelines or reflecting self identification, neuropsychologists should also attend to gender, age, education, SES, language, acculturation/ethnic identity, neurotoxic exposures, and geographic/social current and past living situations.

It is critical to carefully listen to what patients describe and to observe patient behavior in order to maximize the attainment of useful clinical information. Although building of rapport is contrary to European American neuropsychologists' 'objective' professional distance, it is an important relationship factor in many cultures.

This volume represents a giant step towards the elimination of neuropsychological misdiagnoses due to misinterpretation and misunderstanding of people who are not members of the dominant culture in U.S. society.

References

Abbott, J. (1997). Injuries and illnesses of domestic violence. *Annals of Emergency Medicine, 29*, 781-785.

Ackerman, R. J. (1996). *Neuropsychological rehabilitation with a middle aged African American woman with multiple sclerosis.* Paper presented at the 104th annual convention of the American Psychological Association, Toronto, Ontario, Canada. Abstract available: http://www.en.com/AfrAmMS.htm.

Ackerman, R. J. (1998). *Women's health: Case study of neuropsychological variables after environmental exposure.* Paper presented at the 106th annual convention of the American Psychological Association, San Francisco.

Ackerman, R. J., & Banks, M. E. (1989). *Ackerman-Banks Neuropsychological Rehabilitation Battery©.* Broadview Heights: ABackans Diversified Computer Processing, Inc.

Ackerman, R. J., & Banks, M. E. (1992a). Classification of Patient Groups Using the Ackerman-Banks Neuropsychological Rehabilitation Battery©. *The Clinical Neuropsychologist, 6*, 333.

Ackerman, R. J., & Banks, M. E. (1992b). *A new approach in rehabilitation assessment: The Ackerman-Banks Neuropsychological Rehabilitation Battery (A-BNRB).* Paper presented at the 16th Annual Postgraduate Course in Rehabilitation of the Brain Injured Child and Adult, Williamsburg.

Ackerman, R. J., & Banks, M. E. (1994a). *Ackerman-Banks Neuropsychological Rehabilitation Battery© Professional Manual* (3rd ed.). Uniontown: ABackans Diversified Computer Processing, Inc.

Ackerman, R. J., & Banks, M. E. (1994b). *What's missing? Neuropsychological issues in women's diagnosis and treatment.* Paper presented at the Psychosocial and Behavioral Factors in Women's Health: Creating an Agenda for the 21st Century conference, Washington, D.C. Abstract available: http://www.en.com/NPdxtx.htm.

Ackerman, R. J., & Banks, M. E. (1995). A neuropsychological case study of musicogenic epilepsy. *Archives of Clinical Neuropsychology, 10*, 286-287. Abstract available: http://www.en.com/musepiNAN94.htm.

Ackerman, R. J., & Banks, M. E. (1996). *A culturally sensitive approach to neuropsychology: Assessment after violence* . Workshop presented at the annual convention Pennsylvania Psychological Association.

Ackerman, R. J., & Banks, M. E. (2000). *Ackerman-Banks Neuropsychological Rehabilitation Battery© Training Manual*. Akron: ABackans Diversified Computer Processing, Inc.

Ackerman, R. J., Banks, M. E., & Corbett, C. A. (1998). When women deal with head injuries. In J. Chrisler & A. Hemstreet (Eds.), *Women in Africa and the African diaspora: Building bridges of knowledge and power. Volume II: Health, human rights, and the environment* (pp. 5-22). Indianapolis: Association of African Women Scholars.

Allen, M. (1994). The dilemma for Women of Color in clinical trials. *Journal of the American Medical Women's Association, 49*, 105-109.

American Psychiatric Association (1987). *Diagnostic and Statistical Manual of Mental Disorders, 3rd Edition, Revised*. Washington, D.C.: American Psychiatric Association.

American Educational Research Association (AERA), American Psychological Association (APA), & National Council on Measurement in Education (NCME) (1999). *Standards for educational and psychological testing*. Washington, DC: AERA Publications.

Ardila, A., Rodriguez-Mendendez, G., & Rosselli, M. (2001). Current issues in neuropsychological assessment with Hispanics/Latinos. In F. R. Ferraro (Ed.), *Minority and cross-cultural aspects of neuropsychological assessment* (pp. 161-179). Lisse, The Netherlands: Swets & Zeitlinger Publishers.

Banks, M. E. (1999). *Rehabilitation issues with victims of violence*. Paper presented at Rehabilitation Psychology 2000: Science & Practice. Abstract available: http://www.en.com/abackans/abrp0399.html.

Banks, M. E. (2000a). *Culturally competent psychology: Gender and aging considerations*. Paper presented at the 108th annual convention of the American Psychological Association, Washington, D.C.

Banks, M. E. (2000b). *Culturally relevant neuropsychological assessment and rehabilitation for African Americans*. Paper presented at the 108th annual convention of the American Psychological Association, Washington, D.C.

Banks, M. E., & Ackerman, R. J. (1991). *Interpretation report for the Ackerman-Banks Neuropsychological Rehabilitation Battery©* [Computer program and documentation]. Broadview Heights: ABackans Diversified Computer Processing, Inc.

Banks, M. E., & Ackerman, R. J. (1995). *Basic brain functions and structures©* [patient feedback software and educational book]. Uniontown: ABackans Diversified Computer Processing, Inc.

Banks, M. E., & Ackerman, R. J. (1996a). *Health issues for women: A rehabilitation neuropsychological profile*. Paper presented at the Traumatic Brain Injury: Models and Systems of Care Conference, Washington, DC. Abstract available: http://www.en.com/abackans/NPRape.htm

Banks, M. E., & Ackerman, R. J. (1996b). *Neuropsychological assessment for rehabilitation: Focus on ethnicity and cultural diversity*. Paper presented at the Traumatic Brain Injury: Models and Systems of Care Conference, Washington, D.C. Abstract available: http://www.en.com/abackans/EthRehab.htm.

Banks, M. E., & Ackerman, R. J. (1997). Ethnogeriatric issues in neuropsychologic assessment and rehabilitation, *Topics in Geriatric Rehabilitation, 12*, 47-61.

Banks, M. E., Ackerman, R. J., and Corbett, C. A. (1995). Feminist neuropsychology: Issues for physically challenged women. In J. Chrisler & A. Hemstreet (Eds.), *Variations on a Theme: Diversity and the Psychology of Women*. Lincoln: University of Nebraska Press.

Bylsma, F. W., Ostendorf, C. A., & Hofer, P. J. (2001). Challenges in providing neuropsychological and psychological services in Guam and the Commonwealth of the Northern Marina Islands. In F. R. Ferraro (Ed.), *Minority and cross-cultural aspects of neuropsychological assessment* (pp. 145-157). Lisse, The Netherlands: Swets & Zeitlinger Publishers.

Campbell, J. C., & Soeken, K. L. (1999). Women's responses to battering over time: An analysis of change. *Journal of Interpersonal Violence, 14,* 21-40.

Collins, M. W., Grindel, S. H., Lovell, M. R., Dede, D. E., Moser, D. J., Phalin, B. R., Nogle, S., Wasik, M., Cordry, D., Daugherty, M. K., Sears, S. F., Nicolette, G., Indelicato, P., & McKeag, D. B. (1999). Relationship between concussion and neuropsychological performance in college football players, *Journal of American Medical Association, 282,* 964-970.

Covington, D. L., Maxwell, J. G., Clancy, T. V., Churchill, M. P., & Ahrens, W. L. (1995). Poor hospital documentation of violence against women. *The Journal of Trauma: Injury, Infection, and Critical Care, 38,* 412-416.

Cross, W. E. (1994). Nigrescence theory: Historical and exploratory notes. *Journal of Vocational Behavior, 44,* 119-123.

Dennis, R. E., Key, L. J., Kirk, A. L., & Smith, A. (1995). Addressing domestic violence in the African American community. *Journal of Health Care for the Poor and Underserved, 6,* 284-298.

Dick, M., B., Teng, E. L., Kempler, D., Davis, D. S., & Taussig, I. M. (2001). The Cross-Cultural Neuropsychological Assessment Battery (CCNB): Effects of age, education, ethnicity, and cognitive status on the performance of healthy and cognitively impaired older adults. In F. R. Ferraro (Ed.), *Minority and cross-cultural aspects of neuropsychological assessment* (pp. 17-41). Lisse, The Netherlands: Swets & Zeitlinger Publishers.

Diller, L. (1992). *Stroke rehabilitation: Advances and prospects.* Invited centennial lecture presented at the 100th annual convention of the American Psychological Association, Washington, D.C.

Echemendia, R. J., & Julian, L. (2001). Neuropsychological assessment of Latino children. In F. R. Ferraro (Ed.), *Minority and cross-cultural aspects of neuropsychological assessment* (pp. 181-203). Lisse, The Netherlands: Swets & Zeitlinger Publishers.

Escandell, V. A. (2001). Cross-cultural neuropsychology in Saudi Arabia. In F. R. Ferraro (Ed.), *Minority and cross-cultural aspects of neuropsychological assessment* (pp. 299-325). Lisse, The Netherlands: Swets & Zeitlinger Publishers.

Fastenau, P. S., Evans, J. D., Johnson, K. E., & Bond, G. R. (2001). Multicultural training in clinical neuropsychology. In F. R. Ferraro (Ed.), *Minority and cross-cultural aspects of neuropsychological assessment* (pp. 345-373). Lisse, The Netherlands: Swets & Zeitlinger Publishers.

Ferraro, F. R., Bercier, B. B., Holm, J., & McDonald, J. D. (2001). Preliminary normative data from a brief neuropsychological test battery in a sample of Native American elderly. In F. R. Ferraro (Ed.), *Minority and cross-cultural aspects of neuropsychological assessment* (pp. 227-240). Lisse, The Netherlands: Swets & Zeitlinger Publishers.

Fillenbaum, G. G., Unverzagt, F. W., Ganguli, M., Welsh-Bohmer, K.A., & Heyman, A. (2001). The CERAD neuropsychology battery: Performance of representative community and tertiary care samples of African-American and European-American elderly. In F. R. Ferraro (Ed.), *Minority and cross-cultural aspects of neuropsychological assessment* (pp. 45-62). Lisse, The Netherlands: Swets & Zeitlinger Publishers.

Gardiner, J. C., Tansley, D. P., & Ertz, D. J. (2001). Native Americans: Future directions. In F. R. Ferraro (Ed.), *Minority and cross-cultural aspects of neuropsychological assessment* (pp. 241-261). Lisse, The Netherlands: Swets & Zeitlinger Publishers.

Golden, C. J., Purisch, A. D., & Hammeke, T. A. (1985). *Luria-Nebraska Neuropsychological Battery: Forms I and II manual.* Los Angeles: Western Psychological Services.

Gouvier, W. D., Pinkston, J. B., Santa Maria, M. P., & Cherry, K. E. (2001). Base rate analysis in cross-cultural clinical psychology: Diagnostic accuracy in the balance. In F. R. Ferraro (Ed.), *Minority and cross-cultural aspects of neuropsychological assessment* (pp. 375-386). Lisse, The Netherlands: Swets & Zeitlinger Publishers.

Greenfeld, L. A., Rand, M. R., Craven, D., Klaus, P. A., Perkins, C. A., Ringel, C., Warchol, G., Maston, C., & Fox, J. A. (1998). *Violence by intimates: Analysis of data on crimes by current or former spouses, boyfriends, and girlfriends.* (Bureau of Justice Statistics Statistics Factbook; NCJ-167237). Washington, D.C.: National Institute of Justice.

Gutierrez, G. (2001). The empirical development of a neuropsychological screening instrument for Mexican-Americans. In F. R. Ferraro (Ed.), *Minority and cross-cultural aspects of neuropsychological assessment* (pp. 205-224). Lisse, The Netherlands: Swets & Zeitlinger Publishers.

Hartman, D. E. (1995). *Neuropsychological toxicology: Identification and assessment of human neurotoxic syndromes.* (2nd ed.). New York: Pergamon Press.

Hartman, D. E. (1998). Missed diagnoses and misdiagnoses of environmental toxicant exposures. *Psychiatric Clinics of North America, 21,* 659-670.

Helms, J. E., & Piper, R. E. (1994). Implications of racial identity theory for vocational psychology. *Journal of Vocational Behavior, 44,* 124-138.

Kelly, J. P. (1999). Traumatic brain injury and concussion in sports. *Journal of the American Medical Association, 282,* 989-991.

Koss, M. P., Ingram, M., & Pepper, S. (1997). Psychotherapists' role in the medical response to male-partner violence. *Psychotherapy, 34,* 386-396.

Kyriacou, D. N., Angelin, D., Taliaferro, E., Stone, S., Tubb, T., Linden, J. A., Muelleman, R., Barton, E., & Kraus, J. F. (1999). Risk factors for injury to women from domestic violence. *New England Journal of Medicine, 341,* 1892-1898.

Lamberty, G. (2001). Traditions and trends in neuropsychological assessment. In F. R. Ferraro (Ed.), *Minority and cross-cultural aspects of neuropsychological assessment* (pp. 3-15). Lisse, The Netherlands: Swets & Zeitlinger Publishers.

Lezak, M., (1995). *Neuropsychological assessment* (3rd ed.). New York: Oxford University Press.

Lichtenberg, P. A., Ross, T. P., Youngblade, L., & Vangel, S. J., Jr. (1998). Normative studies research project test battery: Detection of dementia in African American and European American urban elderly patients. *Clinical Neuropsychologist, 12,* 146-154.

Luria, A. R. (1973). *The working brain: An Introduction to neuropsychology.* New York: Basic Books.

Luria, A. R. (1980). *Higher cortical functions in man* (2nd ed.). New York: Basic Books.

Manly, J.J., & Jacobs, D. M. (2001). Future directions in neuropsychological assessment with African Americans. In F. R. Ferraro (Ed.) *Minority and cross-cultural aspects of neuropsychological assessment* (pp. 79-96). Lisse, The Netherlands: Swets & Zeitlinger Publishers.

Manly, J. J., Miller, S. W., Heaton, R. K., Byrd, D., Reilly, J., Velásquez, R. J., Saccuzzo, D. P., Grant, I. (1998). The effect of African-American acculturation on neuropsychological test performance in normal and HIV-positive individuals. *Journal of the International Neuropsychological Society, 4,* 291-302.

Markstrom-Adams, C., & Adams, G. R. (1995). Gender, ethnic group, and grade differences in psychosocial functioning during middle adolescence. *Journal of Youth & Adolescence, 24,* 397-417.

Marsh, C. E. (1993). Sexual assault and domestic violence in the African American community. *The Western Journal of Black Studies, 17,* 149-155.

Matarazzo, J. D. (1992). Psychological testing and assessment in the 21st Century. *American Psychologist, 47,* 1007-1018.

Matser, E. J. T., Kessels, A. G., Jordan, B. D., Lezak, M. D., & Troost, J. (1999). Chronic traumatic brain injury in professional soccer players. *Neurology, 51,* 791-796.

Matser, E. J. T., Kessels, A. G., Lezak, M. D., Jordan, B. D., & Troost, J. (1999). Neuropsychological impairment in amateur soccer players. *Journal of the American Medical Association, 282,* 971-973.

Miles, G. T. (2001). Neuropsychological assessment of African Americans. In F. R. Ferraro (Ed.), *Minority and cross-cultural aspects of neuropsychological assessment* (pp. 63-77). Lisse, The Netherlands: Swets & Zeitlinger Publishers.

Monahan, K., & O'Leary, K. D. (1999). Head injury and battered women: An initial inquiry. *Health & Social Work, 24,* 269-278.

Muelleman, R. L., Lenaghan, P. A., & Pakieser, R. A. (1996). Battered women: Injury locations and types. *Annals of Emergency Medicine, 28,* 486-492.

Murai, T., Hadano, K., & Hamanaka, T. (2001). Current issues in neuropsychological assessment in Japan. In F. R. Ferraro (Ed.), *Minority and cross-cultural aspects of neuropsychological assessment* (pp. 99-127). Lisse, The Netherlands: Swets & Zeitlinger Publishers.

Poreh, A. (2001). Neuropsychological and psychological issues associated with cross-cultural and minority assessment. In F. R. Ferraro (Ed.), *Minority and cross-cultural aspects of neuropsychological assessment* (pp. 329-343). Lisse, The Netherlands: Swets & Zeitlinger Publishers.

Powell, J. W., & Barber-Ross, K. D. (1999). Traumatic brain injury in high school athletes. *Journal of the American Medical Association, 282,* 958-963.

Raj, A., Silverman, J. G., Wingood, G. M., & DiClemente, R. J. (1999). Prevalence and correlates of relationship abuse among a community-based sample of low-income African American women. *Violence Against Women, 5,* 272-291.

Reidy, T. J., Bowler, R. M., Rauch, S. S., & Pedroza, G. I. (1992). Pesticide exposure and neuropsychological impairment in migrant farm workers. *Archives of Clinical Neuropsychology, 7,* 85-95.

Salmon, D. P. , Galasko, D., & Wiederholt, W. C. (2001). Neuropsychological assessment of dementia on Guam. In F. R. Ferraro (Ed.), *Minority and cross-cultural aspects of neuropsychological assessment* (pp. 129-144). Lisse, The Netherlands: Swets & Zeitlinger Publishers.

Strickland, T. L., D'Elia, L. F., James, R., & Stein, R. (1997). Stroop color-work performance of African Americans. *Clinical Neuropsychologist, 11,* 87-90.

Trask, H. K. (2000). Keynote presentation. Presented at Color of Violence: Violence Against Women of Color conference at University of California, Santa Cruz.

Valciukas, J. A. (1991). *Foundations of environmental and occupational neurotoxicology.* New York: Van Nostrand Reinhold.

Whaley, A. L. (1998). Issues of validity in empirical tests of stereotype threat theory. *American Psychologist, 53,* 679-680.

Williams, R. W., & Bowman, M. L. (2001). Current issues in neuropsychological assessment with rural populations. In F. R. Ferraro (Ed.), *Minority and cross-cultural aspects of neuropsychological assessment* (pp. 265-284). Lisse, The Netherlands: Swets & Zeitlinger Publishers.

Wolfe, N. (2001). Cross-Cultural neuropsychology of aging and dementia: An update. In F. R. Ferraro (Ed.), *Minority and cross-cultural aspects of neuropsychological assessment* (pp. 285-297). Lisse, The Netherlands: Swets & Zeitlinger Publishers.

CONTRIBUTORS
ADDRESS LIST

Rosalie J. Ackerman, Ph.D.
Research and Development Division
ABackans Diversified Computer Processing, Inc.
566 White Pond Drive
Suite C#178
Akron, OH 44320-1116

Alfredo Ardila, Ph.D.
Memorial Regional Hospital
3501 Johnson Street
Hollywood, FL 33021

Martha E. Banks, Ph.D.
Research and Development Division
ABackans Diversified Computer Processing, Inc.
566 White Pond Drive
Suite C #178
Akron, OH 44320-1116

Brian J. Bercier, M.A.
Department of Psychology
University of North Dakota
Box 8380
Grand Forks, ND 58202-8380

Gary R. Bond, Ph.D.
Department of Psychology
(LD 124)
402 N. Blackford Street
Indiana University — Purdue University Indianapolis (IUPUI)
Indianapolis, IN 46202-3275

Michelle L. Bowman, B.A.
Department of Psychology
State University of New York at Potsdam
Potsdam, NY 13676

Frederick W. Bylsma, Ph.D.,
Department of Psychiatry
University of Chicago
5841 South Maryland Avenue
MC 3077
Chicago, IL 60637

Katie E. Cherry, Ph.D.
Department of Psychology
Louisiana State University
Baton Rouge, LA 70803

Deborah S. Davis, M.A.
School of Social Ecology
University of California
Irvine, CA 92697-4285

Malcolm B. Dick, Ph.D.
Institute for Brain Aging and Dementia
Room 1100
Gottschalk Medical Plaza Bldg.
University of California
Irvine, CA 92697-4285

Ruben J. Echemendia, Ph.D.
Department of Psychology
The Pennsylvania State University
314 Moore Bldg.
University Park, PA 16802

Vincent A. Escandell, Ph.D.
Department of Neurosciences
PON Box 3354 MBC 6
King Faisal Specialist Hospital and Research Center
Riyadh, Saudi Arabia 11211

Dewey J. Ertz, Ph.D.
Manlove Psychiatric Group
636 St. Anne Street
Rapid City, SD 57701

Jovier D. Evans, Ph.D.
Indiana University — Purdue University Indianapolis (IUPUI)
Indianapolis, IN 46202-3275

Philip S. Fastenau, Ph.D.
Department of Psychology
(LD 124)
402 N. Blackford Street
Indiana University — Purdue University Indianapolis (IUPUI)
Indianapolis, IN 46202-3275

F. Richard Ferraro
Department of Psychology
Box 8380
University of North Dakota
Grand Forks, ND 58202-8380

Gerda G. Fillenbaum, Ph.D.
Center for the Study of Aging and
Human Development
Duke University Medical Center
Durham, NC 27710

Douglas Galasko, M.D.
Department of Neurosciences
University of California at
San Diego
9500 Gilman Drive (0948)
La Jolla, CA 99852
and Neurology Service
San Diego Veterans Affairs Medical
Center
San Diego, CA

Mary Ganguli, M.D., M.P.H.
School of Medicine and
Department of Epidemiology
Graduate School of Public Health
University of Pittsburgh
Pittsburgh, PA 19807

James C Gardiner, Ph.D.
MHS-S VA Black Hills
13 Comanche Road
Fort Meade, SD 57741-1099

Wm. Drew Gouvier, Ph.D.
Department of Psychology
224 Audubon
Louisiana State University
Baton Rouge, LA 70803

Guadalupe Gutierrez, Ph.D.
Chicano Studies Department
Arizona State University
Box 812002
Tempe, AZ 85287-3802

Kazuo Hadano, M.D.
Department of Psychogeriatrics
National Institute of Mental Health
Ichikawa, Japan

Toshihiko Hamanaka, M.D.
Department of Psychiatry
Nagoya City University
Nagoya, Japan

Albert Heyman, M.D.
Division of Neurology
Department of Medicine
Duke University Medical Center
Durham, NC 27710

Pamina J. Hofer, Ph.D.
Private Practice
Guam and University of Guam
Guam

Jeffrey Holm, Ph.D.
Department of Psychology
University of North Dakota
Box 8380
Grand Forks, ND 58202-8380

Diane M. Jacobs, Ph.D.
Gertrude H. Sergievsky Center
Columbia University College of Phy-
sicians and Surgeons
630 West 168th Street
P&S Box 16
New York, NY 10032

Kathy E. Johnson, Ph.D.
Department of Psychology
(LD 124)
402 N. Blackford Street
Indiana University — Purdue
University Indianapolis (IUPUI)
Indianapolis, IN 46202-3275

Laura Julian, B.A.
Department of Psychology
The Pennsylvania State University
314 Moore Bldg.
University Park, PA 16802

Daniel Kempler, Ph.D.
Department of Otolaryngology
Keck School of Medicine and School
of Gerontology
University of Southern California
1200 N. State Street
Los Angeles, CA 90033

Greg J. Lamberty, Ph.D.
ABPP-CN
Noran Neurological Clinic
910 Medical Place
Suite 210
910 East 26th Street
Minneapolis, MN 55404

J. Douglas McDonald, Ph.D.
Department of Psychology
University of North Dakota
Box 8380
Grand Forks, ND 58202-8380

Jennifer Manly, Ph.D.
Gertrude H. Sergievsky Center
Columbia University College of Physicians and Surgeons
630 West 168th Street
P&S Box 16
New York, NY 10032

Gary T. Miles, Ph.D.
Department of Veterans Affairs
Palo Alto Health Care System
3801 Miranda Avenue
Palo Alto, CA 94304

Toshiya Murai, M.D.
Department of Psychiatry
Faculty of Medicine
Kyoto University
Shogoin-Kawaharacho 54
Kyoto 606-8507, Japan

Catherine A. Ostendorf, M.A.
Private Practice
Chicago, IL

James B. Pinkston, B.A.
Department of Psychology
Louisiana State University
Baton Rouge, LA 70803

Amir Poreh, Ph.D.
Department of Psychology
Hebrew University of Jerusalem
Mt. Scopus
Jerusalem, 91905, Israel

Gerardo Rodriguez-Menendez, Ph.D.
Carlos Albizu University
2173 NW 99 Avenue
Miami, FL 33166

Monica Rosselli
Florida Atlantic University
2912 College Avenue
Davie, FL 33314

David P. Salmon, Ph.D.
ADRC
Florence Riford Clinic
Department of Neurosciences
University of California at San Diego
9500 Gilman Drive (0948)
La Jolla, CA 99852

Michael P. Santa Maria, B.A.
Department of Psychology
Louisiana State University
Baton Rouge, LA 70803

I. Maribel Taussig, Ph.D.
4251 Gulf Shore Blvd.
N. Suite 11-C
Naples, FL 34103

Dennis P. Tansley, Ph.D.
MHS-S VA Black Hills
13 Comanche Road
Fort Meade, SD 57741-1099

Evelyn L. Teng, Ph.D.
Department of Neurology
Keck School of Medicine
University of Southern California
LAC+USC Medical Center
GNH 5641
Los Angeles, CA 90033

Frederick W. Unverzagt, Ph.D.
Department of Psychiatry
Indiana University School of Medicine
Indianapolis, IN 46202-5266

Kathleen A. Welsh-Bohmer, Ph.D.
Department of Psychiatry and Behavioral Sciences and Bryan Alzheimer's
Disease Research Center
Duke University Medical Center
Durham, NC 27710

Wigbert C. Wiederholt, M.D.
ADRC
Florence Riford Clinic
Department of Neurosciences
University of California at
San Diego
9500 Gilman Drive (0948)
La Jolla, CA 99852

Richard W. Williams, Ph.D.
State University of New York at
Potsdam
Flagg Hall, 153
Potsdam, NY 13676

Nicola Wolfe, Ph.D.
Adjunct Faculty
California School of Professional
Psychology (CSPP)
Alliant University
1005 Atlantic Avenue
Alameda, CA 94501

SUBJECT INDEX

AUTHOR INDEX

STUDIES ON NEUROPSYCHOLOGY, DEVELOPMENT, AND COGNITION

1. *Fundamentals of Functional Brain Imaging: A Guide to the Methods and their Applications to Psychology and Behavioral Neuroscience.* Andrew C. Papanicolaou
   1998. ISBN 90 265 1528 6 (hardback)

2. *Forensic Neuropsychology: Fundamentals and Practice.* Edited by Jerry J. Sweet
   1999. ISBN 90 256 1544 8 (hardback)

3. *Neuropsychological Differential Diagnosis.* Konstantine K. Zakzanis, Larry Leach and Edith Kaplan
   1999. ISBN 90 256 1552 9 (hardback)

4. *Minority and Cross-Cultural Aspects of Neuropsychological Assessment.* Edited by F. Richard Ferraro
   2002. ISBN 90 256 1830 7 (hardback)

5. *Ethical Issues in Clinical Neuropsychology.* Edited by Shane S. Bush and Michael L. Drexler
   2002. ISBN 90 256 1924 9 (hardback)